The
Intensive Care
Manual

NOTICE

Medicine is an ever-changing science. As new research and clinical experience broaden our knowledge, changes in treatment and drug therapy are required. The editors and the publisher of this work have checked with sources believed to be reliable in their efforts to provide information that is complete and generally in accord with the standards accepted at the time of publication. However, in view of the possibility of human error or changes in medical sciences, neither the editors nor the publisher nor any other party who has been involved in the preparation or publication of this work warrants that the information contained herein is in every respect accurate or complete, and they are not responsible for any errors or omissions or for the results obtained from use of such information. Readers are encouraged to confirm the information contained herein with other sources. For example and in particular, readers are advised to check the product information sheet included in the package of each drug they plan to administer to be certain that the information contained in this book is accurate and that changes have not been made in the recommended dose or in the contraindications for administration. This recommendation is of particular importance in connection with new or infrequently used drugs.

The Intensive Care Manual

MICHAEL J. APOSTOLAKOS, M.D.

ASSOCIATE PROFESSOR OF MEDICINE
DIRECTOR, ADULT CRITICAL CARE
UNIVERSITY OF ROCHESTER SCHOOL OF MEDICINE AND DENTISTRY

PETER J. PAPADAKOS, M.D.

ASSOCIATE PROFESSOR OF ANESTHESIOLOGY AND SURGERY
DIRECTOR, DIVISION OF CRITICAL CARE MEDICINE
UNIVERSITY OF ROCHESTER SCHOOL OF MEDICINE AND DENTISTRY
PROFESSOR OF RESPIRATORY CARE
STATE UNIVERSITY OF NEW YORK
GENESEE COMMUNITY COLLEGE

McGRAW-HILL
MEDICAL PUBLISHING DIVISION

New York   Chicago   San Francisco   Lisbon   London   Madrid   Mexico City
Milan   New Delhi   San Juan   Seoul   Singapore   Sydney   Toronto

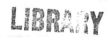
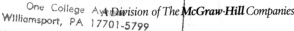

McGraw-Hill

A Division of The McGraw·Hill Companies

The Intensive Care Manual

1234567890 DOC DOC 0987654321

ISBN 0-07-006696-5

This book was set in Minion by Pine Tree Composition.
The editors were Michael P. Medina and Regina Y. Brown.
The production supervisor was Richard Ruzycka.
The interior designer was Joan O'Connor.
The cover designer was Aimee Nordin.
RRD/Crawfordsville was printer and binder.
This book is printed on recycled, acid-free paper.

Library of Congress Cataloging-in-Publication Data

The intensive care manual / [edited by] Michael J. Apostolakos.
     p. ; cm.
  Includes bibliographical references and index.
  ISBN 0-07-006696-5
    1. Critical care medicine—Handbooks, manuals, etc. I. Apostolakos, Michael J.
  [DNLM: 1. Critical Care—methods—Handbooks. 2. Emergencies—Handbooks. WB 39
  I598 2001]
  RC86.8 .I586 2001
  616'.028—dc21

                                                              00-046609

This book is dedicated to our loving wives,
Cindy and Susan
and
our children,
Yianni, Kenny, and Yanni.

Contents

Contributors

CHAPTER 4:

APPROACH TO MECHANICAL VENTILATION

ANTHONY P. PIETROPAOLI, MD

Assistant Professor of Medicine
Medical Director, Respiratory Care
Pulmonary and Critical Care Unit
University of Rochester Medical Center
Rochester, NY

CHAPTER 5:

APPROACH TO RENAL FAILURE

ANDREW B. LIEBOWITZ, MD

Associate Professor of Anesthesiology
Director, Surgical ICU
Mount Sinai Hospital
New York, NY

CHAPTER 6:

APPROACH TO INFECTIOUS DISEASE

DOUGLAS SALVADOR, MD

Resident in Internal Medicine
University of Rochester School of Medicine and Dentistry
Strong Memorial Hospital
Rochester, NY

ROBERT F. BETTS, MD

Professor of Medicine
University of Rochester School of Medicine and Dentistry
Strong Memorial Hospital
Rochester, NY

CHAPTER 7:

APPROACH TO NUTRITIONAL SUPPORT

PAMELA R. ROBERTS, MD, FCCM

Associate Professor of Anesthesiology/Critical Care
Department of Anesthesiology/Critical Care
Wake Forest University School of Medicine
Winston-Salem, NC

CHAPTER 8:

APPROACH TO CARDIAC ARRHYTHMIAS

ANDREW CORSELLO, MD

Instructor in Medicine
University of Rochester School of Medicine and Dentistry
Rochester, NY

JOSEPH M. DELEHANTY, MD

Associate Professor of Medicine

Director, Cardiovascular ICU
University of Rochester Medical Center
Rochester, NY

DAVID HUANG, MD

Assistant Professor of Medicine
University of Rochester Medical Center
Rochester, NY

CHAPTER 9:

APPROACH TO ACUTE MYOCARDIAL INFARCTION: DIAGNOSIS AND MANAGEMENT

SETH M. JACOBSON, MD

Fellow in Cardiovascular Disease
University of Rochester
Rochester, NY

JOSEPH M. DELEHANTY, MD

Associate Professor of Medicine
Director, Cardiovascular ICU
University of Rochester Medical Center
Rochester, NY

CHAPTER 10:

APPROACH TO ENDOCRINE DISEASE

DAVID KAUFMAN, MD

Assistant Professor of Surgery, Anesthesia, Internal Medicine
and University of Rochester Medical Center Medical Humanities

Director, Surgical Intensive Care Unit
Rochester, NY

CHAPTER 11:

APPROACH TO GASTROINTESTINAL PROBLEMS IN THE INTENSIVE CARE UNIT

JAMES R. BURTON, JR., MD
Resident in Internal Medicine
Department of Medicine
University of Rochester
School of Medicine and Dentistry
Strong Memorial Hospital
Rochester, NY

THOMAS A. SHAW-STIFFEL, MD, CM, FRCPC, FACP
Associate Professor of Medicine
Director of Hepatology
University of Rochester Medical Center
Rochester, NY

CHAPTER 12:

APPROACH TO HEMATOLOGIC DISORDERS

JANICE L. ZIMMERMAN, MD, FCCM, FCCP, FACP
Professor of Medicine
Director, Department of Emergency Medicine
Ben Taub General Hospital
Houston, TX

CHAPTER 13:

APPROACH TO COMA

CURTIS BENESCH, MD
Assistant Professor of Neurology
University of Rochester Medical Center
Rochester, NY

CHAPTER 14:

APPROACH TO SEDATION
AND AIRWAY MANAGEMENT IN THE ICU

PETER J. PAPADAKOS, MD, FCCP, FCCM
Associate Professor of Anesthesiology
Professor of Respiratory Care SUNY
University of Rochester Medical Center
Rochester, NY

Preface

The ICU Manual was developed as a bedside reference for house officers, fellows, and attendings who care for patients in ICUs. The book is organized in organ-specific chapters. This was done to increase the utility of and simplify the use of this manual. The organ specific approach parallels the way patients in the ICU are cared for. This approach enables the clinician to organize the diagnosis and management of complicated critically ill patients. The book has numerous illustrations, tables, and figures to ease information transfer. A variety of authors, each with their own areas of expertise, were utilized to improve the book's perspective and overall character. We feel you will find the ICU Manual informative and helpful in your care of critically ill patients.

Good luck.

CHAPTER 1

The Critically Ill Patient: Overview of Respiratory Failure and Oxygen Delivery

MICHAEL J. APOSTOLAKOS

INTRODUCTION

The care of the critically ill patient is complex and, at times, overwhelming. Many organ systems may be affected simultaneously. Each of these organ systems and the approach to their dysfunction is discussed in subsequent chapters. This chapter focuses on respiratory failure (hypoxemic and hypercapnic) and oxygen delivery: the underlying concepts are central to what we do in the intensive care unit (ICU).

RESPIRATORY FAILURE

Respiratory failure may be divided into two broad categories: hypoxemic (type 1) and hypercapnic (type 2). Hypoxemic respiratory failure is defined as a partial pressure of oxygen in arterial blood (Pao_2) of less than 55 mm Hg when the fraction of inspired oxygen (Fio_2) is 0.60 or more. Hypercapnic respiratory failure is defined as a partial pressure of carbon dioxide in arterial blood ($Paco_2$) of more than 45 mm Hg. Disorders that initially cause hypoxemia may be complicated by respiratory pump failure and hypercapnia (Table 1–1). Conversely, diseases that produce respiratory pump failure are frequently complicated by hypoxemia resulting from secondary pulmonary parenchymal processes (e.g., pneumonia) or vascular disorders (e.g., pulmonary embolism).

Hypoxemia

Hypoxemia may be broadly divided into four major categories.

1. Hypoventilation and low Fio_2
2. Diffusion limitation
3. Ventilation/Perfusion ($\dot{V}/\dot{Q}$) mismatch
4. Shunt

TABLE 1–1 Common Causes of Hypoxemia and Hypercapnia

Hypoxemia

Pneumonia
Acute respiratory distress syndrome (ARDS)
Pulmonary embolism
Congestive heart failure (CHF)

Hypercapnia

Muscle weakness
Factors that increase CO_2 production (e.g., fever, sepsis, trauma)
Airway obstruction

HYPOVENTILATION AND FIO_2 Hypoventilation and a low FIO_2 are rare causes of hypoxemia in ICU patients. Hypoventilation should be suspected as the cause of hypoxemia in patients with an elevated $PaCO_2$. Oversedation or hypercapnic respiratory failure are common causes of this condition. Low FIO_2 should not be a cause of this condition unless there is an inadvertent oxygen disconnection on a patient receiving oxygen. Hypoventilation and a low FIO_2 may be separated from the other causes of hypoxemia in that they are the only ones associated with a normal alveolar-aterial (A-a) oxygen gradient.

The alveolar-arterial (A-a) gradient is the difference between PAO_2 and PaO_2. The A-a gradient may be calculated from the following equation:

$$A-a \text{ gradient} = FIO_2(PB - PH_2O) - \frac{PaCO_2}{R} - PaO_2$$

Where

      FIO_2 is the fraction of inspired oxygen

      PB is the barometric pressure

      PH_2O is the partial pressure of water

      R is the respiratory quotient

The A-a gradient is normally less than 10 mm Hg on room air. In adults over age 65, normal values may extend up to 25 mm Hg.

Case Example

An example of the usefulness of calculating the A-a gradient is demonstrated in the following case: A 21-year-old patient was admitted to the ICU from the emergency department (ED) with a drug (narcotic) overdose. On presentation to the ED, the respiratory rate was 4/min. Initial arterial blood gas (ABG) values were pH, 7.1; $PaCO_2$, 80 mm Hg; PaO_2, 40 mm Hg; O_2 sat, 70%. The patient was intubated and transferred to the ICU. To calculate the patient's A-a gradient from the equation previously given (Normal value is 10 mm Hg or less on room air):

    A-a gradient = .21 (747 mmHg – 47 mmHg) – 80 mmHg/.8 – 40 mmHg
          = 147 mmHg – 100 mmHg – 40 mmHg = 7 mmHg

The normal A-a gradient value supports the hypothesis that this patient's hypoxemia was caused solely by hypoventilation and that no other cause of hypoxemia, such as pneumonia, needs to be investigated. The normal A-a gradient value separates this category of hypoxemia from the other three categories.

DIFFUSION LIMITATION Diffusion limitation is a rare cause of hypoxemia in ICU patients. The alveolar capillary unit has about 1 second in which to exchange

(a)

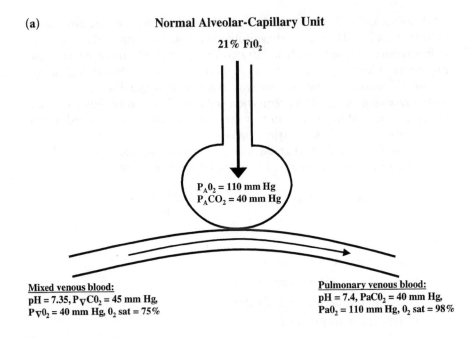

Normal Alveolar-Capillary Unit

21% FIO_2

$P_AO_2 = 110$ mm Hg
$P_ACO_2 = 40$ mm Hg

Mixed venous blood:
pH = 7.35, $P_VCO_2 = 45$ mm Hg,
$P_VO_2 = 40$ mm Hg, O_2 sat = 75%

Pulmonary venous blood:
pH = 7.4, $PaCO_2 = 40$ mm Hg,
$PaO_2 = 110$ mm Hg, O_2 sat = 98%

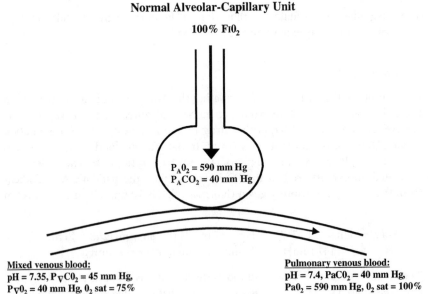

Normal Alveolar-Capillary Unit

100% FIO_2

$P_AO_2 = 590$ mm Hg
$P_ACO_2 = 40$ mm Hg

Mixed venous blood:
pH = 7.35, $P_VCO_2 = 45$ mm Hg,
$P_VO_2 = 40$ mm Hg, O_2 sat = 75%

Pulmonary venous blood:
pH = 7.4, $PaCO_2 = 40$ mm Hg,
$PaO_2 = 590$ mm Hg, O_2 sat = 100%

FIGURE 1–1 Physiology of oxygenation in lung under normal circumstances (a), during $\dot{V}/\dot{Q}$ mismatch (b), and shunt (c).

(b)

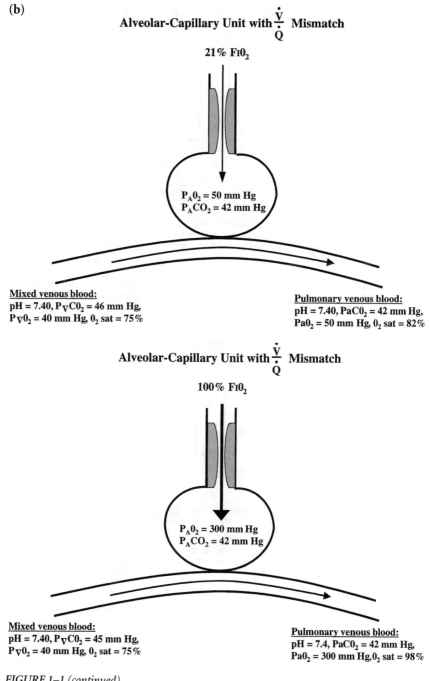

Alveolar-Capillary Unit with $\dfrac{\dot{V}}{\dot{Q}}$ Mismatch

21% F$_{IO_2}$

$P_AO_2 = 50$ mm Hg
$P_ACO_2 = 42$ mm Hg

Mixed venous blood:
pH = 7.40, $P_{\bar{V}}CO_2 = 46$ mm Hg,
$P_{\bar{V}}O_2 = 40$ mm Hg, O_2 sat = 75%

Pulmonary venous blood:
pH = 7.40, $PaCO_2 = 42$ mm Hg,
$PaO_2 = 50$ mm Hg, O_2 sat = 82%

Alveolar-Capillary Unit with $\dfrac{\dot{V}}{\dot{Q}}$ Mismatch

100% F$_{IO_2}$

$P_AO_2 = 300$ mm Hg
$P_ACO_2 = 42$ mm Hg

Mixed venous blood:
pH = 7.40, $P_{\bar{V}}CO_2 = 45$ mm Hg,
$P_{\bar{V}}O_2 = 40$ mm Hg, O_2 sat = 75%

Pulmonary venous blood:
pH = 7.4, $PaCO_2 = 42$ mm Hg,
$PaO_2 = 300$ mm Hg, O_2 sat = 98%

FIGURE 1–1 (continued)

(c)

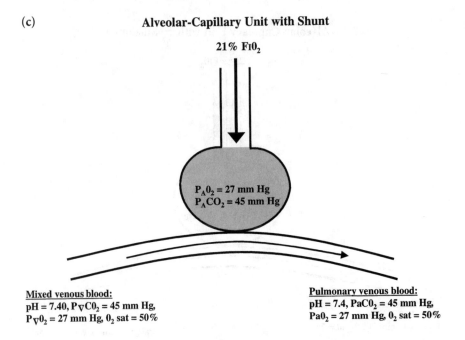

Alveolar-Capillary Unit with Shunt

21% FIO_2

P_AO_2 = 27 mm Hg
P_ACO_2 = 45 mm Hg

Mixed venous blood:
pH = 7.40, $P_{\overline{V}}CO_2$ = 45 mm Hg,
$P_{\overline{V}}O_2$ = 27 mm Hg, O_2 sat = 50%

Pulmonary venous blood:
pH = 7.4, $PaCO_2$ = 45 mm Hg,
PaO_2 = 27 mm Hg, O_2 sat = 50%

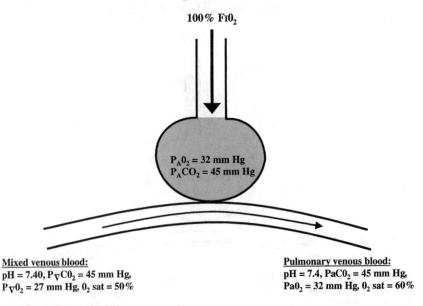

Alveolar-Capillary Unit with Shunt

100% FIO_2

P_AO_2 = 32 mm Hg
P_ACO_2 = 45 mm Hg

Mixed venous blood:
pH = 7.40, $P_{\overline{V}}CO_2$ = 45 mm Hg,
$P_{\overline{V}}O_2$ = 27 mm Hg, O_2 sat = 50%

Pulmonary venous blood:
pH = 7.4, $PaCO_2$ = 45 mm Hg,
PaO_2 = 32 mm Hg, O_2 sat = 60%

FIGURE 1–1 (continued)

carbon dioxide for oxygen. This normally occurs within the first 0.3 second. This leaves approximately 0.7 second as a buffer, which protects against hypoxemia during exercise (which increases cardiac output and decreases time available for gas exchange) or when necessary to overcome diseases that cause diffusion limitation. Except for severe end-stage lung disease (e.g., fibrosis, emphysema), this is a rare occurence and, therefore, a rare cause of acute hypoxemia. Diffusion limitation, in general, is handled by the pulmonary specialist over a long period.

VENTILATION/PERFUSION MISMATCH Ventilation/perfusion ($\dot{V}/\dot{Q}$) mismatch is the most common cause of hypoxemia seen in the ICU. Only perfusion with reduced or absent ventilation leads to hypoxemia. Ventilation without perfusion is simply dead-space ventilation, and by itself, does not lead to hypoxemia. If severe, ventilation without perfusion may lead to carbon dioxide retention. To understand this completely, call to mind the following equations:

$$\dot{V}_{\hat{E}} = \dot{V}_D + \dot{V}_A$$
$$Pa_{CO_2} = k \times \dot{V}_{CO_2}/\dot{V}_A$$

Where

$\dot{V}_E$ is total minute ventilation

$\dot{V}_D$ is dead space minute ventilation

$\dot{V}_A$ is alveolar minute ventilation

$\dot{V}_{CO_2}$ is carbon dioxide production

Normally $\dot{V}_D$ and $\dot{V}_A$ are 30% and 70%, respectively, of minute ventilation. k is a constant and $\dot{V}_{CO_2}$ can generally be considered constant. Therefore, Pa_{CO_2} is inversely proportional to $\dot{V}_A$ (i.e., $Pa_{CO_2} \sim 1/\dot{V}_A$). This becomes important when adjusting ventilator settings.

SHUNT A shunt is simply one extreme of ventilation/perfusion mismatch in which there is perfusion but absolutely no ventilation. Because of this, unoxygenated blood is shunted from the right side of the heart back to the left side of the heart causing profound hypoxemia. As there is absolutely no ventilation to this shunted area, increasing the FiO_2 will not improve the oxygenation. This is how $\dot{V}/\dot{Q}$ mismatch may be separated from shunt in that $\dot{V}/\dot{Q}$ mismatch will improve with increasing FiO_2, but shunt will not. It should be noted that there are intrapulmonary shunts caused by underlying lung disease such as pneumonia, but there are also extra pulmonary shunts, most commonly a patent foramen ovale. When there is a patent foramen ovale and right-sided heart pressure is increased, blood can be shunted across the atria from the right side of the heart to the left side of the heart causing shunt and hypoxemia. This can be diagnosed by a contrast echocardiogram.

ASSESSMENT OF HYPOXEMIA When assessing hypoxemia, an understanding of the normal physiology of the lung is necessary (Figure 1–1a). The pulmonary artery is the only artery in the body that delivers unoxygenated blood. A normal ABG obtained from the pulmonary artery is pH, 7.35, P_{CO_2}, 45 mm Hg, P_{O_2}, 40 mm Hg, and O_2 sat, 75%. The P_{AO_2} is approximately 110 mm Hg (obtained from the A-a gas equation) and alveolar P_{ACO_2} is 40 mm Hg. A perfectly matched alveolar-capillary unit produces pulmonary venous blood with a pH of 7.4, P_{CO_2}, 40 mm Hg; P_{O_2}, 110 mm Hg; and O_2_{SAT}, 100%. However, "normal" ABG values obtained peripherally yield about: pH, 7.4; Pa_{CO_2}, 40 mm Hg; Pa_{O_2}, 95 mm Hg; O_2 sat, 98%. The difference between the pulmonary venous and the arterial blood values is the result of an anatomic shunt. Approximately 2% of venous return from the systemic circulation is to the left side of the circulation, without going through the pulmonary circuit. Two major contributors to this shunt are the bronchial circulation and the thebesian veins of the heart. A combination of 98% of pulmonary venous blood and 2% shunted (systemic venous) blood yields normal peripheral ABG values.

Ventilation/perfusion ($\dot{V}/\dot{Q}$) mismatch leads to hypoxemia when perfused alveolar units have reduced oxygen levels in the alveolar space because of reduced ventilation, which is generally the result of some obstruction (e.g., bronchiolar edema or mucus related to infection, bronchospasm secondary to asthma). $\dot{V}/\dot{Q}$ mismatch, however, may be overcome by an increase in F_{IO_2} (Figure 1–1b). Shunt is simply the extreme of $\dot{V}/\dot{Q}$ mismatch, in which there is no ventilation but perfusion persists. (Remember that ventilation without perfusion is dead-space ventilation). Shunt is not overcome by an increase in F_{IO_2} (Figure 1–1c).

TREATMENT OF HYPOXEMIA Quite simply, there are two major ways to improve oxygenation:

1. Increase F_{IO_2}
2. Increase mean airway pressure

Increasing F_{IO_2} is simple and can only be done one way. Increasing mean airway pressure can be done a multitude of ways. An increase in mean airway pressure improves oxygenation by recruiting partially or fully collapsed alveoli, thus better matching ventilation to perfusion and reducing shunt. The easiest way to increase mean airway pressure is to increase positive end-expiratory pressure (PEEP). Inverse ratio ventilation also increases MAP by increasing the normal inspiratory-expiratory ratio from 1:2 to 1:1 or 2:1.[1] This change keeps the positive pressure in the chest for a longer time. Some believe that this technique simply adds to the PEEP by not allowing enough time for exhalation. This has led to the term "sneaky PEEP" being used in reference to IRV. High-frequency ventilation and oscillating ventilation are "high-tech" ways of increasing mean airway pressure and oxygenation.[2] Two less commonly used ways to improve oxygenation—prone positioning and inhaled nitric oxide—work by improving $\dot{V}/\dot{Q}$ matching.[3,4]

Hypercapnia

In addition to oxygenation, the other major function of the respiratory system is ventilation (carbon dioxide removal). At a constant rate of carbon dioxide production ($\dot{V}CO_2$), $PaCO_2$ is determined by the level of alveolar ventilation. The relationship between $\dot{V}A$, $\dot{V}CO_2$, and $PaCO_2$ is:

$$\dot{V}_A = k \times \dot{V}CO_2/PaCO_2$$

Where

    $\dot{V}_A$ is alveolar minute ventilation

    k is a proportionality constant

    $\dot{V}CO_2$ is rate of CO_2 production

When $\dot{V}CO_2$ is constant, the patient's $PaCO_2$ is inversely proportional to the $\dot{V}_A$ in a linear fashion.

Remember that:

$$\dot{V}_E = \dot{V}_D + \dot{V}_A$$

Where

    $\dot{V}_E$ is total minute ventilation

    $\dot{V}_D$ is dead space minute ventilation

    $\dot{V}_A$ is alveolar minute ventilation

Normally dead space ventilation is approximately 30% of total ventilation. This, however, can increase in certain conditions, such as chronic obstructive pulmonary disease (COPD) or acute respiratory distress syndrome (ARDS). At times, dead space ventilation may approach 70% or more of total ventilation. If this occurs, the relative amount of $\dot{V}_A$ is reduced and total ventilation must be increased, if PCO_2 is to be maintained. When this demand cannot be met, hypercapnia ensues. Abnormalities of the airways or alveoli (as described above) increase the demand and the metabolic rate or elevates respiratory quotient ($RQ = \dot{V}CO_2/\dot{V}O_2$) (Table 1–1).

The other aspect of the supply-and-demand equation that can lead to hypercapnia is when the supply side is adversely affected. The supply side is made up of the neuromuscular system. Normally, the respiratory system can sustain approximately 50% of the maximum voluntary ventilation (MVV). This is called the maximal sustainable ventilation (MSV). A 70-kg adult, under basal conditions, has a total ventilation of approximately 6 L/min, a MSV of 80 L/min, and a MVV of 160 L/min. When certain conditions intervene (Table 1–1), the body's ability to supply increases in ventilation is compromised, and therefore, hypercapnia can occur. This may lead to respiratory failure.

OXYGEN DELIVERY

Oxygenation is simply one factor in oxygen delivery, which is one of the most important aspects to understand in the care of critically ill patients. Oxygen is required by all cells in the human body for oxidative phosphorylation (energy production). If inadequate oxygen is delivered, anaerobic metabolism ensues. This less effective means of energy production results in acidosis and eventual cell death. The inadequate delivery of oxygen to tissues, with resultant organ dysfunction and death, is referred to as the shock state (see chapter 3).

The determinants of oxygen delivery ($\dot{D}O_2$) are:

$$\dot{D}O_2 = \text{Cardiac output} \times CaO_2$$

Where

CaO_2 is the concentration of oxygen in the arterial blood

The CaO_2 is divided between the oxygen that is bound to hemoglobin and the oxygen that is dissolved in the blood and is described by:

$$CaO_2 = O_2 \text{ saturated in Hb} + O_2 \text{ dissolved in plasma}$$
$$CaO_2 = (O_2 \text{ sat} \times \text{Hb (g/dL)} \times 1.34) + PaO_2 \times 0.003$$

Assuming a PaO_2 of 100 mm Hg, an O_2 sat of 100%, and a hemoglobin level of 14 g/dL, the concentration of oxygen in the blood is:

$$\frac{17.8 \text{ mL}}{dL} + \frac{0.3 \text{ mL}}{dL} = \frac{18.1 \text{ mL}}{dL}, \text{ or } \frac{181 \text{ mL}}{L}$$

Assuming a cardiac output of 6 L/min, the average $\dot{D}O_2$ is 1000 mL/min, or indexed to a body surface area of 1.7 m^2, approximately 600 mL/min/m^2. From the above equations, it is readily apparent that the major determinants of oxygen delivery are cardiac output, hemoglobin level and oxygen saturation. PaO_2 is only important in that it determines the oxygen saturation. That is to say, the amount of oxygen dissolved in the blood is small compared with that bound to hemoglobin.

The oxyhemoglobin (HbO_2) dissociation curve helps in understanding important aspects of the oxygen content of blood (Figure 1–2). From the S-shaped curve, it can be seen that there is not consistent affinity for hemoglobin at all levels of PO_2. This property of hemoglobin is called cooperativity. Each molecule of hemoglobin can bind four molecules of oxygen. With each molecule that is bound, hemoglobin's affinity for oxygen increases at each of the other binding sites. The curve also shows that with normal hemoglobin, a PO_2 of 60 mm Hg correlates with an oxygen saturation of 90%, a PO_2 of 40 mm Hg (venous blood) correlates with an oxygen saturation of 75%, and a PO_2 of 27 mm Hg correlates with an oxygen saturation of 50%. There are several factors that alter affinity (Figure 1–2): increased body temperature, decreased pH, an increased level of

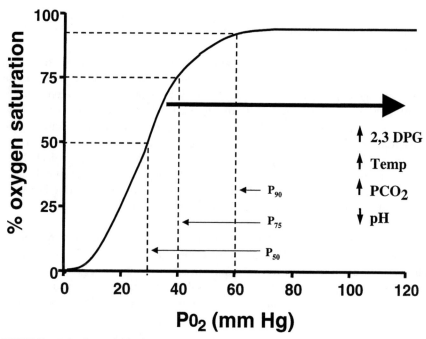

FIGURE 1–2 Oxyhemoglobin dissociation curve. Note parameters, which shift curve to right and thus favor unloading oxygen.

2,3-diphosphoglycerate (2,3 DPG), and an increased P_{CO_2}, all shift the oxyhemoglobin dissociation curve to the right (indicating a decreased affinity to bind oxygen). The opposite conditions shift the curve to the left and favor binding of oxygen.

In summary, the three major determinants of oxygen delivery are cardiac output, oxygen saturation, and hemoglobin level. Pa_{O_2} is only important in that it determines oxygen saturation.

OXYGEN CONSUMPTION

Under normal circumstances, our bodies use approximately 25% of delivered oxygen. The Fick equation describes this oxygen consumption ($\dot{V}_{O_2}$) as:

$$\dot{V}_{O_2} = \text{Cardiac output} \times (Ca_{O_2} - Cv_{O_2})$$

Where

Cv_{O_2} represents the content of oxygen in the venous blood

The venous blood, however, is only 75% saturated, with a Pv_{O_2} of approximately 40 mm Hg. By using the equations above, this calculates to an oxygen concentration of approximately 136 mL/L. The oxygen consumption calculates to approximately 250 mL/min. This results in an oxygen extraction ratio ($\dot{V}O/\dot{D}O_2$) of approximately 25%.

As can be seen in the graph in Figure 1–3, under normal circumstances this oxygen consumption is not dependent on delivery, only the oxygen extraction ratio changes with alterations in oxygen delivery. However, as oxygen delivery continues to fall, a critical value of extraction is reached, in which no further oxygen can be extracted. Oxygen delivery is inadequate to meet cellular demand and anaerobic metabolism ensues. This is the shock state, which is more fully described in chapter 3. Although it was originally thought that during critical illness this pathologic supply dependency extended beyond what was believed to be adequate restoration of circulation (Figure 1–3), this theory was exposed to be mathematical coupling and the goals of restoration of perfusion have been adjusted accordingly.

Also, oxygen delivery, under most circumstances, is most affected by changes in cardiac output (i.e., a 25% change correlates with a 25% change in oxygen delivery). The other factors (hemoglobin level, oxygen saturation, PaO_2) affect oxygen delivery in a less drastic fashion, unless there are extreme circumstances (i.e., very low hematocrit). The amount of oxygen dissolved in the blood is so small in

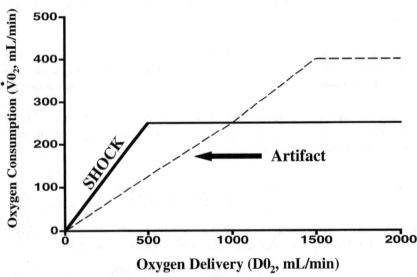

FIGURE 1–3 *Oxygen consumption versus oxygen delivery. Normal conditions (bold line). Under most conditions (flat part of curve), oxygen consumption is not dependent on delivery. However, if oxygen delivery decreases to a certain point, consumption becomes dependent on delivery, and patient goes into shock. Dashed line represents artifact of previously held theory, which suggested that during certain pathologic conditions, oxygen consumption was dependent on delivery far past normal resuscitation goals; this theory has been largely debunked.*

comparison to that bound to hemoglobin that it can almost be ignored. Practically, the PaO_2 is only important in that it determines the oxygen saturation, a much more important determinant.

SUMMARY

This chapter focuses on the important aspects of the two types of respiratory failure and on oxygen consumption and delivery. Understanding these important factors is vital in the care of critically ill patients and serves as a foundation of your knowledge base in critical care medicine.

REFERENCES

1. Morris AH, Wallace CJ, Menlovet RL, et al. Randomized clinical trial of pressure-controlled inverse ratio ventilation and extracorporeal CO_2 removal for adult respiratory distress syndrome. *Am J Respir Crit Care Med* 1994; 149:295–305.
2. Riphagen S, Bohn D. High frequency oscillatory ventilation. *Int Care Med* 1999; 25:1459–1462.
3. Dellinger RP, Zimmerman JL, Taylor RW, et al. Effects of inhaled nitric oxide in patients with acute respiratory distress syndrome: Results of a randomized phase II trial. *Crit Care Med* 1998; 26:15–23.
4. Papazian L, Bregeon F, Gaillat F, et al. Respective and combined effects of prone position and inhaled nitric oxide in patients with acute respiratory distress syndrome. *Am J Respir Crit Care Med 1998* ; 157:580–585.
5. Grippi MA. Respiratory failure: An overview. In Fishman AP, Elias JA, Fishman JA, et al., eds. *Fishman's pulmonary diseases and disorders,* 3rd ed. New York: McGraw-Hill 1998:2525–2535.

CHAPTER 2

Approach to Intravascular Access and Hemodynamic Monitoring

JAMES E. SZALADOS

INTRODUCTION

Care of critically ill patients requires vascular access for either therapeutic delivery of fluids and pharmaceutical agents or for diagnostic hemodynamic monitoring. By definition, critically ill patients are physiologically unstable and, therefore, may need medical interventions aimed at supporting one or more functionally compromised organ systems and gauging the response to therapy. Vascular access is the therapeutic cornerstone that facilitates these measures. All patients who meet admission criteria to critical care units (CCUs) should have a secure vascular access site, even if they are not currently receiving intravenous therapy, because of the potential need for unanticipated emergent interventions. The need for and choice of vascular access lines must be continuously weighed against the costs and risks of complications.

Sterile and Aseptic Technique

Sterile technique is fundamental to procedural medicine; training in its clinical application is vital and must precede procedural training. Infection of indwelling catheters and cannulae (i.e., "line infections") significantly affect patient morbidity and mortality and the duration and cost of hospitalization. The average cost of a line infection in a critically ill patient is $12,000 to $15,000 (1999). Insertion sites at which there is a potential for infection, such as cellulitis or abscess, must be avoided; sites at which there is a likelihood of contamination, such as the groin, should be used with caution. Intertriginous areas, such as the groin, may be colonized with fungi, such as *Candida albicans*, and insertion through such cutaneous colonization may result in subsequent hematogenous spread of pathogens. Sebum, the exocrine secretion of sebaceous glands in the skin, is an excellent growth medium for microorganisms; because of this, the skin should be cleansed with either 70% alcohol or povidone iodine, or both. The shaving of local hair before procedures is not recommended, because it may cause cuts and abrasions, and depilatories are not practical. Cannulation of the jugular veins in males results in a higher incidence of infection than use of the subclavian site, primarily because of overgrowth with facial hair and local accumulation of sebum. The jugular venous site also poses a risk for salivary contamination.

Sterile isolation of the proposed insertion site and the equipment from potential inadvertent contamination by either the operator or the unprepared surroundings is accomplished by the appropriate use of sterile gloves and drapes, plus gowns, caps, and masks, where indicated. Wide draping and preparation of the site are especially important when inexperienced practitioners are involved in the procedure. Vigilance and careful attention to suspected breaches in sterile technique are vital. For elective procedures, the cost-benefit analysis of suspected breaches in technique favors starting over, since the cost of time and supplies is negligible in comparison to the cost of infection. Because it is tacitly understood that access lines placed emergently are inherently more likely to be contaminated, all access catheters placed in the field, and probably even those placed in the emergency department, should be removed and reinserted at new sites once the patient is stabilized in the ICU. Aseptic technique differs from sterile technique mainly in the use of clean, but not necessarily sterile, gloves and drapes. Aseptic technique is most often applied in the insertion of peripheral intravenous catheters, and in some institutions, arterial cannulae.

The barriers to infectious communication, which protect the patient from the operator and the surroundings and are referred to as "sterile technique," can also protect the operator from infection by the patient. When sterile or nonsterile gloves, shields, or gowns are used to prevent the transmission of infection from the patient to medical personnel, these barriers are referred to as "universal precautions." The fundamental assumption of universal precautions is that all patients may be unrecognized carriers of infection. Transmissible infections that can be acquired during vascular access procedures include those communicated by close proximity with an infected individual, such as cutaneous and respiratory infections and blood-borne infections transmissible through inadvertent needlestick injury. Although the risk of transmission per event is relatively low, the implications of infection may be devastating. Infections, such as hepatitis B and C viruses, human T-cell lymphotropic virus (HTLV), human immunodeficiency virus (HIV), and perhaps unrecognized others, pose considerable risk to health care workers who regularly work with sharp objects contaminated with human body fluids.

At least 20 different pathogens have been shown to be transmitted by needlestick injury. The risk of transmission of viral hepatitis is greatest. The risk of acquiring HIV infection is estimated to be 0.4% for a single percutaneous exposure to body fluid from an HIV-infected patient. Since vascular access cannot be initiated without the use of sharp cannulae designed for cutaneous penetration and these cannulae have, by definition, come into contact with patient body fluids, they represent a significant hazard to health care providers and support staff. Injuries involving hollow needles bear a greater risk of disease transmission than injury from surgical needles. Inadvertent needlestick injuries occur in as many as 80% of inexperienced practitioners. Needlestick injuries tend to be highly underreported; it is estimated that 25% of all injuries are documented. Occupational health guidelines are readily available and should be adhered to in the event of inadvertent needlestick injury. In addition, it is the responsibility of the operator to ensure that all sharp objects used during a procedure have been accounted for and properly disposed of; this helps to avoid injury to others.

The ubiquitous use of latex gloves as a barrier to infection has resulted in an increased prevalence of sensitization in both patients and health care providers, and consequently, in local and systemic allergic reactions. The incidence of latex allergy in the general population is estimated at 1%; in health care workers, at 7% to 10%; and in chronically ill patients who have procedures done periodically (such as those with myelodysplastic disease, urologic abnormalities, or cerebral palsy), at 28% to 67%. The incidence of sensitization to latex increases with the frequency of exposure, especially exposure to products with a high protein content. During manufacturing, latex is washed and dried in a process known as leaching, which removes the water-soluble protein allergens. However, the protein content of latex gloves has been shown to vary 1000-fold among gloves from the same manufacturer and 3000-fold among gloves from different manufacturers.

Inhalation of latex particles in the cornstarch dust that coats some latex gloves is a common route for sensitization. Since allergic reactions to latex may be life-threatening, a high index of suspicion is important. Identification of patients at risk, early recognition of reactions, and implementation of treatment protocols have helped decrease latex-related morbidity. Alternatives to latex gloves and tourniquets are readily available; however, some latex elements are neither replaceable or widely recognized.

The vascular catheters that are routinely used in the ICU are constructed of plastic polymers, such as polyurethane, polyethylene, polytetrafluoroethylene (Teflon), or siliconized polypropylene, and are impregnated with barium or tungsten salts to confer radiologic opacity and facilitate confirmation of their position. Because all indwelling vascular catheters have been shown to develop a thin film of thrombin after insertion, which may facilitate bacterial adherence and catheter colonization,[1] some catheters are impregnated with heparin or bonded with heparin or antibiotics. Since *Staphylococcus epidermidis* and *S. aureus* are the most common organisms isolated from line cultures, the use of catheters that incorporate ionically bonded cefazolin, silver sulfadiazine, chlorhexidine, and other bonded antibacterial agents have led to a decrease in the incidence of bacterial line contamination.[2] Although plastic catheters are foreign intravascular bodies and, therefore, susceptible to hematogenous bacterial contamination, most catheters become infected through translocation of percutaneous bacteria along the insertion tract. Thus, catheters (Broviac, Hickman) inserted for long-term use are tunneled subcutaneously between the cutaneous and vascular insertion sites and often include an antimicrobial cuff to decrease the incidence of cutaneously initiated infection. Routine surveillance of the insertion site is necessary for the early detection of infection (e.g., erythema, exudate).

The use of antimicrobial ointments and occlusive dressings is not uniformly recommended because of the potential for skin maceration and accumulation of sebum and moisture, which promote bacterial growth and line infection. Sterile gauze secured with hypoallergenic tape and changed every 48 hours is the currently recommended standard of care. Catheters may also be infected hematologically when systemic bacteremia occurs. In these cases, catheter cultures reveal organisms such as *Enterococcus* species, *Enterobacter* species, and *Streptococcus pneumoniae*, among others.

The gut motor hypothesis suggests that bacterial translocation across the gut occurs during times of hypoperfusion and that such secondary bacteremia can reinforce or perpetuate the inflammatory response syndrome. If the specific organism can be isolated in culture, it may suggest the source. Diagnostic criteria for catheter tip–related systemic infection include positive results on culture of both the catheter tip and blood.[3] Catheter-tip infection is confirmed by the presence of more than 15 colony-forming units (CFU) in semiquantitative culture analysis or more than 100 CFU/mL in quantitative cultures, which are isolated from the catheter tip only.

Catheter-related septicemia occurs when catheter tip infection is accompanied by isolation of the same organism in blood drawn from a site other than the infected catheter. Antibiotic therapy must be considered whenever bacteremia is present and specifically tailored to the specific organism and its antibiotic sensitivity profile. Mitigating circumstances, such as the presence of prosthetic heart valves, artificial joints, and pacemaker leads, must be considered when the treatment options for line infection are considered.

Catheter infection without systemic bacteremia is probably best treated by immediate removal of the catheter and administration of systemic antibiotic agents. Catheters are foreign bodies and cannot be effectively sterilized by systemic antibiotic therapy. Therefore, catheters in place during active systemic infection should be removed or changed once bacteremia is controlled, because bacteria may subsequently be embolized to the lung or periphery or induce a local infection, such as phlebitis or endocarditis.

Choice of Catheter

The rate of flow through tubes and catheters is described by the Poiseuille-Hagen formula, which states that flow is directly proportional to radius and inversely proportional to length and viscosity of the fluid. Resistance is the mathematical inverse of flow. The formula is expressed by:

$$Q = \frac{\pi r^4}{8\mu L}$$

Where

Q is rate of flow

r is the catheter's internal radius

μ is the viscosity of fluid running through the catheter

L is the catheter length[A7]

From this relationship, it is clear that a short peripheral catheter may be a better choice than an identical gauge, longer, centrally placed catheter. The Advanced Cardiac Life Support protocol of the American Heart Association advocates the preferential use of antecubital venous cannulation in cardiac resuscitation. The flow through an introducer sheath, or cordis, is much greater than flow through any lumen of a multilumen central line. The transfusion of red blood cells should be through catheters of a least 20-gauge to prevent hemolysis; the rate of flow of transfusing blood can be significantly improved by dilution with saline, thereby decreasing viscosity.

The size of a catheter can be expressed in either gauge or French units, which are measures of external diameter. Gauges range from 14 to 27 with the smallest numerical label corresponding to the largest outside diameter. French sizing is usually reserved for catheter bores larger than 14-gauge, such as introducer sheaths for pulmonary artery catheters or pacing wires. Mathematically, French size is defined as the outside catheter diameter in millimeters multiplied by three.

A large variety of catheters are available for venous cannulation and the specific choice of catheter should be based on the intended purpose. Access to the central circulation is indicated for the administration of medication, nutrition, blood, and fluid or for the continuous or intermittent monitoring of biochemical or physiologic parameters. The administration of hyperosmotic or vasoactive compounds or the rapid infusion of large volumes is best accomplished by access into central veins. All vasoactive drugs should be infused into central venous catheters. These veins can be cannulated using a variety of single-lumen or multilumen catheters. Triple- and quadruple-lumen catheters are available and are used to isolate multiple infusions or to simultaneously monitor central filling pressure. However, since flow rate is limited by length, shorter, large-lumen introducer sheaths (Nos. 6 through 9 Fr) are better for volume resuscitation and may also serve as conduits for the insertion of either multilumen or pulmonary artery catheters.

Since high rates of flow are better maintained when flow is laminar rather than turbulent, removal of the side port of an introducer catheter and its acute angle of connection increases flow rate. Dialysis catheters are a type of central venous catheter inserted specifically for dialysis access; however, some models incorporate a third lumen for the administration of medications or pressure monitoring. Dialysis catheters are placed using techniques and sites analogous to other central venous cannulae (e.g., subclavian, jugular, and femoral veins). Insertion of temporary pacemaker wires is a common ICU procedure and requires an appropriately sized introducer catheter, pacing wires, and a generator. Similarly, arteries are catheterized for monitoring or for the introduction of diagnostic and therapeutic technology, such as cardiac catheterization or intra-aortic balloon counterpulsation. However, arterial catheters are not used for the administration of either medication or fluids. Inadvertent administration of caustic medications into arteries is associated with serious complications, such as vasospasm, with consequent ischemia and arterial embolism.

Stasis predisposes to coagulation and, therefore, intravascular catheters are flushed regularly, either with sterile fluids or anticoagulant solution.[4] Pressure transducers are designed to maintain catheter patency by continual infusion of flushing solution at the rate of 3 mL/hr. The use of anticoagulants in venous transducer lines helps maintain patency, whereas the use of anticoagulants in arterial transducer fluid is no longer standard. Common anticoagulants used in venous flushing solutions are heparin (100 U/mL) or sodium citrate 1.4% solution. The key disadvantage of heparinized flushing solutions is heparin-induced thrombocytopenia (HIT), and rarely, systemic anticoagulation in patients with impaired heparin clearance. Polytetrafluorethylene catheters are less thrombogenic, but more rigid, and are thus favored for arterial cannulation.

The Seldinger technique is a method of vascular cannulation that is guide wire–assisted and allows the introduction of progressively more sophisticated catheters over a guide wire after small-bore vascular access has been accomplished; the technique can be modified for either arterial or venous cannulation. The passage of a flexible-tip (J-wire) guide wire through a small needle or cannula into a vessel makes the subsequent passage of larger catheters over a guiding wire both easier and safer.

Monitoring

Vascular access is also used for monitoring, which is one aspect of data collection. The greater the complexity of the individual patient, the greater the need for additional data for appropriate case analysis and decision making. Invasive monitoring must be considered to be an extension of data collection along a continuum and should only be used when the added value it brings is both necessary and justified. For monitoring to have utility and effectiveness, the monitor must detect a physiologically useful signal, respond rapidly to physiologic change, process the data into a user-friendly format, visually display the data, and perhaps also display data trends. For monitoring to positively affect patient care, the practitioner must be able to interpret the data in the clinical setting, separate data from artifact, and conceptualize the physiologic, biochemical, or pharmacologic basis for the changes observed. Provider education and knowledge have a tremendous effect on patient outcome when technology such as the pulmonary artery catheter is used in critical care diagnostic and therapeutic decision making. The prevalence of unrecognized erroneous data being unquestioningly incorporated into decision making may be the root cause of outcome studies that question the utility, safety, and efficacy of the pulmonary artery catheter. Practitioners must personally participate in all aspects of data collection, including monitor and transducer offset and calibration and waveform interpretation, and they must readily question results that do not appear to fit the clinical picture.

Catheters are used to monitor physiology and biochemistry. Physiologic monitoring can include the monitoring of oxygen saturation of blood, or blood flow, but most commonly refers to the monitoring of intravascular pressure. For pressure monitoring to be possible via indwelling vascular catheters, weak pressure signals must be transformed into electrical signals by pressure transducers. The catheter must be connected to a noncompliant tubing filled with a continuous column of fluid. Because fluid is noncompressible, it reliably carries pressure signals to a transducer. The transducer is composed of an internal diaphragm within a saline container. The transducer diaphragm is connected to an electrical resistance bridge, the Wheatstone bridge, in such a way that motion of the diaphragm modulates an electrically applied current.

The sensitivity of the transducer system can be described as the change in applied current that occurs in response to a given pressure change; the value is usually 5 μV/V per millimeter of mercury. Offset, or zero calibration, must occur before accurate pressure data can be obtained. Offset is obtained by "zeroing" the transducer to air. The principle of signal transduction applies equally to arterial and venous pressure monitoring. Pressure is electronically recorded in millimeters of mercury (or torr), whereas convention manometry transduces pressure in centimeters of water (cm H_2O). Either unit can be converted to the other by using the definition of 1 mm Hg being equal to pressure measured in centimeters of water divided by 1.36.

The pressure data is only valid if the height of the transducer corresponds to the "phlebostatic axis," or the level of the right atrium. A transducer that is set too low reads a pressure that is falsely high; a transducer that is set too high reads a pressure that is falsely low.

Analgesia and Sedation

Patient comfort requires consideration of local or systemic analgesic and anxiolytic medications. Although systemic anxiolytics or analgesics may result in diminution of sympathetic tone, which can cause precipitous hemodynamic compromise in acutely ill patients, local analgesics are usually well tolerated. Systemic narcotic analgesics, such as morphine or fentanyl, with or without adjunctive use of anxiolytic-amnesics, such as midazolam, lorazepam, or propofol, can facilitate patient tolerance and thereby increase the safety of bedside procedures. Local anesthetic infiltration is usually adequate if used in sufficient quantity and dosage, although some patients do not tolerate either positioning or draping without systemic anxiolytics. Infiltration with local analgesia must include both cutaneous and deep structures. Periosteum is exquisitely sensitive and must be well anesthetized during subclavian vein cannulation. Lidocaine, in a concentration of 1% to 2%, is most frequently used, and the inclusion of epinephrine, 1:100,000 to 1:200,000, may decrease cutaneous bleeding. However, local anesthetics combined with epinephrine must never be injected in the proximity of arteries, especially end arteries without collateral flow, because vasospasm can rapidly precipitate distal ischemia.

Informed Consent

Whenever possible, preparation for invasive procedures should include a discussion of the indications, risks, and alternatives with the patient or patient's family. Informed consent, which includes mention of the most common complications and their operator-specific occurrence rates, should be routinely documented briefly in the patient medical record. In the perioperative period, operative consent usually includes provisions for the placement of anticipated and unanticipated access lines, but this does not waive the responsibility of the practitioner to discuss planned interventions with the patient or family. Specific procedural signed consent is not usually obtained for vascular access procedures in the operating room or the ICU, but again, it is prudent practice to discuss, if not specifically seek, consent for planned interventions that are associated with risk. On the other hand, the nature of the ICU often necessitates that interventions take place quickly to be effective, and detailed discussions may be impossible. Vascular access that is deemed medically essential for the level of care requested by the patient or family may be done in the absence of consent and, under some circumstances, in the presence of patient dissent. Patients who have received analgesic or anxiolytic medications may be confused or sedated and amnesic and therefore unable to properly provide informed consent. The principle of informed consent may be waived under emergent conditions and the doctrine of implied consent invoked. Under implied consent, the patient, by seeking out the health care system, implicitly consents to emergent procedures that are deemed medically necessary. Documentation in the chart of the need for and the expected benefit of procedures performed emergently without consent is prudent practice.

ARTERIAL CANNULATION

Arteries are most often cannulated for the purposes of continuous monitoring of blood pressure or blood chemistry analysis or for the facilitation of therapeutic interventions, such as intra-aortic balloon counterpulsation (IABP)or for continuous arteriovenous hemofiltration (CAVH). IABP and CAVH are very specific indications for vascular cannulation and are not discussed further.

Monitoring of Blood Chemistry

To obtain samples for specific blood chemistry analyses, such as measurements of arterial blood gases, arterial lactate, and general hematologic and chemical profiles, plastic catheters can be safely percutaneously inserted into superficial arteries. Arterial catheters are less likely than central venous catheters to be contaminated by infused substances, since arterial catheters are not used for fluid and medication administration. In addition, blood can be drawn from an arterial cannula with less effort and in less time than from venous catheters, although this is generally insignificant. The presence of an arterial cannula is independently correlated with the frequency of arterial blood specimen collection and analysis and therefore with the cost of care. In addition, routine monitoring of blood chemistries can phlebotomize the patient at a relative rate of one unit of packed red blood cells per week. Finally, venous blood gas analysis is a very good indicator of pH and partial pressure of carbon dioxide in blood. When coupled with pulse oximetry, venous blood gas analysis is both safe and cost-effective under most but not all circumstances.

Continuous intravascular blood gas monitoring is now technologically feasible. Photochemical sensors, optical electrodes, convert changes in blood gas partial pressure into changes in light absorption or emission through the use of photochemical dyes. However, this technology remains limited by problems with calibration and durability.

Monitoring of Systemic Arterial Pressure

Indirect measurement of arterial pressure can be accomplished by means of either palpation, auscultation (Riva-Rocci method, Korotkoff sounds), oscillometry, plethysmography, or Doppler transduction. The most commonly used indirect arterial monitoring device for determination of automatic mean arterial blood pressure, called the "Dinamap," is based on the principles of oscillometry and is the only such technique for determination of this pressure. Mean arterial blood pressure can be mathematically derived from measured systolic blood pressure (SBP) and diastolic blood pressure (DBP) by using the following equation:

$$MAP = \frac{SBP + (2 \times DBP)}{3}$$

Where

MAP is mean arterial pressure

The mean arterial pressure correlates with the static pressure of blood in the arterial circuit and is an important index of perfusion. Pulse pressure is the mathematical difference between the systolic and diastolic blood pressure values and reflects both the ventricular stroke volume and vascular compliance.

The inability to obtain reliable blood pressures with a cuff in patients who are obese, lack appropriate cuff application sites, have arrhythmias, or in situations in which there is high risk for hemodynamic instability are indications for the direct measurement of arterial pressure. Insertion of an arterial cannula is the most reliable method of blood pressure monitoring. In general, the arterial cannula reflects a more accurate diastolic blood pressure than does an occlusive cuff; however, the mean blood pressure measurements should be very similar.

Choice of Site and Technique and Their Potential Complications

The radial artery is the most frequently chosen site for arterial cannulation; however, the ulnar, brachial, axillary, femoral, and dorsalis pedis arteries are well described alternatives.[5] The choice of site is based on anatomic availability, arterial patency, absence of local infection, coagulation status, and, as always, a risk-benefit analysis. Raynaud's disease is a relative contraindication to arterial cannulation. The proximity of the ulnar artery to the ulnar nerve, the relative difficulty of immobilizing the elbow joint during brachial artery cannulation, and the predisposition of the dorsalis pedis artery to occlusion by thrombosis makes these sites less favorable than the radial or femoral arteries.

Adequate collateral circulation is vital to safety and, therefore, should be demonstrated and documented before the procedure. Allen's test can be used to evaluate the adequacy of collateral ulnar flow before radial artery cannulation, but it is not definitive and therefore is controversial. Following manual occlusion of both the radial and ulnar arteries, a normal (negative) test result is a return of color to the digits within 14 seconds or less after release of pressure on the ulnar artery. In rare instances, it may be necessary to perform a surgical arterial cutdown. Daily checks of distal perfusion should be routinely documented.

Arterial catheters, like all monitoring catheters, except those used for intracranial pressure monitoring, provide a continuous infusion of anticoagulant and intravenous fluid under pressure. The use of either heparinized or citrated saline is equally acceptable. Arterial catheters are routinely flushed manually after sampling; saline is infused into the artery under pressure (250 to 300 mm Hg). During flushing, the perfusion area of the artery is often observed to visibly blanch. Flushing must be limited to short duration because the pressure of fluid easily exceeds arterial pressure, so retrograde flow and passage of catheter debris into the aortic arch is possible with continued flushing. The risk of such a significant retrograde flow is most likely with catheters placed closest to the central arteries, such as brachial and axillary artery catheters. The left upper extremity arteries as a site for arterial cannulation may be preferable to the right side; the right hand is dominant in the majority of patients. The technique of arterial cannulation optimally requires palpation of the artery, manual fixation of the artery, and catheter-over-needle (and possibly Seldinger technique) luminal insertion. Blood return and waveform confirm the proper placement of the arterial catheter.

Complications of arterial cannulation are relatively rare (Table 2–1). Although arterial access sites are less likely to become infected than are venous cannulae because of higher local oxygen tension, insertion should be accomplished in a sterile manner. The incidence of infection increases with increasing duration of cannulation. The rate of infection significantly increases when surgical cutdown is used.

TABLE 2–1 **Complications of Arterial Cannulation**

Hematoma

Nerve injury

Heparin-induced thrombocytopenia

Blood loss from diagnostic tests

Arterial thrombosis

Digit loss

Cutaneous necrosis

Embolization, proximal or distal

Pseudoaneurysm

Infection

Retroperitoneal hemorrhage

Arteriovenous fistula

Inadvertent intra-arterial drug injection

Inadvertent disconnection and hemorrhage

False readings

Systemic infection from contaminated flushing solution or sampling syringes is also possible. Finally, seeding of intravascular foreign bodies in patients with documented bacteremia is expected; the foreign body becomes a secondary source of infection after the presenting bacteremia has been controlled. Catheters should be removed if pain, discoloration, or systemic signs of catheter sepsis develop, and the duration of arterial cannulation should be limited to 7 days, or less if possible.

Arterial Waveform Analysis and Artifact

The monitor typically displays both a continuous arterial waveform and a numerical value for systolic, diastolic, and mean arterial pressure. Visual assessment of the waveform is essential to the interpretation of the numerical value, because artifact can be inferred from the waveform only. The transducer must be level with the heart, brain, or organ in which perfusion is considered most vital; however, in supine critically ill patients, this is usually not an issue. In general, the transducer should be placed at the uppermost anatomic level of circulatory concern; for example, in a sitting neurosurgical patient, the transducer is most commonly placed at the level of the circle of Willis.

The mean arterial blood pressure is the driving pressure for arterial blood flow and is continuously calculated by dividing the integrated area under the arterial pressure waveform by the duration of the cardiac cycle. Blood pressure in blood vessels depends both on the flow rate, or cardiac output (CO), and the total peripheral (systemic vascular) resistance (TPR):

$$MAP = CO \times TPR$$

Where

MAP is mean arterial pressure

CO is cardiac output

TPR is total peripheral resistance

The most obvious and direct implication of this mathematical relationship is that arterial blood pressure is a very poor indicator of blood flow and resultant organ perfusion. Since pressure can remain constant within the limits of the accepted normal values because of vasoconstrictive reflexes and despite substantial reductions in flow, blood pressure changes generally signal loss of protective reflexes and may be the effects of, for example, pharmaceutical interventions, diabetes-related dysautonomia, and shock.

Arterial waveform data can also be used to infer more subtle information about cardiovascular function. Regular variations in the beat-to-beat blood pressure numbers and waveform on inspiration suggest intravascular volume depletion. A wide pulse pressure similarly suggests intravascular volume depletion and may also indicate underlying aortic insufficiency. The initial upstroke and peak amplitude of the arterial waveform is produced by the ejection of blood from the left ventricle and, therefore, implies contractility information, and the rate of downstroke in the arterial waveform allows inferences regarding systemic vascular resistance.

The blood pressure measured by an intra-arterial cannula depends to some extent on the properties of the vessel cannulated. The arterial pressure waveform is susceptible to artifacts, such as catheter whip and damping, which influence the validity of the pressure data. Catheter whip, or systolic amplification, occurs when arterial pressure waves are reflected back to the catheter tip from points of constriction, branching, or noncompliant arterial walls. Reflection of pressure waves off arterial walls can distort pressure waveforms, causing overreading of systolic pressure. Peripheral catheters are more susceptible to systolic amplification because the velocity of blood flow increases gradually as the blood pulse moves peripherally, since the walls of the large arteries are more compliant and absorb energy. The systolic pressure increases and the systolic wave narrows progressively as the arterial pressure wave is measured more peripherally, and systolic amplification of the waveform increases as the compliance of the arteries decreases peripherally.

Spontaneous oscillation is a characteristic of fluid-filled transducer systems. The resonant frequency of a transducer system is the inherent oscillation frequency produced by a pressure signal introduced into the system. Mechanical transducers absorb some of the energy of the systems they monitor and release of some of this energy. This causes a vibration to occur at the natural resonance frequency specific to the system.

Damping is the tendency for the vibration, or oscillation, to stop and is a function of compliance, air, tube length, tube coiling, connections in the tubing, and stopcocks. Air in the form of bubbles in the flush solution is very compressible and absorbs a great deal of energy, resulting in significant damping. Excessive damping results in an underestimation of the systolic blood pressure and an overestimation of the diastolic blood pressure, whereas the opposite is true for underdamped systems. Mean pressure is only minimally affected by damping. The resonant frequency can be quantitatively determined using the "flush formula,"[6] in which the frequency (in hertz) equals the paper speed (in millimeters per second) divided by the distance (in millimeters) between oscillation waves. The more closely matched a pressure signal is to the resonant frequency of the system, the greater the likelihood of signal amplification, which defines the underdamped system. An underinflated pressure bag causes an artifactual drop in the blood pressure reading. A transducer that has fallen to the floor causes the displayed blood pressure to be greatly elevated.

Pulse Oximetry

The adjunctive use of pulse oximetry in CCUs has added an additional level of monitoring, which allows the saturation of arterial blood to be measured directly using the law of Beer-Lambert and the principle of reflectance spectrophotometry.

The mandated use of pulse oximetry during anesthesia has greatly improved anesthesia safety; ideally therefore, pulse oximeters should be used on all critically ill patients. However, pulse oximetry alone is not considered an appropriate early warning of apnea, because significant desaturation may not occur for 15 minutes or more in patients with a normal functional residual capacity who are breathing pure oxygen. Furthermore, the pulse oximeter does not indicate the adequacy of ventilation. Clinically detectable cyanosis does not occur until the oxygen saturation of arterial blood reaches 80% or less.

Oxyhemoglobin reflects more red light than does reduced hemoglobin, whereas both hemoglobins reflect infrared light identically. Adult blood usually contains four types of hemoglobin: oxyhemoglobin (HbO_2), methemoglobin (MetHb), reduced hemoglobin (Hb), and carboxyhemoglobin ($HbCO_2$). However, except in pathologic conditions, methemoglobin and carboxyhemoglobin occur only in very low concentrations.

Pulse oximeters emit light only at only two wavelengths, 660 nm (red light) and 940 nm (near-infrared light). Reduced hemoglobin absorbs approximately 10 times more light, at a wavelength of 660 nm, than does oxyhemoglobin; at a wavelength of 940 nm, the absorption coefficient of oxyhemoglobin is greater than that of reduced hemoglobin. Signal processing based on a calibration curve determines the saturation of the arterial blood as it pulses past the probe. The pulse oximeter has substantially affected the use of ABG analysis for the determination of oxygenation saturation alone.

The SaO_2 displayed by the pulse oximeter is correctly referred to as the SpO_2, to differentiate it from the SaO_2 obtained by ABG analysis and is represented by the following equation:

$$SpO_2 = \frac{HbO_2}{HbO_2 + Hb} \times 100$$

Where

SpO_2 is Saturation of Hb with O_2 measured by pulse oximetry

HbO_2 is oxyhemoglobin concentration in blood

$HbO_2 + Hb$ is total hemoglobin concentratin in blood

Using the oxyhemoglobin dissociation curve, an SpO_2 of 90% corresponds to a PaO_2 of approximately 60 mm Hg and an SpO_2 of 75%, to a PaO_2 of 40 mm Hg. The SpO_2 measured by pulse oximetry can be expected to be within 2% of the value for hemoglobin saturation of blood measured by a co-oximeter. Anemia does not interfere with the accuracy of the SpO_2 as long as the hematocrit remains above 15%. The heart rate on the oximeter must correlate with the true heart rate for the SpO_2 to be considered accurate. The SpO_2 is falsely elevated in the presence of carboxyhemoglobinemia and the SpO_2 falsely reads 85% when significant methemoglobinemia is present.

Methemoglobinemia may occur more frequently in septic critically ill patients than previously recognized, since methemoglobin is generated in the presence of nitrites, which are a by-product of the nitric oxide pathway. In addition, since the pulse oximeter requires pulsatile flow, placement of the probe on the index finger or thumb of a patient with a radial arterial cannula serves as an early warning of ischemia in the radial artery distribution. The accuracy of the pulse oximeter is greatly reduced when the arterial oxygen saturation falls below 75%.

CENTRAL VENOUS CATHETERIZATION

The central veins are the major veins that drain directly into the right heart. Indications for central venous cannulation include a need for both access and monitoring (Table 2–2). The approaches to the central circulation can be classified on the basis of whether the inferior or superior vena cava is used. Venous air embolism is a possibility whenever the venous system is opened to atmospheric pressure above the level of the right atrium, or phlebostatic axis. Inadvertent entrainment of air through a 14-gauge catheter can occur at a rate of 90 mL/sec and produce a fatal air embolism in less than 1 second. Air embolism is most likely to occur during hypovolemia and spontaneous respiration when the hydrostatic pressure in the right side of the heart falls significantly below atmospheric pressure during early inspiration. The probability of air embolism is diminished, but not eliminated, by placing the patient in Trendelenburg's (head down) position for superior vena cava (SVC) cannulation and reverse Trendelenburg's (head up)

TABLE 2–2 Indications for Central Venous Cannulation

Access for rapid infusion of fluid

Long-term access required

Monitoring of cardiac function
• Preload
• Cardiac output
• Mixed venous saturation

Drug administration
• Vasoactive medications
• Highly osmotic or irritant drugs
• Hyperalimentation
• Chemotherapy
• Long-term antibiotics

Long-term inotropic medications (outpatient inotropic therapy)

Dialysis access

Temporary transvenous pacing wire placement

Aspiration of air emboli

Jugular venous bulb monitoring

position for femoral inferior vena cava (IVC) cannulation. Venous air embolism is best treated by aspiration of the air from the heart, but immediate temporizing measures include placing the patient in the left lateral decubitus Trendelenburg's position, increasing preload cautiously, and using aggressive inotropic support. Embolization of catheter fragments or the guide wire most often indicate serious deviation from proper technique. Difficulty in obtaining successful venipuncture is most often the result of poor anatomic landmarks, previous phlebitis or thrombosis, or distortion of anatomy by surgery or trauma. The complications of central venous cannulation are many, including those based in the patient's anatomic variability, inadvertent complications despite maintaining the standard of care, a breach in technique, and operator inexperience. Complications of central vein cannulation are listed in Table 2–3.

Approaches to the Central Venous Circulation

INFERIOR VENA CAVAL ACCESS The IVC is accessed via the femoral vein, which lies medial to the palpable femoral artery and below the inguinal ligament in the femoral triangle (Figure 2–1). Radiographic confirmation of subsequent catheter placement is not necessary. The primary advantage to the femoral venous access site is the relatively low rate of insertion-related complications, making it a good choice for emergent high-volume infusion. However, higher rates of catheter infection have been reported at this site, especially when the catheter is being used for total parenteral nutrition, and higher rates of deep venous thrombosis (DVT), especially in trauma patients, may outweigh the potential advantages. During cardiopulmonary resuscitation, thoracic compressions may increase inferior vena caval pressure, prolonging the circulation time of drugs to the heart. The femoral vein should not be cannulated for volume infusion in trauma patients if abdominal or pelvic venous injury or hepatic trauma is suspected or if surgical clamping of the IVC is anticipated. In the presence of known or suspected DVT, the femoral approach should be used with great caution, since instrumentation of the vein may dislodge thrombi proximally. The occurrence of DVT after prolonged instrumentation of the femoral venous system, especially in patients who are immobile as a result of trauma or who are in hypercoagulable states, is another consideration before planning femoral vein access.

SUPERIOR VENA CAVAL ACCESS The SVC is accessed directly via the subclavian, internal jugular, or external jugular veins (Figure 2–2) and indirectly via the antecubital veins. The proximity of these veins to major arteries in the neck and thorax and the possibility of pneumothorax reflect the more common complications of these approaches.

Since the catheters and guide wires are of sufficient length to reach the right atrium and ventricle, arrhythmias caused by mechanical stimulation of the heart are common. Transient ectopy is very common and need not be treated. However, the ability to immediately recognize and treat ventricular tachyarrhythmias

TABLE 2–3 **Complications of Central Venous Cannulation**

Hematoma

Microshock

Pneumothorax

Hemothorax

Chylothorax: Left internal jugular (LIJ) approach

Arterial puncture from cannulation

Subcutaneous infiltration: proximal port

Data misinterpretation

Perforation
• Superior vena cava
• Right atrium
• Right heart (tamponade)

Arrhythmias
• Bundle branch block
• Ectopy
• Ventricular tachycardia

Nerve injury
• Brachial plexus
• Stellate ganglion
• Phrenic nerve
• Recurrent laryngeal

Emboli
• Air
• Clot
• Catheter fragment
• Guide wire
• Systemic embolization
   1. patent foramen ovale
   2. arterial cannulation

Thrombosis
• Vein
• Aseptic thrombotic endocarditis
• Catheter-related infections
   1. Puncture site
   2. Catheter: colonization or infection
   3. Suppurative thrombophlebitis
   4. Endocarditis

Pulmonary artery catheter
• Pulmonary artery rupture
• Catheter knotting
• Valvular injury of the external jugular valve or tricuspid valve
• Pulmonary infarction
• Chordae tendineae rupture

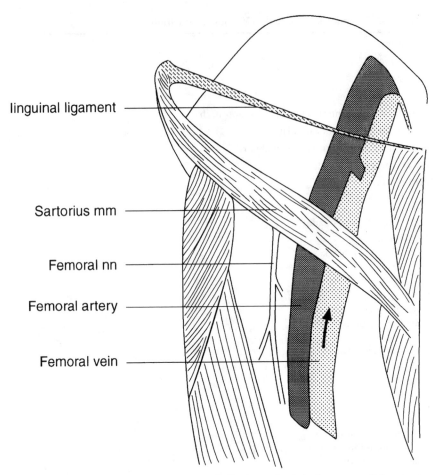

linguinal ligament

Sartorius mm

Femoral nn

Femoral artery

Femoral vein

FIGURE 2–1 Anatomy of the femoral triangle. The femoral vein is the most medial neurovascular structure within the femoral triangle. The palpable landmark is the femoral artery. The base of the inverted triangle is the inguinal ligament; the vastus intermedius (laterally) and the adductor longus (medially) are the muscular boundaries. The femoral nerve lies laterally and must be avoided. The arrow represents the direction of flow in the femoral vein.

is necessary; therefore, continuous monitoring of the electrocardiogram (ECG) during central venous access is highly recommended.

The tip of central venous catheters should lie in the SVC and not in the right atrium, where the catheter tip can perforate or erode into the pericardium, or in the right ventricle, where stimulation of conduction pathways can lead to paroxysmal arrhythmias and conduction block. Perforation of the SVC and right atrium have resulted in mortality rates that approach 70% and 100%, respectively.

SUBCLAVIAN VEIN CANNULATION The subclavian vein is the preferred site for central venous cannulation (Figure 2–2), since it is a large vein with relatively

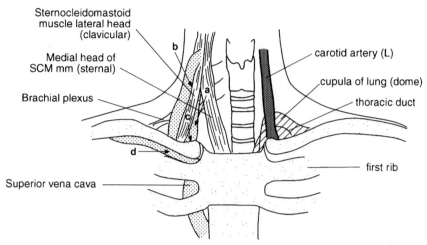

FIGURE 2–2 Anatomical landmarks for superior vena cava access. The internal jugular vein lies under the lateral head (clavicular) of the sternocleidomastoid (SCM) muscle and can be approached anteriorly (a) or posteriorly (b). The vulnerable structures include the carotid artery, brachial plexus cords, the dome of the pleura, and on the left side, the thoracic duct. A superior approach to the subclavian artery is possible in the base of the anterior cervical triangle (c). The subclavian vein passes under the medial aspect of the clavicle and can be accessed there (d); see text.

constant anatomy and is the vein most likely to be patent, even during profound hypovolemia since the vein is tethered to the surrounding dense connective tissue. The subclavian vein crosses under the clavicle, medial to the midclavicular line. The vein is most often entered at the junction of the outer one-third and medial two-thirds of the clavicle, with the needle parallel to the clavicle and directed at the sternal notch. The subclavian vein is the direct continuation of the axillary vein as it passes over the first rib and under the clavicle. The veins run anterior to the anterior scalene muscle, which separates the vein from the subclavian artery and pleura. The subclavian vein and internal jugular veins join at the thoracic inlet to form the brachiocephalic vein, which drains directly into the SVC. The left side is somewhat preferable for right heart catheterization because the angulation from the right subclavian vein into the right side of the heart is more acute. In experienced hands, the incidence of pneumothorax is no greater with the subclavian approach than it is with the internal jugular approach.

INTERNAL JUGULAR VEIN CANNULATION The internal jugular vein passes under the clavicular (lateral) head of the sternocleidomastoid muscle as the most lateral structure in the carotid sheath. Since the internal jugular vein lies posterior to the muscle belly, it can be accessed from either a medial (anterior) approach or a lateral (posterior) approach (Figure 2–2). The use of portable ultrasonography to guide internal jugular vein cannulation is becoming increasingly common and has obvious benefits in those patients in whom the palpation of anatomic landmarks is not possible.

The risk of inadvertent carotid artery puncture is always present and is slightly higher with the anterior approach and during periods of hypotension. Carotid puncture with a small-gauge needle carries a low risk of morbidity; hematoma and plaque embolization are relatively rare. Cannulation of the internal carotid artery with a large-bore catheter may provoke serious hemorrhage and may require emergent vascular surgery consultation. A foreign body in the carotid artery carries a high risk of embolic (e.g., air, clot) cerebrovascular complication: definitive therapy must not be delayed. The left internal jugular approach carries a risk of injury to the thoracic duct and resulting chylothorax. The indirect disadvantages of jugular venous cannulation include limited neck mobility and patient discomfort, proximity to oral and tracheostomal secretions, and overgrowth of the insertion site by facial hair in males, predisposing these catheters to contamination and infection.

EXTERNAL JUGULAR VEIN CANNULATION The external jugular vein is an alternative jugular approach to the central venous system. The advantages of external jugular cannulation are a low risk of pneumothorax, minimal risk of carotid artery puncture, and easy control of bleeding. However, these advantages are outweighed by the difficulty in accessing the highly mobile and collapsible vein, in anchoring catheters, in passing the guide wire and catheter through a venous valve (which may be made incompetent after catheterization), and the risk of venous injury at the acutely angled junction of the internal and external jugular veins. The external jugular approach is not recommended for routine critical care central venous access.

PERIPHERALLY INSERTED CENTRAL CATHETERS A reasonable alternative to direct access to major veins is the use of a peripherally inserted central catheter (PICC) or long-arm central catheter; however, these are more applicable for patients who need long-term care than patients in the CCU. These catheters are inserted into the brachial or cephalic veins in the antecubital area and then threaded into the SVC, where the proper position is confirmed either radiographically or electrocardiographically. Anesthesiologists routinely place special long-arm central catheters, which have multiple aspiration ports, in patients for neurosurgical procedures to facilitate aspiration of air embolism, to monitor central venous pressure (CVP), and to administer some medications. The PICC catheter is used mainly for long-term antibiotic or chemotherapy administration.

Central Venous Pressure Monitoring

CVP can be transduced at any point in the central venous system, including the IVC; however, the reliability and validity of the IVC is affected by intra-abdominal pathology. The phlebostatic axis is at the level of the tricuspid valve or right atrium in a supine patient; this is where intravascular pressure reaches zero and is independent of body habitus. Although changes in posture can be expected to affect the reference pressure at the phlebostatic axis by less than 1 mm Hg, the CVP is a less accurate indicator of filling pressures when it is measured in the lateral or upright position, because of venous pooling. The CVP is most often used as an approximation of preload and reflects a balance between venous return and right-sided cardiac output. Under normal conditions, the right side of the heart is composed of a thin wall of myocardium and is more compliant than the more muscular left side of the heart. Since CVP measures intravascular pressure and not transmural pressure, which is the actual determinant of ventricular preload, its validity as an index of preload is influenced by pulmonary variables, such as intrathoracic pressure, and by cardiac variables, such as cardiac compliance.

Central filling pressures, such as the CVP, pulmonary artery wedge pressure (PAWP), and pulmonary capillary wedge pressure (PCWP), are measured at end-expiration, when the relative intrathoracic pressure is zero (i.e., it equals atmospheric pressure), and therefore intravascular pressure equals transmural pressure. High levels of positive pressure ventilation, which affect the CVP, should never be discontinued to determine a "more accurate" CVP. In instances where the CVP is thought to be falsely elevated by intrathoracic pressure, an alternative form of preload assessment should be considered or esophageal manometry should be used to estimate transthoracic pressure. The transthoracic pressure can then be subtracted from the CVP to provide a better estimate of preload.

Graphic depiction of the CVP (also the PCWP and left atrial pressure) waveforms consists of three positive wave deflections (a, c, and v) and two descents (x and y) (Figure 2–3). The a wave is the increase in venous pressure that is generated by atrial contraction. The c wave occurs when the atrioventricular valve (tricuspid or mitral) is displaced into the atrium during isovolumetric ventricular contraction. The v wave reflects the increase in atrial pressure that occurs as venous return begins to fill the atrium during isovolumetric relaxation, while the atrioventricular valves are still closed. The x descent corresponds to ventricular ejection, as the emptying ventricle draws down on the floor of the atrium and decreases the CVP. The y descent occurs as the atrioventricular valve opens and blood enters the ventricle during ventricular diastole.

The importance of these waveforms lies in their ability to reflect on pathophysiologic processes. Absence of the a wave occurs in atrial fibrillation, in which case the x descent may also be absent. Amplified, or "cannon," a waves occur in the presence of stenosis of the atrioventricular (mitral) wave. Both the x and y descents are exaggerated in the presence of constrictive pericarditis, whereas cardiac tamponade magnifies the x descent and abolishes the y descent.

In the presence of atrioventricular valve incompetency, free transduction of ventricular pressure during ventricular contraction generates large "cannon" V waves that are pathognomonic for regurgitant flow, especially mitral regurgita-

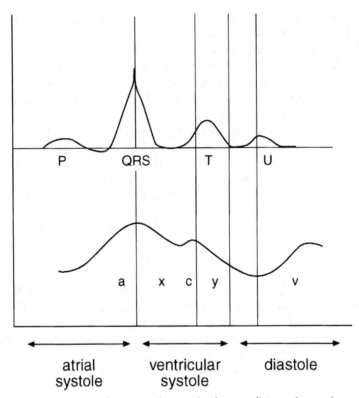

P   QRS   T   U

a   x   c   y   v

atrial
systole
ventricular
systole
diastole

FIGURE 2–3 *The CVP wave form as it relates to the electrocardiogram (see text).*

tion. In the case of the CVP, pulmonary hypertension increases right ventricular afterload, decreases right ventricular compliance, and accentuates the *v* waveform depicted on the monitor.

PULMONARY ARTERY CATHETER

The pulmonary artery catheter (PAC), or Swan-Ganz catheter, provides a more accurate measure of left ventricular preload; however, it also is subject to operator bias and misinterpretation.[7,8] The pulmonary artery catheter was originally introduced in 1970 by Swan and Ganz, whose names are still attached to the catheter today. The importance of basing clinical interventions on judicious interpretation of the data obtained from the PAC cannot be overemphasized.[9,10] Although the discipline of critical care medicine is to a large extent rooted in use of the PAC, recent suggestions that the use of the PAC in clinical medicine is associated with increased morbidity and mortality may reflect, in large part, decisions made on the basis of inaccurate data alone, without sufficient consideration of the underlying physiologic principles.

Pulmonary Artery Catheter Placement

The PAC is passed into the central venous circulation through an introducer catheter, or cordis, and is then passed sequentially through the great veins, the right atrium, right ventricle, pulmonary outflow tract, and into a pulmonary artery. A 1.5-mL silastic balloon allows catheter placement to be flow-directed, because the balloon tip of the catheter, inflated during catheter passage, facilitates placement in the pulmonary outflow tract. Fluoroscopic assistance during placement may be indicated if a transvenous pacemaker has been placed recently, selective pulmonary artery catheterization is necessary, or anatomic abnormalities, such as Eisenmenger's complex, exist.

Catheterization of the right side of the heart carries the additional risks of arrhythmias, intravascular coiling and knotting, and vascular perforation. Continuous waveform analysis of the pressures transduced at the PAC tip allows subjective assessment of the location of the catheter tip. Progression of the catheter tip through the right side of the heart must be monitored by transduced waveform analysis (Figure 2–4).

Since the placement of the catheter is flow-directed, advancement of the catheter incrementally with each heartbeat facilitates appropriate passage. Catheter advancement without concomitant waveform progression strongly correlates with placement in the IVC or coiling within the right heart chambers. When the catheter

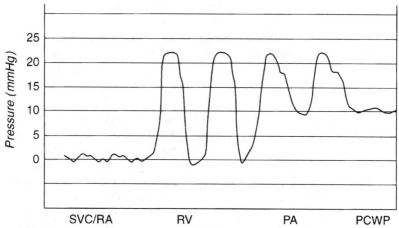

FIGURE 2–4 *Waveform analysis during pulmonary artery catheterization. The pressures transduced sequentially include the superior vena cava (SVC) and right atrium (RA) which are typical CVP readings. Entry into the right ventricle (RV) is marked by a rise in the systolic component. The characteristic rise in diastolic pressure signals entry into the pulmonary artery (PA). With the balloon inflated, 'wedge' positioning of the balloon tip is signaled by a flattening of the PA waveform. Deflation of the pulmonary artery balloon in the wedge position should be accompanied by a return to the PA waveform, as blood flow resumes past the catheter tip.*

reaches the distal pulmonary artery, the diastolic pressure characteristically rises. Further advancement of the catheter causes the waveform to flatten and signifies that the "wedge" position has been reached; at this point, the balloon occludes the flow of blood past the catheter tip. "Pseudo-wedging" may occur if the catheter is caught underneath the pulmonary valve or trabeculae or between papillary muscles. In this case, waveform flattening occurs prior to pulmonary artery waveform identification. Deflation and reinflation of the balloon is critical, since distal migration of the catheter tip occurs frequently. If slow inflation of the balloon results in a continued rise of the transduced pressure to high levels, the catheter tip is either "overwedged" in the pulmonary capillary, which carries a high risk of pulmonary artery rupture, or the balloon has herniated past the tip of the catheter, where pressure transduction occurs. Suspicion of "overwedging" requires that inflation attempts be immediately abandoned, the catheter withdrawn a short distance into the pulmonary artery, and the wedge position re-ascertained by slow re-advancement of the catheter.

The Physiology and Analysis of Pulmonary Catheter Data

PULMONARY CAPILLARY WEDGE PRESSURE AND CARDIAC FUNCTION
The pressure determined from this "wedge" waveform at end-expiration is the PCWP, and may be used as an index of left atrial pressure, and by further extrapolation, the left ventricular end-diastolic pressure. However, true left ventricular preload is actually ventricular wall tension caused by ventricular end-diastolic filling volume, which stretches myocardial sarcomeres.

The relationship of ventricular performance to isometric preload is Starling's law of the heart, and the resulting graphic depiction of this relationship is referred to as a Starling curve (Figure 2–5). Interpretation of the data obtained from use of the PAC is based on the Starling curve and is the foundation for cardiovascular critical care.

A fundamental concept of cardiac physiology is that optimal preload develops a tension on the muscle, which causes the overlap of actin and myosin in the myocyte to approximate 2.2 μm. Otherwise, and more practically stated, optimal preload is that precontraction load, or tension, that optimizes ventricular performance. In graphic terms, optimal preload is the volume that produces ventricular distension nearing the apex of the Starling curve, maximally increasing cardiac contractile function. Overdistention of the sarcomeres beyond 3.0 μm causes a decrease in contractile performance and a negative slope in the Starling curve. Since the pulmonary artery catheter measures pressure, the corresponding volume preload can be inferred only if compliance remains constant during the period of measurement (i.e., compliance = volume/ pressure).

The pulmonary artery catheter has as its greatest utility the ability to depict a mathematical and graphic relationship between cardiac filling pressure and cardiac performance. Data is most reliable when it is directly measured, and mathematical manipulation sequentially introduces error. The use of indexed values,

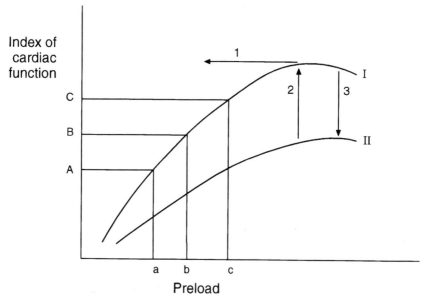

FIGURE 2–5 *Curvilinear depiction of Starlings law of the heart: The Starling curve relates preload (CVP, PCWP, LVEDP, or LVEDV) to cardiac function (EF, SV, CO) and forms the basis of cardiovascular critical care since both dependent and independent variables can be tracked using a PAC. The incremental increases in preload (a, b, c) are accompanied by corresponding increases in cardiac function (A, B, C). Therapeutic interventions can change the variables. Diuresis decreases preload (1), inotropes increase cardiac function at any given filling pressure (2), and the use of beta or calcium channel blockers can inhibit contractility and move the patient's cardiac function between curves I and II.*

standardized to body surface area (i.e., cardiac index = cardiac output/body surface area) facilitates the comparison of hemodynamic variables among patients. However, if the data is used primarily to predict trends over time, indexing provides little added benefit.

The principle on which the use of the PCWP as a measurement of left ventricular preload rests on is the assumption that inflation of the balloon in the wedge position within the pulmonary artery obstructs blood flow around the catheter tip and creates a static column of blood that is contiguous to the left atrium and, at end diastole before mitral valve closure, with the left ventricular end-diastolic pressure. Since catheter placement is flow-directed, the balloon usually carries the PAC tip to zone 2 of West, where the hydrostatic pressure in the pulmonary artery (P_{pa}) exceeds alveolar (P_A) pressure, which exceeds pulmonary venous (P_{pv}) pressure $(P_{pa} > P_A > P_{pv})$, or to zone 3 of West, where $P_{pa} > P_{pv} > P_A$ (Figure 2–6). Since the mean airway pressure in zones 1 and 2 is intermittently greater than pulmonary venous pressure, collapse of the vasculature causes inability to transduce accurate intravascular pressure. The reliability of the PCWP is greatest

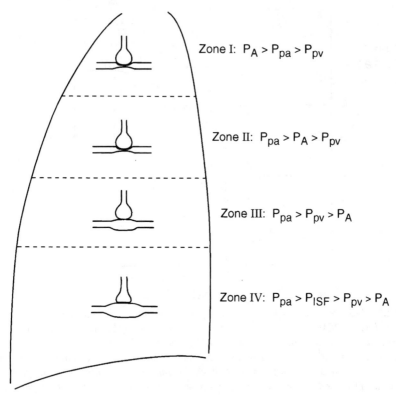

Zone I: $P_A > P_{pa} > P_{pv}$

Zone II: $P_{pa} > P_A > P_{pv}$

Zone III: $P_{pa} > P_{pv} > P_A$

Zone IV: $P_{pa} > P_{ISF} > P_{pv} > P_A$

FIGURE 2–6 West zones of the lung. West zones relate ventilation and perfusion. Flow is greatest in dependent zones, partially governed by gravity. Ventilation/perfusion ratio is greatest toward the apex of the lung. In order to best reflect cardiac function, the tip of the PAC should lie in zone 3 or 4.

when the catheter tip is in zone 3 or 4, since only in these zones is there a continual column of uninterrupted blood between the catheter tip and the left atrium. High mean airway pressure and hypovolemia are the most common causes of relatively decreased zones 3 and 4 of the lung.

The risks and difficulties inherent in repeated efforts at repositioning guided by lateral chest radiographs is not practical, cost-effective, or safe. Instead, the catheter is assumed to be in zone 3 or 4, unless there is a marked transduction of pulmonary pressures on the pulmonary artery and PCWP waveforms.

Airway PEEP increases the proportion of zones 1 and 2 relative to zone 3 because of alveolar recruitment. The probability that the catheter tip lies in zone 3 or 4 is higher if a change in PCWP is less than half the incremental change in PEEP, and if the pulmonary artery diastolic (PAD) pressure is slightly higher than the PCWP. The true PCWP may be approximated using the formula:

$$PCWP = PCWP_M - 0.5(PEEP - 10)$$

Where

PCWP$_M$ is the measured PCWP at any level of PEEP

Because the PCWP, analogous to the CVP, reflects a balance between blood return to the left side of the heart and the ejection of blood in the left ventricle by cardiac pumping function, it is not in itself an absolute. Elevated PCWP may indicate either fluid overload or decreased cardiac contractility. The PCWP does not reflect the volume of extracellular fluid. During myocardial ischemia, decreased ventricular compliance and impaired contractility reduce the ability of the left side of the heart to maintain an effective forward flow of blood, which is reflected in decreased stroke volume and ejection fraction, causing the measured PCWP to become elevated at any given preload. The appropriate therapeutic intervention at this time, active decrease of preload or active increase in contractility, requires both more data regarding cardiac output and previous training and experience. The accuracy of the PCWP as an indicator of left ventricular end-diastolic pressure (LVEDP) is compromised in a number of pathophysiologic conditions in addition to the cardiopulmonary interactions described earlier.[11] Mitral stenosis results in left atrial end-diastolic pressure and PCWP that are higher than LVEDP, an artifact caused by impaired left atrial ejection. The presence of "cannon" v waves on the pressure tracing can aid diagnosis of this condition.

Large atrial masses, such as myxomas or mural thrombi, may falsely increase atrial pressures by decreasing atrial compliance and falsely elevate the PCWP. In aortic regurgitation, the PCWP underestimates the LVEDP because the mitral valve closes before left ventricular filling is completed. Regurgitant flow across the aortic valve continues to increase LVEDP and cannot be measured unless the mitral valve has also become incompetent. The CVP is always lower than the PCWP, except when pulmonary vascular resistance is substantially elevated, in which case CVP is higher than PCWP, or in the case of tamponade, in which the two pressures are equal. Pericardial tamponade restricts the filling of all cardiac chambers and results in the pathognomonic condition known as "equalization of pressures," in which CVP, mean pulmonary artery pressure, and PCWP are equal. The PCWP and the pulmonary artery diastolic pressure are usually similar if the heart rate is less than 90 beats per minute.

PULMONARY CAPILLARY WEDGE PRESSURE AND ADULT RESPIRATORY DISTRESS SYNDROME The PCWP is a useful guide to both pulmonary capillary filtration pressure and left ventricular filling pressure. The determination of the PCWP is often emphasized as a diagnostic tool in the differentiation of cardiogenic and noncardiogenic pulmonary edema. The diagnosis of ARDS rests on the PCWP determination; however, patients with ARDS are usually receiving ventilation using PEEP. The relationship of actual and measured PEEP has been discussed in the preceding section. Pulmonary capillary transmembrane fluid flux is described by Starling's law, which defines the equilibrium between hydrostatic and osmotic forces across a capillary membrane:

$$F = [(P_i - P_o) - (COP_i - COP_o)] \times K$$

Where

    F is transmembrane fluid flux

    P_i is hydrostatic pressure within artery

    P_o is hydrostatic pressure outside the capillary

    COP_i is intravascular oncotic pressure

    COP_o is extravascular oncotic pressure

    K is the filtration coefficient

or

$$P_{cap} = PCWP + 0.4 \, (P_a - PCWP)$$

Where

    P_{cap} is pulmonary capillary filtration pressure

    P_a is pulmonary artery pressure

Elevation of the pulmonary capillary hydrostatic pressure in the presence of left ventricular failure favors transudation of fluid across the basement membrane and into the alveoli. When the volume of fluid overcomes the maximal lymphatic clearance, pulmonary edema occurs, manifested by a widening of the alveolar-arterial oxygen gradient and decreased lung compliance. Since a great many other factors can produce an identical picture (e.g., inflammation, high levels of negative alveolar pressure, hypoalbuminemia), the PCWP aids the differential diagnosis. Low or normal levels of PCWP in the presence of clinically determined pulmonary edema is a major criterion for the diagnosis of ARDS.

CARDIAC OUTPUT MEASURED BY THERMODILUTION In addition to intracardiac pressure measurements, the PAC also enables the measurement of cardiac output by thermodilution.[12] A thermistor at the tip of the PAC continually measures the temperature of the blood in the pulmonary artery as it flows past the catheter tip. Injection of a known quantity of fluid at a known temperature into the right atrium allows the change in the temperature of the mixed blood as it flows past the thermistor to be plotted as a function of time, as shown in Figure 2–7. The differentiated rate of change (dT/dt) is proportional and the integrated area under the curve is inversely proportional to the cardiac output. Thermodilution is a modification of an indirect indicator dye (indocyanine green) dilution technique in which the flow is equal to the amount of dye injected divided by the integral of the instantaneous concentration of dye in sampled arterial blood over time. The determination of cardiac output using the Fick equation predates the PAC but nonetheless requires right heart catheterization. The Fick equation is:

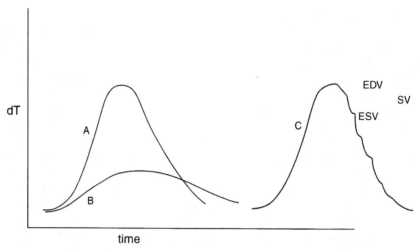

FIGURE 2–7 Thermodilution cardiac output curves. The curves represent a change in temperature detected by the thermistor at the PAC tip as a mixed injectate of known temperature flows past. The curve with the greatest change in temperature (dT) per unit of time has the lower area under the curve but has the greatest cardiac output associated with it (A and B). Curve C depicts a thermodilution curve as sensed by a rapid response thermistor capable of determining end–diastolic volume (EDV) and subsequent volume changes (ESV) as the right ventricle empties. The ejection fraction (EF) is the EDV-ESV, which is the stroke volume SV, divided by EDV.

$$CO = \frac{\dot{V}o_2}{Cao_2 - Cvo_2}$$

Where

    CO is cardiac output

    $\dot{V}o_2$ is whole body O_2 consumption

    Cao_2 is content of O_2 in arterial blood

    Cvo_2 is content of O_2 in venous blood

This equation is now most commonly used as a method of calculating $\dot{V}o_2$ when the cardiac output is measured directly, using the PAC. Thermodilution cardiac output determination is the currently accepted standard of practice and adds greatly to the utility of the PAC. Although room temperature injectates are reliable in most patients, the signal-to-noise ratio is more favorable with cold injectates, especially in patients with low body temperature or low cardiac output. Variation of the cardiac output with phases of the respiratory cycle suggest that either measurements be timed to coincide with the same respiratory phase or an average value be used to predict trends. In clinical situations, trends which occur over time during the care of a patient are always more valuable than absolute numerical values.

The thermodilution cardiac output as determined by the PAC is subject to artifactual inaccuracies based on the method used. Since the determination of cardiac output is directly based on the temperature change sensed by the thermistor at the catheter tip, smaller changes in temperature produce a falsely elevated level of cardiac output. Smaller temperature changes, which artifactually elevate the derived cardiac output, can occur with the use of less injectate than necessary or warmer-than-measured injectate (after a long wait at room temperature before injection of cold saline) and in the presence of right-to-left cardiac shunts. On the other hand, the most common cause of artifactually decreased cardiac output is tricuspid regurgitation, which allows a prolonged mixing time of blood and injectate, resulting in prolonged transit time in the right side of the heart and a decrease of the temperature change with time. A rate of injection that is too slow also gives a falsely low value for cardiac output. Left-to-right shunts may make thermodilution cardiac output unmeasurable. Finally, rapid infusion of fluids may dilute the injectate and also render the cardiac output measurement inaccurate.

DERIVED CARDIAC INDEXES Cardiac performance interpretation must be based on the fundamentals of cardiac physiology. The amount of blood ejected from each ventricle per heartbeat is the stroke volume (SV). The output of the left ventricle per unit time is the cardiac output (CO). CO can also be expressed as a function of heart rate and stroke volume:

$$CO\ (L/min) = HR\ (beats/min) \times SV\ (mL/beat)$$

Where

CO is cardiac ouput

HR is heart rate

SV is stroke volume

Cardiac performance can then be expressed as a measure of the chronotropic and inotropic states of the heart. Chronotropy, or heart rate, is the effective balance of vagal and sympathetic tone in the resting heart rate. Inotropy, or contractility, is the sum of the tension generated by preload and the sum of contractility influences, including sympathetic effects on membrane receptors, channels, and intracellularly mediated contractility. However, CO also depends on the impedance, or resistance, to flow. This resistance is referred to as afterload and is low in the pulmonary arterial circulation right ventricular afterload and high in the aortic and systemic arterial circulation left ventricular afterload. Thus, afterload is most commonly referred to as either pulmonary vascular resistance (PVR) or systemic vascular resistance (SVR), although afterload is truly more complicated than vascular resistance alone. Although afterload is crucially important to cardiac performance, it can only be measured experimentally in heart-lung preparations ex-vivo. The PAC cannot measure afterload or SVR but does allow an inference based on measured ventricular performance.

Mathematically, vascular resistance on the pulmonary and systemic circulations can be expressed as derivatives of Ohm's law, which states that current is electromotive force divided by resistance, or flow equals pressure divided by resistance. Rearrangement to solve for vascular resistance produces:

$$PVR = \frac{MAP - PCWP}{CO \times 80}$$

$$SVR = \frac{MAP - CVP}{CO \times 80}$$

Where

MAP is mean arterial pressure

CVP is central venous pressure

CO is cardiac output

Alternatively, ventricular afterload can be expressed as the myocardial wall tension during ejection as defined by the Laplace equation. Note that the CO and vascular resistances are thus mathematically inversely proportional. CO is measured and vascular resistance is calculated, lending greater credence to the treatment of CO. A more direct estimate of aortic resistance is based on the relationship:

$$R\,(aortic) = \frac{arterial\ pulse\ pressure}{SV}$$

Where

R (aortic) is aortic resistance

SV is stroke volume

Note that the Poiseuille-Hagen formula suggests that resistance is also indirectly influenced by viscosity (hematocrit). Furthermore, patients with arteriovenous shunting typically have decreased baseline SVR. Further manipulation of measured data can potentially increase the inferences possible PAC monitoring; however, these manipulations must be interpreted with caution. The data which is directly obtained from the PAC (i.e., CVP, PCWP, CO, Svo_2)can be combined with ECG information and manipulated mathematically to derive additional indexes of hemodynamic function (Table 2–4). Note however, that since information that is directly measured, such as the CO, has greater validity than derived indices, such as SVR, the former should carry more weight in management decisions.

ASSESSMENT OF CARDIAC PHARMACOLOGIC INTERVENTION The PAC is the gold standard for the clinical assessment of the physiologic response of the

TABLE 2-4 Hemodynamic Formulas and Normal Ranges

Variable	Formula	Normal Range
Cardiac index (CI)	$CI\ (L/min/m^2) = \dfrac{CO\ (L/min)}{BSA\ (m^2)}$	2.8–4.2 L/min/m^2
Stroke volume (SV)	$SV\ (mL\ per\ beat) = \dfrac{CO\ (L/min) \times 1000\ (mL/L)}{HR\ (beats\ per\ min)}$	60–90 mL per beat
Stroke index (SI)	$SI\ (mL\ per\ beat\ per\ m^2) = \dfrac{SV\ (mL\ per\ beat)}{BSA\ (m^2)}$	30–65 mL per beat per m^2
Systemic vascular resistance (SVR)	$SVR\ (dynes/sec/m^2 - 5) = \left(\dfrac{MAP\ (mm\ Hg)\ -\ CVP\ (mm\ Hg)}{CO\ (L/min)}\right) \times 80$	1200–1500 dynes/sec/m^2
Pulmonary vascular resistance (PVR)	$PVR\ (dynes/sec/m^2 - 5) = \left(\dfrac{MPAP\ (mm\ Hg)\ -\ PCWP\ (mm\ Hg)}{CO\ (L/min)}\right) \times 80$	100–300 dynes/sec/m^2
Left ventricular stroke work index (LVSWI)	LVSWI (g-m per beat per m^2) = 0.0136 [MAP (mm Hg) – PCWP (mm Hg)] SI (mL per beat per m^2)	45–60

NOTES: Units are in parentheses in equations.

ABBREVIATIONS: BSA, body surface area; CO, cardiac output; HR, heart rate; MAP, mean arterial pressure; CVP, central venous pressure; MPAP, mean pulmonary artery pressure; PCNP, pulmonary capillary wedge pressure.

critically ill patient to therapeutic intervention (Figure 2–5). Because of this mode of assessment, pharmacologic intervention that affects cardiac performance can be specifically, and often selectively, directed at preload, chronotropy, inotropy, or afterload.

Preload is increased by the administration of fluids that replenish or expand intravascular volume, such as blood products, colloids, or crystalloid (Figure 2–5a,b,c). Effective decreases in preload can be accomplished relatively by venodilating agents, such as low-dose nitrates or morphine, or definitively through diuresis (Figure 2–5, *arrow 1*). Chronotropy can be increased by vagolytic agents, such as atropine sulfate or related compounds, indirect and direct sympathomimetic agents, or artificial electrical pacing. Indirect sympathomimetic agents are those compounds, such as ephedrine, which trigger the release of epinephrine from sympathetic nerve terminals, and direct sympathomimetic agents are the epinephrine analogs, such as isoproterenol, which acts directly on the β_1-receptors to increase heart rate. Heart rate is also indirectly regulated by the carotid baroreceptors and possibly also by atrial stretch receptors (Bainbridge reflex). Inotropy can be decreased (Figure 2–5, *arrow 3*) indirectly through the blockade of β_1-receptors or calcium antagonists and directly through depression of excitation-contraction coupling at the subcellular level. Recently, the identification and demonstration of physiologically active myocardial β_3-receptors[13] that exert negative effects on the inotropic state of the human heart have opened a new and exciting potential avenue of therapeutics based on the selective stimulation and blockade of this receptor. Inotropy can likewise be augmented (Figure 2–5, *arrow 2*) with indirect and direct β_1-receptor stimulation by means of sympathomimetic agents, with inhibition of the membrane-based transtubular sodium-potassium ATPase pump by means of digitalis glycosides (which increase calcium flux into the myocytes), with manipulation of the serum-ionized calcium concentration relative to intracellular calcium concentration by means of administration of intravenous calcium salts, and by means of the inhibitors of phosphodiesterase (PDE), such as aminophylline, and specifically the inhibition of PDE-3 by amrinone and milrinone. Afterload can be increased by the generalized stimulation of sympathetic tone, administration of vasopressin, or by selective activation of α_1-receptors, which precipitate vasoconstriction. Cold-induced vasoconstriction and increased cardiac afterload are an often-unrecognized cause of increased cardiac workload and therefore a potential cause of cardiac ischemia. However, afterload can be decreased pharmacologically by activators of the nitric oxide pathway, such as sodium nitroprusside; calcium channel blocking agents, such as nicardipine; direct smooth-muscle dilators, such as hydralazine; inhibitors of angiotensin-converting enzyme (ACE), such as captopril; or indirect sympathectomy, affecting central sympathetic outflow.

ASSESSMENT OF CARDIOPULMONARY INTERACTION Cardiac and pulmonary function are highly interdependent, and changes in pleural and intrathoracic pressure, oxygenation, and ventilation exert important effects on pulmonary blood flow and left-sided CO.[14] During spontaneous ventilation, the generation of negative pleural pressure aids in thoracic venous return and augments cardiac diastolic filling. The implementation of positive pressure ventilation by definition prevents the generation of negative intrathoracic pressure. Incremental increases in intrathoracic pressure (e.g., PEEP, mean airway pressure, peak airway pressure) progressively impair the venous return to the right side of the heart (preload) and thereby decrease CO. Transmitted pleural pressure to the compliant right side of the heart diminishes distensibility during diastole and further impairs venous return. Simultaneously, alveolar distention can impinge on pulmonary capillary flow, increase PVR and impose increased afterload. Bowing of the ventricular septum into the left ventricle occurs late as pressures in the right side of the heart increase further.

However, most patients who require high levels of positive airway pressure to maintain adequate oxygenation have alveolar hypoxia, which may increase PVR through hypoxic pulmonary vasoconstriction, further impairing function of the right side of the heart. Conversely, increasing alveolar recruitment and resolution of alveolar hypoxia may, with continued application, improve cardiac function by diminishing the presence of hypoxic pulmonary vasoconstriction. PEEP may decrease left ventricular afterload and, until decreased preload intervenes, transiently increase CO. Since pressures in the right side of the heart with high levels of positive pressure ventilation may not be a reliable indicator of preload, the measurement of CO, mixed venous saturation, or right ventricular ejection fraction is almost always considered a mandatory intervention.

CONTINUOUS CARDIAC OUTPUT AND MIXED VENOUS OXIMETRY CO can be measured at 2- to 3-minute intervals by a catheter that includes a thermal filament at the level of the right ventricle. CO determinations at frequent regular intervals allow "continuous" CO monitoring. In addition, injectate fluid load and operator variability are reduced and changes in physiologic state more rapidly detectable.

CO is proportional to the saturation of mixed venous blood; the higher the CO the greater the saturation of mixed venous blood. Fiberoptic technology allows some PACs to measure the saturation of hemoglobin in the blood as it flows past the PAC tip in the pulmonary arteries, using the principle of reflectance spectrophotometry. Mixed venous blood is blood that includes blood return from all organs, including the heart via the thebesian veins, just before reoxygenation in the pulmonary capillaries. In catheters that are not equipped with fiberoptic systems capable of measuring the hemoglobin saturation directly, blood can be slowly aspirated from the distal port of the PAC and submitted for ABG analysis. Sepsis causes a decrease in both peripheral $\dot{V}o_2$ and arteriovenous shunting, which is reflected as an increase in the Svo_2. Variables that contribute to Do_2 (e.g., anemia, hypovolemia, cardiogenic shock, arterial hypoxemia, carboxyhemoglobinemia) all cause a decrease in the Svo_2. Pathologic left-to-right intracardiac shunting produces an increase in the amount of oxygenated blood in the right ventricle and thus an increase in the Svo_2 and a grossly inaccurate (arteriovenous) O_2 gradient.

PULMONARY ARTERY CATHETERS AND VOLUMETRIC RIGHT VENTRIC-
ULAR EJECTION FRACTION A variant of the conventional PAC uses a rapid response thermistor, capable of determining right ventricular end-systolic volumes
(ESV) and end-diastolic volumes (EDV), and thereby makes possible the calculation of the right ventricular ejection fraction (RVEF) (Figure 2–7c), expressed as
RVEF = ESV/EDV.[15] This particular catheter therefore combines measured volumetric and pressure data to increase the sensitivity and reliability of the PAC in
the assessment of biventricular function.

There is evidence to suggest that patients admitted to the ICU with significant
right ventricular dysfunction that cannot be predicted with conventional PAC
monitoring.[16] The diagnostic superiority of right ventricular end-diastolic volume (RVEDV) measurement over measurements of urine output, CVP, and
PCWP has been repeatedly suggested in patients with burns, sepsis, and trauma.
The effect of high positive airway pressures, especially PEEP, disparately affects
the thin walled right ventricle. The effect of increasing PEEP on right ventricular
afterload and the coincident increase in RVEDV and depression of RVEF is best
assessed by using the volumetric catheter. Filling pressures thus are more likely to
be overestimated in the presence of undetected right heart dysfunction. Advantages to RVEF-based cardiac performance evaluation has not been demonstrated
in cardiac patients. The RVEF catheter loses accuracy in the presence of arrhythmias or tricuspid valve regurgitation.

OXYGEN KINETICS AND PULMONARY ARTERY CATHETERS One of the
most important applications of the PAC is information regarding whole body
oxygen delivery ($\dot{D}o_2$) and volume of oxygen uptake ($\dot{V}o_2$). The caveat that $\dot{D}o_2$
and $\dot{V}o_2$ are systemic indexes not applicable to individual tissue beds should not
detract from their utility as gross measures of the adequacy of resuscitation. The
primary determinant of $\dot{D}o_2$ is cardiac output; therefore, an incremental change
in cardiac output (CO) is more important to $\dot{D}o_2$ than an equal incremental
change in Cao_2 or its comprised variables.

$$\dot{D}o_2 = Cao_2 \times CO$$
$$\dot{D}o_2 = \{((Hb) \times 1.34 \times Sao_2) + (Pao_2 \times 0.0031)\} \times CO$$

Oxidative phosphorylation is a more efficient pathway for substrate metabolism than anaerobic glycolysis and generates more adenosine triphosphate (ATP)
per mole of glucose, 36 moles in comparison to 2 moles, respectively. ATP provides cellular bioenergy for enzymatic pathways. For oxidative phosphorylation
to predominate, $\dot{D}o_2$ must at least match $\dot{V}o_2$. Oxygen delivery that is inadequate
to meet metabolic demand, or the metabolic requirement for oxygen (MRo_2),
defines the state of shock. Since $\dot{D}o_2$ depends primarily on cardiac output (CO),
shock states are classified based on the underlying pathophysiologic mechanism
that causes the compromise in CO. Progressive mismatches between $\dot{D}o_2$ and $\dot{V}o_2$
are manifested first by a decreasing mixed venous oxygen saturation, an excess of
systemic lactate, and metabolic acidosis. Under normal conditions $\dot{D}o_2$ exceeds

$\dot{V}o_2$ significantly, and there is a range over which decreases in $\dot{D}o_2$ have no detectable metabolic consequences. Compensation in this range occurs through modulation of the oxygen extraction ratio (O_2ER). The O_2ER is the ratio of $\dot{V}o_2$ to $\dot{D}o_2$ and represents the fraction of delivered oxygen that is taken up into the tissues, usually in the range of 20% to 30%.

$$O_2ER = \frac{\dot{V}o_2}{\dot{D}o_2 \times 100}$$

Maximal oxygen extraction occurs when the O_2ER approximates 50% to 60%. At this point, known as the point of critical oxygen delivery, the $\dot{V}o_2$ becomes dependent on $\dot{D}o_2$ (supply-dependent $\dot{V}o_2$), a state also known as dysoxia. Lactate production increases progressively as this mismatch increases. This can be depicted in a relationship (Figure 2–8) that has great conceptual utility,[17] but remains controversial despite many years of application.[18] However, since plasma lactate level represents a balance between production and extraction in tissues, such as the liver, lactate may not be detectable despite increases in production. Lactate excess may also be a result of endotoxin inhibition of pyruvate dehydro-

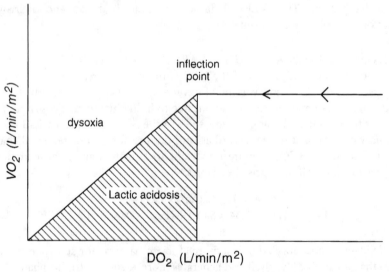

FIGURE 2–8 *The theoretical relationship between oxygen delivery ($\dot{D}O_2$) and oxygen uptake ($\dot{V}O_2$): Gradual decrease in $\dot{D}O_2$ has little or no detectable effect on $\dot{V}O_2$ since compensation occurs by icnreased peripheral extraction. Further decrease in $\dot{D}O_2$ to the inflection point causes the $\dot{V}O_2$ to become pathologically flow dependent and a state of dysoxia occurs in which there is a change from oxidative to anaerobic metabolism. Pathologic supply dependency is heralded by the development of lactic acidosis. Although theoretically useful, the relationship is controversial because mathematical coupling can occur when both $\dot{V}O_2$ and $\dot{D}O_2$ are measured using the same device (PAC), and it does not account for possible metabolic alterations induced by inflammatory mediators which may alter $\dot{V}O_2$ at the tissue and cellular levels.*

genase and thiamine deficiency.[19] The point of critical oxygen delivery is probably much higher than normal in critically ill patients, possibly because the tissue MRo_2 level is increased by metabolic stress.

ECHOCARDIOGRAPHIC AS]SESSMENT OF CARDIAC FUNCTION

More recently, minimally invasive and noninvasive measures of cardiac performance have achieved some measure of popularity. Transesophageal echocardiography (TEE) is the best established of these and has greater applicability in the ICU patient because of thoracic pathophysiology, which often limits the size of acoustic windows available to transthoracic echocardiography (TTE).[20] Esophageal or gastric placement of the ultrasound TEE transducer results in close proximity of the transducer to the heart and, therefore, minimal image degradation by air interfaces. TEE in two and three dimensions (2-D, 3-D) provides real-time visualization of ventricular dimensions in diastole and systole, Doppler imaging of flow, and computer-assisted calculation of ejection fraction.[21] Doppler imaging has great value in the imaging of valvular heart disease, pulmonary blood flow, hepatic blood flow, and intracardiac shunts and can be either color-flow Doppler or pulsed Doppler. TEE is extremely valuable in the diagnosis of mechanical obstruction of cardiac function, such as pericardial fluid and tamponade, atrial myxoma, pulmonary embolus, and prosthetic valve failure. TEE may also aid in the early bedside evaluation of suspected thoracic artery aneurysm or dissection, as an adjunct to arteriography. In addition, segmental wall-motion abnormalities are significantly more sensitive and earlier indicators of ischemia than are changes in the PCWP or the ECG. The value of adjunctive information obtained echocardiographically in the specific setting of the ICU is well documented and TEE skills are important, if not vital, tools for the hemodynamic management of critically ill patients.

THORACIC BIOIMPEDANCE PLETHYSMOGRAPHY AND ESOPHAGEAL DOPPLER TECHNOLOGY

The use of thoracic impedance plethysmography is a noninvasive alternative to using invasive vascular cannulation solely for the purposes of diagnostic measurements. This technique is based on changes in the electrical impedance of the thoracic cavity that occur with changes in thoracic blood volume throughout the cardiac cycle. An alternating current of small amplitude (2.5 to 4.0 mA) traverses the chest at a frequency of 70 to 100 kHz. Four (transmitter-sensor) pairs of cutaneous electrodes determine the impedance to current flow. Since respiratory variations occur at a lower frequency than cardiac variations, the effect of respirations can be eliminated. Stroke volume (SV) is determined mathematically, based on the specific resistivity of blood, thoracic length, basal thoracic impedance, ventricular ejection time, and the maximum rate of impedance change during systolic upstroke. The SV correlates with the impedance change over a cardiac cycle. Cardiac output can be readily derived from the SV by the equation CO = SV × HR, where HR is heart rate. Additional indices, such as ejection velocity index, ventricular ejection time, and thoracic fluid index, can assist in more subtle evaluation of cardiac function. Since bioimpedance estimates the pulsatile component of SV, conditions in which the flow is more continuous than pulsatile (e.g., sepsis, hemodilution) may artifactually lower the calculated CO. The use of bioimpedance plethysmography is very limited in the presence of arrhythmias. Since plethysmography requires an estimated CVP, its utility can be greatly increased if the CVP is directly measured by an invasive method. Thoracic bioimpedance overestimates CO: (1) if the CVP is lower than estimated, (2) in the presence of low cardiac flow, (3) when inotropes are used, and (4) in the presence of aortic insufficiency. Thoracic bioimpedance underestimates CO in the presence of sepsis, hypertension, and intracardiac shunts. In general, bioimpedance has utility in the intermittent, short-term, or initial evaluation of cardiovascular function in the critically-ill patient but is severely limited in continuous and intensive long-term management.

An alternative to thoracic bioimpedance plethysmography is transesophageal Doppler monitoring. Monitoring of cardiac function with Doppler technology estimates the velocity of blood flow in the descending aorta and mathematically derives correlates of CO and afterload. The esophageal doppler may incorporate M-mode ultrasound technology to standardize the placement of the doppler probe with respect to aortic diameter. Since the esophageal Doppler method relies mainly on direct measurement and less on assumption, the thoracic Doppler probe shows promise in the care of critical care patients.

MUCOSAL TONOMETRY

The mucosal tonometer is a potentially useful method for the assessment of tissue-specific perfusion. Tonometer technology has been applied to the esophageal and gastric mucosa, the mucosa of the rectum, and the sublingual oral mucosa. Although the monitoring site varies, the technology and the physiologic principles are the same. The central role of the gastrointestinal tract postulated in the gut motor hypothesis is as an initiator and perpetuator of bacteremia and inflammatory mediator release.[22] The splanchnic circulatory system is among the first to be affected by systemic shock, and splanchnic hypoperfusion continues for a time after systemic variables (e.g., blood pressure, HR, urine output, lactic acid level, CO) have been restored to normal.[23] Local acidosis resulting from hypoperfusion and dysoxia can be quantitatively estimated using the Henderson-Hasselbach equation, the measured arterial bicarbonate, and the CO_2 inside a silastic balloon, which theoretically reflects tissue P_{CO_2}. Although mucosal tonometry represents a technology in evolution and is therefore controversial, it has tremendous potential as a measurable and tissue-specific endpoint for resuscitation.

$$pHi = 6.1 + log_{10} \frac{\text{arterial } Hco_3}{\text{saline } Pco_2 \times 0.03}$$

Where pHi = intracellular pH

Hco_3 = bicarbonate

saline Pco_2 = partial pressure of carbon dioxide in the saline balloon

CAPNOGRAPHY

Although capnography is readily available in the CCU, its application as an adjunctive tool for hemodynamic monitoring is not well appreciated. The capnograph detects, measures, and depicts the respiratory flow of CO_2 during expiration. The presence of CO_2 in exhaled gas is an indicator of ventilation (and endotracheal tube placement) and pulmonary perfusion. Quantitative measure of the concentration of CO_2 at end-expiration, known as the end-tidal CO_2 (CO_2ET), is both a measure of ventilation and perfusion. In instances where perfusion is thought to be constant, titration of ventilation to the CO_2ET can optimize ventilation. However, during steady-state ventilation, alterations in the CO_2ET signify changes in cardiac output and resultant changes in pulmonary perfusion. In fact, the presence of CO_2ET in the early phases of cardiac resuscitation are associated with improved outcome.

SUMMARY

A fundamental indication for admission to the ICU is the availability of specialized technology and personnel to facilitate rapid intervention for diagnosis and therapy.

The cost of monitoring must be continuously weighed against the potential benefit and risk. Costs may be direct, such as acquisition costs of equipment, or indirect, such as the additional personnel time that must be committed to maintenance, data acquisition and recording, and treatment of complications. If expensive technology cannot be demonstrated to positively affect patient outcome, justification of its use becomes increasingly difficult. To a large extent, it is vital to recognize that monitoring provides data that only becomes meaningful when properly interpreted and used for timely and appropriate intervention.

REFERENCES

1. Gosbell IB. Central venous catheter-related sepsis: Epidemiology, pathogenesis, diagnosis, treatment and prevention. *Int Care World* 1994;11:54.

2. Kamal GD, Pfaller MA, Rempe LE, et al. Reduced intravascular catheter infection by antibiotic bonding: A prospective, randomized, controlled trial. *JAMA* 1991;265:2364.
3. Curtas S, Tramposch K. Culture methods to evaluate central venous catheter sepsis. *Nutr Clin Pract* 1991;6:43.
4. Randolph AG, Cook DJ, Gonzales CA, et al. Benefit of heparin in central venous and pulmonary artery catheters: A meta-analysis of randomized clinical trials. *Chest* 1998;113:165.
5. Seneff M. Arterial line placement and care. In Rippe JM, Irwin RS, Fink MP, eds. *Procedures and techniques in intensive care medicine.* Boston: Little, Brown, 1995:15.
6. Kleinman B, Powell S, Kumar P, et al. The fast flush test measures the dynamic response of the entire blood pressure monitoring system. *Anesthesiology* 1992;77:1215.
7. Iberti TJ, Fischer EP, Leibowitz AB, et al. A multicenter study of physicians' knowledge of the pulmonary artery catheter. *JAMA* 1990;264:2928.
8. Connors AF, Speroff T, Dawson NV, et al. The effectiveness of right heart catheterization in the initial care of critically ill patients. *JAMA* 1996;276:889.
9. American Society of Anesthesiologists task force on pulmonary artery catheterization. *Anesthesiology* 1993;78:380.
10. Pulmonary Artery Catheter Consensus Conference: Consensus statement. *Crit Care Med* 1997;25:10.
11. Tuman KJ, Carroll GC, Ivankovich AD. Pitfalls in interpretation of pulmonary artery catheter data. *J Cardiothorac Anesth* 1989;3:625.
12. Nishikawa T, Dohi S. Errors in the measurement of cardiac output by hemodilution. *Can J Anaesth* 1993;40:142.
13. Bond RA, Lefkowitz RJ. The third beta is not the charm. *J Clin Invest* 1996;98:241.
14. Diebel LN, Myers T, Dulchavsky S. Effects of increasing airway pressure and PEEP on the assessment of cardiac preload. *J Trauma* 1997;42:585.
15. Ivatury RR, Simon RJ, Islam S, et al. A prospective randomized study of end points of resuscitation after major trauma: Global oxygen transport indices versus organ-specific gastric mucosal pH. *J Am Coll Surg* 1996;183:145.
16. Hoffman MJ, Greenfield LJ, Sugerman HJ, et al. Unsuspected right ventricular dysfunction in shock and sepsis. *Ann Surg* 1983;198:307.
17. Shoemaker WC, Appel PL, Krom HB. Role of oxygen debt in the development of organ failure, sepsis, and death in high-risk surgical patients. *Chest* 1992;102:208.
18. Ronco JJ, Phang PT, Walley KR, et al. Oxygen consumption is independent of changes in oxygen delivery in severe adult respiratory distress syndrome. *Am Rev Respir Dis* 1991;143:1267.
19. Mizock BA, Falk JL. Lactic acidosis in critical illness. *Crit Care Med* 1992;20:80.
20. Porembka DT, Hoit BD. Transesophageal echocardiography in the intensive care patient. *Crit Care Med* 1991;19:826.
21. Feinberg MS, Hopkins WE, Davila-Roman VG, et al. Multiplane transesophageal echocardiographic doppler imaging accurately determines cardiac output measurements in critically ill patients. *Chest* 1995;107:769.
22. Aranow JS, Fink MP. Determinants of intestinal barrier failure in critical illness. *Br J Anaesth* 1996;77:71.
23. Fiddian-Green RG. Gastric intramucosal pH, tissue oxygenation, and acid base balance. *Br J Anaesth* 1995;74:591.

CHAPTER 3

Approach to Shock

PETER J. PAPADAKOS

"In acute diseases, coldness of the extremities is a very bad sign."

HIPPOCRATES, 400 BC

INTRODUCTION

Shock in its various forms presents a very common challenge in the ICU. Over the past decade, we have developed new terminology to better understand shock. In an attempt to develop a common language, a consensus conference of the Society of Critical Care Medicine and the American College of Chest Physicians was held in August 1991 to produce a series of universal definitions for the systemic inflammatory response syndrome (SIRS).This interplay of cellular and systemic responses, which may be modulated by cytokines, may replace the terms septic, cardiogenic, hypovolemic, distributive, and obstructive shock.

This enhanced understanding of the pathophysiology of shock syndromes and SIRS may not only give us a common language but also may aid in the development of treatment protocols. We now understand that the immediate recognition of and institution of treatment for SIRS and shock are paramount in the ICU.

PATHOPHYSIOLOGY

The term "shock" can simply be defined as inadequate tissue perfusion along with cellular hypoxia and oxygen debt, which results in cellular dysfunction and is caused by inadequate systemic oxygen delivery or impairment of cellular oxygen uptake. This can be the result of poor oxygen delivery, maldistribution of blood flow, the effect of cytokines on cell function, a low perfusion pressure, or a combination of these factors.[1-3] The common denominator in all shock states and the earliest manifestation of shock is reduced oxygen consumption (Vo_2). Cellular hypoxia can incite SIRS and multiple organ dysfunction syndrome (MODS). It is obvious that oxygen debt should be rapidly reversed and systemic oxygen delivery and consumption maintained. The oxygen debt is caused by a low flow in hypovolemic or cardiogenic shock, by a cellular or metabolic deficit in septic shock, and by a maldistribution of blood flow in other types of shock.

This decade has lead to an understanding of how various cytokines may be released during shock states and interplay with various organ systems to cause end-organ damage or MODS. Cytokines, for example, nitric oxide (NO), interleukin-2 (IL-2), and tumor necrosis factor (TNF), and their release in various forms of shock may modulate the microvascular and cellular responses of shock. The low flow, or hypovolemia, in some forms of shock may also be responsible for the release of various cytokines. The cytokine cascade in SIRS may account for many of the presenting signs of shock, such as respiratory failure, capillary leak, shunting, redistribution, depressed myocardial function, oxygen uncoupling, and cellular ischemia.

The mediator response in SIRS can be divided into four phases based on the cytokine-cellular response:

1. Induction
2. Triggering of cytokine synthesis
3. Evolution of cytokine cascade
4. Elaboration of secondary mediators with ensuing cellular injury

The events following endotoxin exposure provide a good model for discussion of the phases of SIRS. Endotoxin, shed from bacteria as they multiply or die, is one of the most powerful triggers of SIRS and acts by stimulating phagocytic cells, particularly macrophages, to synthesize TNF-α, which then activates the complement coagulation cascades and also induces endothelial cell activation.

GENERAL PRINCIPLES

The general progression of the SIRS response may be similar or different for each type of shock, and the use of hemodynamic profiles may aid in its classification (Table 3–1). Although certainly not mandated as a management tool, data gathered using a pulmonary artery catheter (PAC) facilitates classification and understanding of the causes of shock. Furthermore, knowledge of these hemodynamic profiles is helpful in the diagnosis and management of shock. New monitors, such as esophageal echocardiographic and esophageal Doppler ultrasonographic hemodynamic monitors, HemoSonic 100 (Arrow International Reading, PA) may give a clinician real-time data on volume status and cardiac contractility, which may eventually prove more helpful than the PAC.

More specific symptoms for each type of shock are shown in Table 3–2. Some older terminology, such as hyperdynamic shock (an increased cardiac output and lowered vascular resistance), early and late shock, and warm and cold shock, are no longer used.

The body's responses to shock may vary according to the cause. For example, distributive shock may be characterized by low cardiac output. This variability may progress in all forms of shock to a set of common organ effects (Table 3–3).

TABLE 3–1 Hemodynamic Profiles of Various Types of Shock

Type of Shock	Pulmonary Artery Occlusion Pressure	Cardiac Output	SVR
Cardiogenic	↑	↓	↑
Hypovolemic	↓	↓	↑
Distributive	↓ or nl	↑ or nl or ↓	↓
Obstructive	↑ or nl or ↓	↓	↑

ABBREVIATIONS: SVR, systemic vascular resistance; ↑, increases; ↓, decreases; nl, normal.

TABLE 3–2 **General Symptoms of Shock**

CNS Changes

- Confusion
- Coma
- Combative behavior
- Agitation
- Stupor

Skin Changes

- Cool
- Clammy
- Warm
- Diaphoresis

Cardiovascular

- Increase or decrease in heart rate
- Arrhythmia
- Angina
- Low, high, or normal cardiac output
- Changes in pulmonary pressure (see Table 3–1)

Pulmonary

- Increased respiratory rate
- Increase or decrease in end-tidal CO_2
- Decrease in O_2 saturation
- Increased pulmonary pressures
- Respiratory failure
- Decreased tidal volume
- Decreased FRC

Renal

- Decreased urine output
- Elevation in BUN and creatinine levels
- Change in urine electrolyte levels

ABBREVIATIONS: CNS, central nervous system; CO_2, carbon dioxide; O_2, oxygen; FRC, functional residual capacity; BUN, blood urea nitrogen.

EVALUATION OF SYMPTOMS

History

The type of shock must be evaluated by reviewing the history of the disease process.

In cardiogenic shock, the patient may have a history of cardiac disease, poor cardiac function, congestive heart failure, myocardial ischemia, or valvular heart disease. In hypovolemic shock, there is usually a history of blood loss, trauma, fluid losses, dehydration, third spacing, or other fluid losses. Distributive shock is usually associated with exposure to an infectious or allergic agent, neurologic events, or a reaction to various immunologic substances. In obstructive shock,

TABLE 3–3 Common Effects of Shock on Organs

Systemic

- Capillary leak
- Formation of microvascular shunts
- Cytokine release

Cardiovascular

- Circulatory failure
- Depression of cardiovascular function
- Arrhythmia

Hematologic

- Bone marrow suppression
- Coagulopathy
- Disseminated intravascular coagulation (DIC)
- Platelet dysfunction

Hepatic

- Liver insufficiency
- Elevation of liver enzyme levels
- Coagulopathy

Neuroendocrine

- Change of mental status
- Adrenal suppression
- Insulin resistance
- Thyroid dysfunction

Renal

- Renal insufficiency
- Change in urine electrolyte levels
- Elevation of BUN and creatinine levels

Cellular

- Cell-to-cell dehiscence
- Cellular swelling
- Mitochondrial dysfunction
- Cellular leak

there may be a history of trauma or a process that leads to a mechanical obstruction of cardiac filling, such as cardiac tamponade.

Early recognition of hypotension and hypoperfusion is essential in prevention and treatment of all types of shock. Hypoperfusion may be the trigger for much of the end-organ dysfunction and cytokine activation. In adults, a drop in systolic blood pressure of more than 40 mm Hg constitutes significant hypotension. Hypoperfusion may be present in the absence of significant hypotension if microcirculatory factors are activated. Shock is usually recognized as hypotension characterized by hypoperfusion abnormalities.

General symptoms are illustrated in Table 3–2 and are a guide for rapid evaluation and treatment.

Hypovolemic Shock

Hypovolemic shock occurs when there is a depletion of fluid in the intravascular space as a result of hemorrhage, vomiting, diarrhea, dehydration, capillary leak, or a combination of these. Capillary leak is common with the activation of the systemic inflammatory response.[1] The hemodynamic findings in hypovolemic shock are decreased cardiac output, decreased pulmonary capillary wedge pressure (PCWP), and an increase in systemic vascular resistance (SVR). The echocardiographic and echodoppler profile is one of decreased right-sided filling, decreased stroke volume, and decreased aortic diameter.

Distributive Shock

The most common cause of distributive shock is septic shock. Other forms of distributive shock are anaphylactic shock, acute adrenal insufficiency, and neurogenic shock. The primary problems are the development of shunts and capillary leak. In distributive shock, there is activation of SIRS and a breakdown of cellular function in the septic process. The hemodynamic profile is characterized by a normal or increased cardiac output with a low SVR and low-to-normal left ventricular filling pressure. The echocardiographic profile is one of low stroke volume and an increase in aortic diameter.

Obstructive Shock

Direct mechanical obstruction to cardiac filling is the keystone of obstructive shock. In obstructive shock, there is depression of the ability to fill the right side of the heart, which may be the result of a fluid collection around the heart, cardiac tamponade, or a massive increase in intrathoracic pressure. In cardiac tamponade, the pressure in the right side of the heart, the pulmonary artery, and the left side of the heart equilibrate in diastole. A drop of more than 10 mm Hg in systolic blood pressure during inspiration, or paradoxical pulse, is an important finding.[4,5] Another form of obstructive shock is tension pneumothorax, in which there is increased intrathoracic pressure with hypotension, resulting from decreased preload.

DIAGNOSTIC TESTING

General laboratory tests should include measurement of blood lactate level (usually secondary to anaerobic metabolism), which is a marker for poor oxygen delivery or use[6] and serum bicarbonate level (a decrease in this level is a marker for metabolic acidosis). There can also be an elevation in blood glucose level and changes in the level of several electrolytes: zinc, magnesium, and calcium; these should be measured.[7] Alterations in renal parameters commonly include an elevation in creatinine and blood urea nitrogen (BUN) levels and changes in urine electrolyte levels. Liver parameters are also affected by shock states; alterations occur in all liver enzyme levels. ABG analysis is one of the most important laboratory tests because it measures the baseline oxygen delivery and utilization, which is the basic problem in shock. The most common findings are hypoxia, metabolic acidosis, and an elevation in Pa_{CO_2}.

Coagulation

The coagulation cascade may be affected by the shock syndrome through activation of SIRS with evidence of disseminated intravascular coagulation (DIC), an increase in fibrin split products, and a fall in fibrinogen and antithrombin III levels. Coagulation factors are also affected by liver failure, with increases in prothrombin time (PT) and activated partial thomboplastin time[8] (APTT).

Hematologic Parameters

In septic or infectious shock, the WBC count can be either high or low. In other forms of shock, bone marrow suppression may lead to decreased production of all hematologic cells. Platelet counts may fall or platelets may not function normally in several forms of shock. Erythropoietin levels also decrease in shock.

Renal Parameters

Oliguria and renal insufficiency are important markers for shock because the kidney is very sensitive to hypoperfusion and cytokine effects.[9] Oliguria may be caused by direct renal injury by cytokines, prerenal volume problems, or postrenal problems. In all critically ill patients, a urine output of less than 0.5 mL/kg per hour is defined as oliguria.

Echocardiography

The addition of echocardiography in the ICU has added greatly to our ability to diagnose and manage various forms of shock. Formal echocardiography requires special training for both the transthoracic and esophageal forms. Over the past few years, an esophageal Doppler echocardiographic probe has been developed that is easy to use and gives data on aortic artery diameter, stroke volume, and cardiac output in real time.[10]

COMPLICATIONS OF SHOCK

The most serious complication of shock is that low tissue perfusion may be an activating factor of SIRS through the release and modulation of cytokines and other vasoactive substances. This low-flow state and cytokine modulation may be at the heart of organ failure and MODS. The two most sensitive organs are the lungs (at risk for ARDS) and the kidneys (at risk for acute renal failure, or ARF). If this low-flow state is not rapidly corrected, other organ dysfunction occurs.[1,2] Metabolic acidosis or lactic acidosis is a sensitive marker for low-flow states, and prolonged elevations of serum lactate level may be markers for increased morbidity and mortality.[6] The cytokine cascade not only modulates vascular tone, but also controls other physiologic functions, such as bone marrow production, cell permiability, and electrolyte regulation, as well as DIC.

DIFFERENTIAL DIAGNOSIS

Distributive Shock

Sepsis, accompanied by capillary leak, shunting, and microvascular changes, is the classic example of distributive shock. Sepsis is a form of distributive shock that occurs as a complication of a severe infection. The various circulatory and cellular events are caused by systemic activation of the inflammatory cascade and release of numerous mediators from tissue, mast cells, and circulating basophils.

Another cause of distributive shock is anaphylaxis, an immediate hypersensitivity reaction, which is mediated by the interaction of immunoglobulin (IgE) antibodies on the surface of most white cells and basophils. Anaphylaxis can be triggered by drugs, especially antibiotics (e.g., beta-lactamase inhibitors, cephalosporins, sulfonamides), and animal toxins (from the stings of hornets, wasps, and bees). Other causes include heterologous serum, such as tetanus antitoxin, snake antitoxin, serums, blood transfusions, immunoglobulins, and vaccine products. Many health care workers and patients are now allergic to latex, which is found in countless products used in health care, industrial preparations, and in the home. There have been multiple deaths and these events are now commonly reported by the lay press; special care must be taken in caring for these patients because latex is commonly used in gloves, IV tubing, and many other products.

Anaphylactoid reactions are very similar to anaphylaxis, but without activation of IgE, and can be caused by a wide range of materials and agents, including ionic contrast media, protamine, opioids, polysaccharide volume expanders (e.g., dextran, hydroxyethyl starch), anesthetics, and muscle relaxants.

Neurogenic shock is another form of distributive shock. It involves loss of peripheral vasomotor control as a result of neurologic dysfunction or injury to the nervous system.

Adrenal gland dysfunction can also trigger distributive shock. Adrenal crisis can be caused by a deficiency of adrenal production of mineralocorticoids and glucocorticoids. It can be triggered or caused by adrenal hemorrhage, trauma, or overwhelming infections, especially fungal infections, such as histoplasmosis, blastomycosis, and coccidioidomycosis. Another increasingly common infection, tuberculosis, can also trigger it. Adrenal crisis is also found in patients with HIV infection, both as a direct cause of HIV or by superinfection by other organisms. Drugs may also cause adrenal dysfunction both by chronic immunosuppression by corticosteroids or by direct effect, such as with antifungal agents.

Trauma, burns, and pancreatitis are all fairly common inciting events that trigger the cytokine cascade, leading to SIRS and distributive shock. Although this condition mimics the signs and symptoms of sepsis, this kind of distributive shock can be generated without an accompanying infection.

Hypovolemic Shock

Causes of hypovolemia that may lead to shock include loss of intravascular volume through dehydration (from low fluid intake, diarrhea, bowel obstruction, sweating, or diabetes insipidus), diuresis (from diuretics or elevated blood glucose levels), capillary leak and third spacing (from burns, sepsis, pancreatitis, or surgical stress), hemorrhage (from trauma, gastrointestinal bleeding, fractures, vascular injuries, ruptured ovarian cysts, ectopic pregnancy, placental abruption, ruptured uterus, placenta previa), and anemia.

Obstructive Shock

Cardiac tamponade and restrictive pericarditis are characteristic of extracardiac obstructive shock. Pulmonary embolism caused by air, amniotic fluid, fat, or vascular clot can cause obstructive shock. Intrathoracic processes, such as pneumothorax, pulmonary hypertension, and diaphragmatic rupture, can all cause increased intrathoracic pressure and a decrease in forward flow of blood.

The diagnosis of pulmonary processes may be made by chest x-ray films. Cardiac processes can be evaluated by rapid echocardiographic examination. Pulmonary embolism can be evaluated by ventilation/perfusion scans, echocardiography, and pulmonary angiography.

Cardiogenic Shock

The most common cause of cardiogenic shock is an acute myocardial infarction (aMI). Myocardial infarction (MI) that affects cardiac valves can present with acute heart failure, as can MI of the left ventricular (LV) wall. Septal infarctions can lead to septal defects. Multiple infarctions can also affect already damaged myocardium, which may lead to rapid failure. Various cardiomyopathies (e.g., viral, alcoholic, infectious) may lead to cardiogenic shock. A post-MI arterial thrombus or aneurysms of the ventricular wall may also precipitate cardiac failure. An MI that is well-tolerated initially but then extends (for hours to days) to involve a large degree of LV myocardium may be the sequence that most frequently leads to shock.

Severely reduced LV contractility induced by ischemia is the fundamental finding in cardiogenic shock. Extensive right ventricular (RV) infarction, which classically accompanies inferior-wall MI, can also present with hypotension.

Cardiogenic shock is assessed by observing the patient's mental status and skin color; by measuring urine output and blood pressure; and by evaluating for diaphoresis, turgor, and tachycardia. Pulmonary congestion is evaluated by auscultation of the lungs for wet sounds (rales) and by the presence of S_3 and S_4 heart sounds. Measuring the levels of cardiac enzymes, myoglobins, and troponins is a rapid screening test and should be done along with evaluation of the ECG. Echocardiography and cardiac catheterization are the current gold standards: echocardiography rapidly shows both the location and extent of cardiac failure.

In cardiogenic shock, forward blood flow is impaired by pump failure; and the typical picture is one of congestive heart failure (CHF), with increased fluid in the lung, pulmonary edema, and hepatic congestion. The hemodynamic picture is one of decreased cardiac output, elevated PCWP, elevated LV filling pressure, and increased SVR. The echocardiographic profile shows decreased cardiac function, wall-motion problems, decreased stroke volume, and decreased aortic diameter.

MANAGEMENT AND THERAPY

Patients suspected to be in shock should be managed in an ICU with close monitoring and skilled nursing. Goals in the care of patients in different types of shock are the same, because the shock syndromes share many characteristics, regardless of their origin.

The basic goal of shock therapy is the restoration of effective perfusion to vital organs and tissue before the onset of cellular injury. This basic therapy entails maintenance of appropriate cardiac function and mean arterial blood pressure. Endpoints as described in Table 3–4 can be used as a general guideline.

Basic resuscitation should include rapid placement of a large-bore intravenous line or a high-flow central line as a route for fluid resuscitation. Protection of the airway through intubation and mechanical ventilation, if needed, can stabilize the patient. In unintubated patients, 2 to 15 L/min of high-flow oxygen is recommended to get oxygen saturation above 92%. To follow renal function, a Foley catheter should be placed early.

Fluid Management

Considerable quantities of fluid are often sequestered at a site of inflammation or lost because of fever, vomiting, or diarrhea. Because shock is greatly intensified when intravascular volume is depleted, fluid replacement is an important component of therapy.

In a series of patients reported by Rackow, both cardiac output and survival were correlated with volume expansion.They demonstrated that increases in oxy-

TABLE 3–4 General Goals for Support of Shock Patients

Hemodynamic Support

- MAP > 60–65 mm Hg
- PCWP = 15–18 mm Hg
- Cardiac index > 2.1 L/min per square meter of body surface area for cardiogenic and obstructive shock
- Cardiac index > 4.0 L/min per square meter of body surface area for septic, traumatic, or hemorrhagic shock

Optimization of Oxygen-Delivery

- Hb level > 10 g/dL
- Arterial oxygen saturation > 92%

Reversal of Organ System Dysfunction

- Maintain urine output > 0.5 mL/kg per hour

ABBREVIATIONS: MAP, mean airway pressure; PCWP, pulmonary capillary wedge pressure; Hb, hemoglobin.

gen consumption correlated with increases in cardiac output and oxygen delivery during fluid challenge of patients in septic shock.

PAC monitoring and the newer technology of echocardiographic Doppler ultrasonography have given the clinician more insight into the shock patient's volume status and can guide therapy to fixed endpoints. This ability to evaluate cardiac function may be an important advantage, because bacterial shock is often associated with impaired LV function.

How much and how fast to give fluids is a matter of great debate. One technique is to give the patient a fluid challenge, ranging from 5 to 20 mL/kg over a period of 10 minutes.[11] The patient is then assessed for hemodynamic response (e.g., blood pressure, heart rate, urine output, mental status) and further fluid is administered based on the patient's response. Alternatively, if the patient has central venous monitoring and the CVP pressure increases by more than 7 mm Hg above the initial pressure, the infusion is discontinued. If the pressure does not exceed the starting pressure by more than 3 mm Hg after 10 minutes of fluid infusion, or if it decreases by 3 mm Hg over a subsequent 10-minute rest period, a second aliquot of fluid is administered over 10 minutes and the "7 to 3 rule" is again applied.[11]

For plasma volume expansion, combinations of physiologic sodium solutions and plasma protein solutions are currently recommended. Albumin use has fallen over the past few years because of high costs and the lack of evidence-based outcome studies that it is superior to crystalloid solutions.[12] Albumin may also induce activation of leukocytes at the endothelium, promoting the inflammatory cascade. Current data using different endpoints, such as mortality, length of ventilation, or renal function, do not show discernable differences between albumin and other colloids and crystalloids.

HYDROXYETHYL STARCHES The advantage of using hydroxyethyl starches (HES) is their prolonged duration in the circulation. The duration of HES as volume replacement is approximately 4 hours, with an intravascular half-life of 8 hours.

HES are natural starches that have undergone hydroxylation and etherification, preventing hydrolysis by alpha-amylase. The main route of elimination of HES is renal, and use of HES should be avoided in patients with renal failure. A new formula of HES with physiologic solution (lactated Ringer's solution) reduces the chloride content and has been shown to have beneficial effects on organ function, with no coagulopathy determined.[13]

DEXTRAN AND GELATIN Use of dextran for volume replacement is vanishing in the United States because of the many side effects caused by these preparations. Gelatins have not been approved for use in the United States because of the high incidence of allergic reactions, but they are used outside the United States.

HYPERTONIC SALINE Hypertonic saline (2500 mOsm/L) increases plasma volume by drawing fluid from the interstitial space.[14] This "one-time" effect is sustained because of other mechanisms attributed to hypertonic saline, namely increased venous constriction and increased cardiac output. Hypertonic saline has added properties that may improve capillary flow and tissue oxygenation, and it now has wide use in neurosurgical and traumatic resuscitation. Hypertonic saline may increase the risk of arteriolar dilation and can theoretically produce or aggravate surgical bleeding.

BLOOD REPLACEMENT Blood and component therapy is the only fluid that can correct anemia and coagulation problems. The optimal hematocrit for ICU patients remains to be determined. If blood transfusion were "risk-free," the current intensive evaluation of transfusion practice would not be taking place. In the ICU, the risk of a blood transfusion–transmitted infection is not a major concern. What is of more consequence for the ICU patient is the evidence accumulating that blood transfusion has a profound negative effect on the immune system. While hemoglobin levels in the 7 to 10 mg/dL range are well tolerated in the "stable, non-stressed" patient, this range might not be optimal for the critically ill patient.

An intriguing new possibility is the use of erythopoietin in the critically ill population. Curwin at Dartmouth Medical Center has presented data that suggests that erythropoietin levels in the critically ill may be inappropriately low and that these patients may not be able to respond to endogenous erythropoietin (unpublished).

CRYSTALLOIDS Physiologic isotonic crystalloid solutions are widely used for volume expansion. Although significant amounts are needed to restore the circulation, in the presence of hypovolemia the kinetics of distribution are altered and the 20% volume expansion may be increased significantly.[15,16]

In the presence of profound shock or massive volume loss, replacement with crystalloid solutions may require five times the volume lost, and the proportion may increase as more fluid is lost. Restoring the macrocirculation to normovolemia does not necessarily restore the microcirculation or improve tissue oxygenation. Edema must always be treated with care. The clinical significance of edema formation is unclear, but theoretically it can reduce oxygen transport.

SUMMARY OF FLUID MANAGEMENT IN SHOCK Fluid replacement with crystalloid solutions is the mainstay of therapy, but this only treats the macrocirculation. Better understanding of the endothelium as an organ has now led to an ongoing investigation into the different effects of fluids used for resuscitation.[17] Perfection of these solutions to enable better microcirculation flow and modulation of the inflammatory response will lead to goal-directed therapy and outcome studies.

Vasoactive Drugs

The effectiveness of multiple vasoactive drugs for the treatment of shock has been studied, but no consensus has been reached. When using vasoactive drugs, however, remember that the goal of this therapy is to increase perfusion to the tissues and not to artificially raise the blood pressure to an arbitrary goal.

There is general agreement that volume control is the first-line treatment for shock. Fluid may stretch the left ventricle, leading to increased cardiac output, and refill the "tank." This leads to increased blood pressure without vasoconstriction, which may actually reduce perfusion.

The four most commonly used vasoactive agents in adult ICUs are dopamine, norepinephrine, phenylephrine, and dobutamine. The dosage ranges for these and other vasoactive drugs used in the ICU are listed in Table 3–5.

In the US, the most commonly used vasopressor in patients with shock is dopamine, which is a naturally occurring precursor of norepinephrine that has different effects at different dosages. These effects, however, do overlap.

TABLE 3–5 **Commonly Administered Vasoactive Intravenous Drugs**

Dopamine, 1–20 μg/kg/min
Norepinephrine, 0.05–2.0 μg/kg/min
Dobutamine, 1–25 μg/kg/min
Epinephrine, 0.05–2.0 μg/kg/min
Phenylephrine, 2–10 μg/kg/min
Isoproterenol, 1–8 μg/min
Amrinone, 5–15 μg/kg per minute, after a 0.75 mg/kg bolus over 5 minutes
Milrinone, 0.375–0.75 μg/kg per minute, after a 37.5–75 mg/kg bolus over 10 minutes

From a dosage of approximately 1 to 3 the direct dopaminergic effect of dopamine is seen. This results in vasodilatation of the renal and splanchnic circulations.[18] The effects seen with the use of higher dosages of dopamine are mainly manifested through the endogenous release of norepinephrine. From 3 to 10 g/kg of body weight per minute, beta$_1$ effects (increased inotropy and chronotropy) predominate. From 10 to 20 g/kg of body weight per minute, alpha$_1$ activity (vasoconstriction) predominates. In patients with shock, lower doses are preferred, with the goal of increasing forward flow and perfusion without inducing vasoconstriction, which may exacerbate ischemia.

Norepinephrine is generally felt to be a second-line agent for shock in the United States; however, in Europe, it is a first-line agent. Norepinephrine has a mixture of beta- and alpha-agonist effects. The higher the dose, the more powerful the vasoconstriction.

Phenylephrine is a selective alpha-agonist and is used to increase blood pressure emergently, but it also decreases the microcirculation, so it cannot be used for long-term resuscitation. As it has no beta effect, it does not cause tachyarrhythmias, and therefore may be useful in the cardiac patient who is prone to such problems.

Dobutamine hydrochloride is a sympathomimetic agent with predominantly beta-adrenergic effects. This drug is not a vasopressor because it does not cause vasoconstriction, but it does increase forward flow. Its use in sepsis has not resulted in improved outcomes; its major use is to increase cardiac output in the failing heart. Dobutamine is not generally recommended in hypotensive patients because it results in reflex vasodilatation, which may manifest as hypotension, especially in volume-depleted patients.

In the treatment of cardiogenic shock with progressive perfusion failure, the ion-dilators, such as amrinone lactate, and dobutamine in combination with a vasopressor may allow cardiac function to improve. In other instances of CHF, there is a good indication for the administration of cardiac glycosides, preferably digoxin.

In summary, the use of vasoactive drugs in shock is directed toward increasing perfusion. Vasopressor agents are used when blood pressure cannot be maintained with fluid alone. Continued monitoring for signs of perfusion inadequacy is necessary while using these agents. Finally, all vasopressor agents with alpha effects must be administered centrally, because if they were to infiltrate, they would cause local necrosis. If infiltration of any other vasopressor agents were to occur, the treatment is phentolamine (an alpha blocker) injected locally into the site of infiltration.

Monoclonal Antibodies

Multiple studies are ongoing in the use of monoclonal agents and receptor blockers to modulate the immune system and the sepsis cascade. At this time bedside application of immunotherapeutic approached for the treatment of shock[19] has not found clinical application.

SUMMARY

Our understanding of shock and SIRS response has evolved to one that is physiologically based. Resuscitation is now based on close monitoring and hemodynamic support and replacement of intravascular volume.

REFERENCES

1. Davies MD, Hagen PO. Systemic inflammatory response syndrome. *Brit J Surg* 1997;84:920–935.
2. Von Rueden TK, Dunham MC. Evaluation and management of oxygen delivery and consumption in multiple organ dysfunction syndrome in multiple organ dysfunction and failure, 2nd ed. In Secor VH, ed. *Mosby Yearbook.* St. Louis, MO: 1996:384–401.
3. Bone RC, et al. Definitions for sepsis and organ failure and guidelines for the use of innovative therapies in sepsis. *Crit Care Med* 1992;20:864–874.
4. Reddy PS, Curtiss EL, O'Toole JD, et al. Cardiac tamponade: Hemodynamic observations in man. *Circulation* 1978;8:265–269.
5. Eisenberg MJ, Schiller NB. Bayes theorem and the echocardiographic diagnosis of cardiac tamponade. *Am J Cardiol* 1991;68:1242–1250.
6. Iberti TJ, Leibowitz AB, Papadakos PJ, et al. Low sensitivity of the anion gap as a screen to detect hyperlactemia in critically ill patients. *Crit Care Med* 1990; 18:275–277.
7. Rose S, Illerhaus M, Wiercinski A, et al. Altered calcium regulation and function of human neutrophils during multiple trauma. *Shock* 2000;13:92–99.
8. Muller-Berghaus G. Pathophysiologic and biochemical events in disseminated intravascular coagulation: dysregulation of procoagulant and anticoagulant pathways. *Seminar Thromb Hemost* 1989;15:58–70.
9. Rasmussen HH, Ibel LS. Acute renal failure: Multivariate analysis of causes and risk factors. *Am J Med* 1982;733:211–218.
10. Cariou A, Mondi M, Luc-Marle J, et al. Noninvasive cardiac output monitoring by aortic blood flow determination: Evaluation of the Sometec Dynemo-3000 system. *Crit Care Med* 1988;12:2066–2072.
11. Packman MI, Rackow EC. Optimum left heart filling pressure during fluid resuscitation of patients with hypovolemic and septic shock. *Crit Care Med* 1983;11:165–169.
12. Cochran Injuries Group, Albumin Reviewers. Human albumin administration in critically ill patients: Systemic review of randomized controlled trials. *Brit Med J* 1998;317:235–40.
13. Treib J, Haass A, Pindur G, et al. All medium starches are not the same: Influence of the degree of hydroxyethyl substitution of hydroxyethyl starch on plasma volume, hemorrheologic conditions, and coagulation transfusion. *Transfusion* 1996;36:450–455.
14. Mattox KL, Maninagas PA, Moore EE, et al. Prehospital hypertonic saline/dextran infusion for post–traumatic hypotension: The USA multicenter trial. *Ann Surg* 1991; 213:482–491.
15. Drobin D. Volume kinetics of Ringer's solution in hypovolemic volunteers. *Anesthesiology* 1999;90:81–91.

16. Funk W, Balinger V. Microcirculatory perfusion using crystalloid or colloid in awake animals. *Anesthesiology* 1995;82:975–982.
17. Britt LD, Weireter LJ, Riblet JL, et al. Complex and challenging problems in trauma surgery. *Surg Clin N Am* 1996;76:645–660.
18. Lund N, DeAsla RJ, Guccione AL, et al. The effect of dopamine and dobutamine on skeletal muscle oxygenation in normoxemic rats. *Cir Shock* 1991;33:164–170.
19. Zeni F, Freeman B, Natanson C. Anti-inflammatory therapies to treat sepsis and septic shock: A reassessment. *Crit Care Med* 1997;25:1095–1100.

CHAPTER 4

Approach to Mechanical Ventilation

ANTHONY P. PIETROPAOLI

INTRODUCTION

Mechanical ventilation is defined as the use of a mechanical device to assist the respiratory muscles in the work of breathing and to improve gas exchange. In this chapter, mechanical ventilation is divided into two techniques: one requiring a tube in the trachea to deliver ventilation (invasive) and another applied with a mask (noninvasive). The indications, objectives, modes, settings, complications, and discontinuation strategies are reviewed for both invasive and noninvasive mechanical ventilation and some disease-specific strategies for invasive mechanical ventilation.

INVASIVE MECHANICAL VENTILATION

Indications

Mechanical ventilation is indicated to support the patient with respiratory failure when adequate gas exchange cannot otherwise be maintained. As reviewed in chapter 1, there are two major categories of acute respiratory failure: hypoxemic (type 1) and hypercapneic (type 2). Patients with either of these often need mechanical ventilation. Many patients present with a mixture of the two types of respiratory failure, and of course, these patients also respond to mechanical ventilation. Invasive mechanical ventilation is often chosen over noninvasive methods when altered mental status or hemodynamic instability accompany acute respiratory failure. The timing of intubation and initiation of mechanical ventilation is a source of controversy, and the decision is often more a matter of art and experience than science. Tracheal intubation is indicated for situations other than provision of mechanical ventilation, such as to provide airway protection and relieve upper airway obstruction.[1] Table 4–1 lists some commonly accepted indications for endotracheal intubation and mechanical ventilation.

Objectives

Mechanical ventilation is supportive and meant to reverse abnormalities in respiratory function, while specific therapies are used to treat the underlying cause of respiratory failure. The physiologic goals of mechanical ventilation are reversal of gas exchange abnormalities, alteration of pressure-volume relationships in the respiratory system, and reduction in the work of breathing.[2] These physiologic goals are interrelated and attain specific clinical results, as shown in Figure 4–1. Other goals in specialized circumstances include allowing use of heavy sedation or neuromuscular blockade and stabilization of the chest wall when injury has disrupted its mechanical function.[2]

TABLE 4–1 Indications for Intubation and Invasive Mechanical Ventilation

- Cardiac arrest
- Respiratory arrest
- Refractory hypoxemia (unresponsive to maximal supplemental oxygen administration and noninvasive ventilatory support)
- Progressive respiratory acidosis (unresponsive to medical therapy, oxygen administration, and noninvasive ventilatory support)
- Symptoms of progressive respiratory fatigue (unresponsive to medical therapy, oxygen administration, and noninvasive ventilatory support)
- Clinical signs of respiratory failure (unresponsive to medical therapy, oxygen administration, and noninvasive ventilatory support)
  - Tachypnea
  - Use of accessory muscles (e.g., sternocleidomastoid, scalene, intercostal, abdominal)
  - Paradoxical inward abdominal movement during inspiration
  - Progressive alteration of mental status
  - Inability to speak in full sentences
- Airway protection (in a patient with an extremely impaired level of consciousness)
- Relief of upper airway obstruction (often manifested by stridor on physical examination)

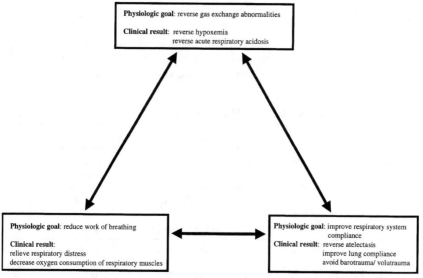

FIGURE 4–1 *Objectives of mechanical ventilation. Interrelationship between physiologic objectives of mechanical ventilation is shown. By accomplishing each of these physiologic objectives, specific clinical goals are met. (Adapted with permission from Slutsky AS. ACCP consensus conference: Mechanical ventilation. Chest 1993; 104(6):1833–1859.*

Modes

Mechanical ventilators were popularized during the polio epidemics of the 1950s. The initial ventilators were primarily negative pressure ventilators, or "iron lungs." Later, positive pressure ventilators gained popularity and today are used almost exclusively. As ventilator technology has progressed, the ways of delivering positive pressure mechanical ventilation have proliferated. In daily practice, however, four basic modes of positive pressure ventilation are most commonly used. These modes can be classified on the basis of how they are *triggered* to deliver a breath, whether these breaths are *targeted* to a set volume or pressure, and how the ventilator *cycles* from inspiration to expiration (Table 4–2).

CONTROLLED MECHANICAL VENTILATION Controlled mechanical ventilation (CMV) is included here only for the purposes of instruction. CMV, or volume control (VC), was the first volume-targeted mode (Figure 4–2a). As its name suggests, it is a pure "control" mode; that is, the minute ventilation ($\dot{V}_E$,) is completely governed by the machine ($\dot{V}_E = V_T \times$ respiratory rate). The physician sets the respiratory rate, tidal volume, inspiratory flow rate, ratio of inspiratory to expiratory time (I:E) fraction of inspired oxygen (F_{IO_2}), and positive end-expiratory pressure (PEEP). In VC, the patient is unable to trigger the ventilator to deliver additional breaths. This mode works well for patients who are unresponsive or heavily sedated, but not for conscious patients, whose respiratory efforts are not sensed by the ventilator, which leads to patient discomfort and increased work of breathing. As a result, this mode has largely been abandoned.

ASSIST-CONTROL VENTILATION This mode is similar to VC mode except that the ventilator senses respiratory efforts by the patient (Figure 4–2b). As in VC, the physician sets a respiratory rate, tidal volume, flow rate, I:E, F_{IO_2}, and

TABLE 4–2 Basic Modes of Mechanical Ventilation

Mode	Trigger	Target	Cycle
Volume control[a]	Ventilator	V_T	Time and V_T
Assist-control[a]	Ventilator ± patient	V_T	Time and V_T
SIMV[a]	Ventilator ± patient	V_T/V_I (SIMV breaths only)	Time and V_T/V_T (SIMV breaths only)
Pressure-control[b]	Ventilator ± patient	Inspiratory pressure	Time
Pressure-support[c]	Patient	Inspiratory pressure	Flow

ABBREVIATIONS: SIMV, synchronized intermittent mandatory ventilation; V_T, tidal volume; ± = with or without.
[a]All volume-targeted modes cycle from inspiration to expiration at the end of inspiratory time, which corresponds to the instant that the V_T is reached. The target V_T is achieved by setting a fixed inspiratory flow for a fixed inspiratory time interval.
[b]In pressure-control mode, the desired pressure is achieved almost immediately after the onset of inspiration. Target pressure is maintained for the duration of set inspiratory time.
[c]In pressure-support mode, the pressure target is maintained until inspiratory flow falls to about 20% of peak flow. Inspiratory time varies from breath to breath.

a.

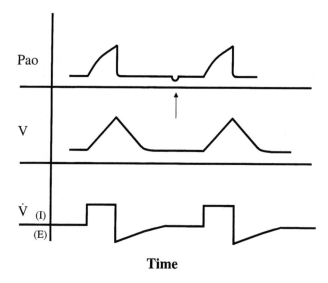

b.

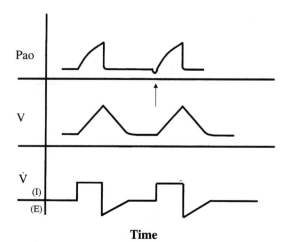

FIGURE 4–2 *Airway opening pressure (Pao), lung volume (V), and inspiratory (I), and ex-*
piratory (E) flow rate (V̇) versus time during mechanical ventilation.
a. Volume control (VC), also known as controlled mechanical ventilation (CMV). During
both breaths shown, defined tidal volume (VT) and inspiratory flow rate are delivered, result-
ing in Pao₂ shown. In this mode, ventilator does not detect patient efforts. A reduction in air-
way pressure from patient effort (arrow) does not result in significant VT or inspiratory flow.
b. Assist-control (AC) ventilation. Notice that ventilator senses decrease in airway pressure
induced by patient effort (indicated by arrow) and delivers same VT and flow in response.

c.

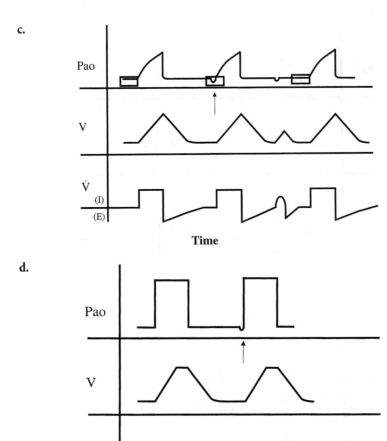

d.

FIGURE 4–2 *(continued)*

c. Synchronized intermittent mandatory ventilation (SIMV). First breath is ventilator-delivered in absence of patient effort. Next, patient effort causes decrease in Pao during synchronization period (boxes), so fully supported breath is delivered. Next effort occurs outside of synchronization period, and patient breathes spontaneously. Resulting volume and pressure are completely patient-generated. Last breath is identical to first, delivered according to set respiratory rate. End of synchronization period coincides with onset of the back-up SIMV breath.

d. Pressure-control (PC) ventilation. Airway pressure is set, and VT and flow rate that result are variable and depend on inspiratory time, airway resistance, respiratory system compliance, and patient effort. In example shown, patient is relaxed. First breath is delivered automatically by ventilator, based on fixed back-up respiratory rate. Second breath is delivered early, when patient lowers airway pressure and triggers ventilator (arrow).

e.

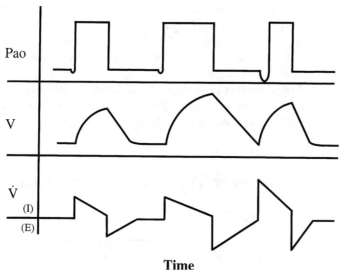

Time

FIGURE 4–2 (continued)

e. Pressure-support (PS) ventilation. Inspiratory pressure is fixed in this mode, as in pressure-control mode. However, this mode is flow-cycled instead of time-cycled. Inspiratory pressure ceases when inspiratory flow rate decreases to about 20% of its peak. VT and flow are determined by inspiratory pressure, airway resistance, respiratory system compliance, and patient effort. First breath shows moderate inspiratory effort. In second example, patient makes a prolonged inspiratory effort, resulting in more prolonged delivery of inspiratory pressure and a larger VT. Third example shows rapid deep breath, resulting in very high peak inspiratory flow rate but short duration of inspiratory pressure. The resulting VT is midway between other two examples. (Modified with permission, from Schmidt GA, Hall JB. Management of the ventilated patient. In Hall JB, Schmidt GA, Wood LDH, eds. Principles of critical care, *2nd ed. New York: McGraw-Hill, 1998:517–535.)*

PEEP. Breaths are delivered automatically, regardless of patient effort ("control"). In assist-control (AC) mode, however, the ventilator detects patient effort and responds by delivering a breath identical to the controlled one ("assist"). The patient can therefore breathe faster than the back-up control rate, but all breaths have the same tidal volume, flow rate, and inspiratory time. So AC mode allows better synchrony between patient and ventilator than VC mode, while still providing a baseline minute ventilation. A more descriptive and accurate name for this mode is "volume-targeted assist-control ventilation." However, the term "AC" is well entrenched and likely will not be replaced by this more cumbersome name.

Like all modes of mechanical ventilation, AC has disadvantages. If the back-up respiratory rate is set too far below the patient's spontaneous rate, exhalation time progressively decreases, since inspiratory time is fixed by the back-up respiratory rate and flow rate. In the extreme, this may result in inadequate time for exhalation (Figure 4–3). As a result, lung volume remains above functional residual capacity (FRC) when the next breath is delivered, a process called dynamic hyperinflation.[2] This increased lung volume is associated with elevation in the alveolar pressure at end-exhalation, or "auto-PEEP" (Figure 4–3). The adverse consequences of these events are discussed later. Another problem occurs when patients with high minute ventilation requirements make persistent inspiratory efforts while a breath is being delivered. If this effort is strong enough, the patient

a. Adequate Time for Complete Exhalation

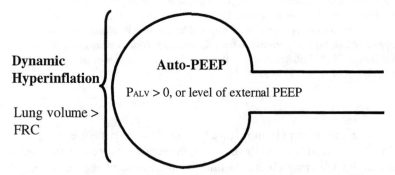

Lung volume = FRC

$P_{ALV} = 0$, or level of external PEEP

b. Inadequate Time for Complete Exhalation

Dynamic Hyperinflation

Auto-PEEP

$P_{ALV} > 0$, or level of external PEEP

Lung volume > FRC

FIGURE 4–3 *Dynamic hyperinflation and auto-PEEP (positive end-expiratory pressure) result from inadequate exhalation time. Simplified schematic shows two lung units, consisting of alveolus and airway, both at end exhalation. In a, there is adequate time for complete exhalation to resting lung volume, or functional residual capacity (FRC). The alveolar pressure is zero, or equal to level of externally applied PEEP. In b, there is inadequate time for exhalation. This occurs when exhalation time is too short and/ or time required to exhale to FRC is pathologically prolonged. Former occurs during mechanical ventilation when inspiratory time is too long or respiratory rate is too high; latter occurs in obstructive lung diseases, like chronic obstructive pulmonary disease (COPD) and asthma. In either case, lung volume remains above FRC at end exhalation (dynamic hyperinflation), resulting in abnormally elevated P_A (auto-PEEP).*

may trigger the ventilator again, a phenomenon known as "breath stacking." This can cause wide swings in airway pressure and increase the risk of barotrauma or ventilator-associated lung injury. Finally, in volume-targeted modes, the inspiratory flow rate is fixed. Many acutely ill patients strive for high inspiratory flow rates. If ventilator delivered air flow is below patient demand, the work of breathing increases as the patient makes futile efforts to augment inspiratory flow.

SYNCHRONIZED INTERMITTENT MANDATORY VENTILATION Like AC mode, synchronized intermittent mandatory ventilation (SIMV) is also a volume-targeted mode and provides a guaranteed $\dot{V}_E$ (Figure 4–2c). For the mandatory breaths, tidal volume and respiratory rate are chosen, guaranteeing a baseline minute ventilation. The practitioner also sets FiO_2, PEEP, and flow rate. As in AC mode, the patient can make inspiratory efforts between the mandatory breaths. If a sufficient effort occurs shortly before the mandatory breath is delivered (a time interval known as the "synchronization period"), a breath identical to the mandatory breath is delivered. If a patient effort occurs outside this synchronization period, the airway pressure, flow rate, and tidal volume are purely patient-generated, and no assistance is provided by the ventilator. While this reduces the likelihood of air-trapping and breath-stacking, it also can increase the work of breathing. Interestingly, if the mandatory respiratory rate is less than approximately 80% of the patient's actual rate, the high level of work expended during the spontaneous breaths will also be expended during the mandatory breaths.[3] This occurs because the respiratory center in the brain has a lag time and is unable to alter its output on a breath-to-breath basis. So if high neurologic output is required for a significant percentage of breaths, that same output will be given for all of the breaths, including those that are delivered by the ventilator. Therefore, attempting to "exercise" the respiratory muscles by setting the SIMV rate at half of the patient's spontaneous rate is counterproductive, because it simply increases the work of breathing and results in respiratory muscle fatigue and weaning failure. To prevent excessive work while still allowing the patient to breath above the SIMV rate, this mode is often combined with pressure-support ventilation, discussed later.

PRESSURE-CONTROL VENTILATION A more accurate name for pressure-control ventilation (PCV) mode is "pressure targeted assist-control ventilation" (Figure 4–2d). The mode is similar to the assist-control mode described above, except that a defined inspiratory pressure (IP) is set, instead of a tidal volume (Figure 4–2d). This allows absolute control over peak pressure delivered by the ventilator, which can have advantages in certain types of lung disease. Other defined settings are similar to assist-control: respiratory rate, I:E ratio, FiO_2, PEEP, and trigger sensitivity. When the ventilator detects patient effort, it delivers a breath identical to the backup-controlled breaths, allowing the patient to breathe faster than the back-up rate. Tidal volume is determined by IP, inspiratory time, airway resistance, respiratory system compliance ($\frac{\Delta V}{\Delta P}$), and patient effort. The delivered volume is predictable if sufficient time is given to allow equalization between the delivered inspiratory pressure and alveolar pressure.[4] If inspiratory time is too short or airway resistance is too high, this equilibration does not occur, resulting in a tidal volume lower than predicted and a decrease in minute ventilation. In response, the patient increases respiratory rate. Paradoxically, the increase in respiratory rate causes a *decrease* in minute ventilation because, as respiratory rate increases, expiratory time also decreases. The result is inadequate time for complete exhalation, dynamic hyperinflation, and auto-PEEP. The resulting decrease in respiratory system compliance reduces the tidal volume attained for the given IP. This is one of the major disadvantages of PCV, and is most often seen in the setting of obstructive lung disease.

Inspiratory flow rate is not fixed in PCV. It varies with IP, inspiratory time, respiratory mechanics, and patient effort. This can be advantageous, because flow rate increases with patient effort, unlike the volume-targeted modes, in which flow rate is fixed. As a result, patients with high minute-ventilation requirements may feel more comfortable on PCV, because they can regulate and increase flow as needed. This variable flow rate has another potential advantage: the flow pattern changes as respiratory system compliance decreases during lung inflation. Thus, flow is high early in inspiration when the system is very compliant and decreases as inflation proceeds and compliance decreases. The result is a lower peak airway pressure and a flow pattern that more closely mimics normal physiology. Whether this leads to any improvements in clinical outcome is unclear.

PRESSURE-SUPPORT VENTILATION The unique feature of pressure-support ventilation (PSV) is that it is flow-cycled instead of time-cycled (Figure 4–2e). So IP ceases when the flow rate drops to about 20% of peak flow rate, and passive exhalation occurs. The practitioner sets pressure-support level, FIO_2 and PEEP. Respiratory rate, inspiratory flow rate, tidal volume, and I:E ratio are determined by the patient's effort and respiratory system mechanics (resistance and compliance). PSV is an "apnea mode," that is, there is no back-up mandatory respiratory rate, so it can only be used for patients with adequate respiratory drive.

PSV is often combined with SIMV. This reduces the work of breathing in comparison to SIMV alone and provides a back-up mandatory minute ventilation not available with PSV alone.

ALTERNATIVE MODES The number of available modes of ventilation has increased rapidly. These include high-frequency ventilation, airway pressure-release ventilation, proportional-assist ventilation, and servo-controlled pressure support modes. A review of these modes is beyond the scope of this chapter, and the reader is referred to in-depth discussions of mechanical ventilation[5] and a recent review article.[6]

Settings

The parameters that need to be set vary, depending on the mode of ventilation used, as demonstrated in Table 4–3. Initial values for the different ventilator settings are shown in Table 4–4.[2]

RESPIRATORY RATE There is a wide range of mandatory ventilator-delivered respiratory rates that can be used. The number varies and is dependent on the minute ventilation goal, which varies with individual patients and clinical circumstances. In general, the range for respiratory rate is between 4/min and 20/min and falls between 8/min and 12/min in most stable patients.[2] In adult respiratory distress syndrome (ARDS), the use of low tidal volumes sometimes necessitates respiratory rates up to 35/min to maintain adequate minute ventilation.[7]

TIDAL VOLUME Evidence is accumulating that tidal volumes should be lower than traditionally recommended, especially in acute respiratory distress syndrome.[7,8,9] When setting tidal volume in volume-targeted modes, a rough estimate for patients with lung disease is 5 to 8 mL/kg of ideal body weight. In patients with normal lungs who are intubated for other reasons, slightly higher tidal volumes can be considered: up to 12 mL/kg of ideal body weight. Tidal volume should be adjusted to maintain a plateau pressure of less than 35 cm H_2O. The plateau pressure is determined by performing an inspiratory-hold maneuver (Figure 4–4*a*), which approximates end-inspiratory alveolar pressure in a relaxed patient.

  Elevation in the plateau pressure may not always increase the risk of barotrauma. This risk rises with transalveolar pressure, which is the alveolar pressure minus the pleural pressure. In patients with chest-wall edema, abdominal distention, or ascites, compliance of the chest wall is reduced. As a result, pleural pressure rises during lung inflation and the rise in transalveolar pressure is lower than

TABLE 4–3 Required Settings for Different Ventilator Modes

Setting	VC	AC	SIMV	PC	PS
Rate	✓	✓	✓	✓	
VT	✓	✓	✓		
IP				✓	✓
TS		✓	✓	✓	✓
Flow rate	✓	✓	✓		
I:E	✓	✓	✓	✓	
FIO₂	✓	✓	✓	✓	✓
PEEP	✓	✓	✓	✓	✓

ABBREVIATIONS: VC, volume control; AC, assist-controlled; SIMV, synchronized intermittent mandatory ventilation; PC, pressure-control; PS, pressure-support; VT, tidal volume; IP, inspiratory pressure; TS, trigger sensitivity; I:E, ratio of inspiratory to expiratory time; FIO₂, fraction of inspired oxygen; PEEP, positive end-expiratory pressure.

TABLE 4–4 **Suggestions for Initial Ventilator Settings**

Parameter	Usual Range	Adjust to Maintain
Rate (breaths/min)	4–20 breaths/min	Patient comfort, pH > 7.25, avoid auto-PEEP
V_T	Lung disease: 5–8 mL/kg Normal: 8–12 mL/kg	Plateau pressure ≤ 35 cm H_2O
IP	10–30 cm H_2O	Plateau pressure ≤ 35 cm H_2O
FIO_2	0.3–1.0%	O_2 sat ≤ 90%, FIO_2 ≤ 0.6%
PEEP	3–20 cm H_2O	Plateau pressure ≤ 35 cm H_2O, O_2 sat ≥ 90%
TS	Pressure: −1–2 cm H_2O Flow −1–3 L/min	Patient triggering ventilator effectively
Flow rate	40–100 L/min	Patient comfort; avoid auto-PEEP
I:E	1:1.5 to 1:3	Patient comfort; avoid auto-PEEP

ABBREVIATIONS: PEEP, positive end = expiratory pressure; V_T, tidal volume; IP, inspiratory pressure; FIO_2, fraction of inspired oxygen; TS, trigger sensitivity; ; I:E, ratio of inspiratory to expiratory time.

occurs with normal chest compliance. In such circumstances, the tidal volume ranges previously discussed should be used.

INSPIRATORY PRESSURE In PCV and PSV, the IP is generally set to keep the plateau pressure at or below 35 cm H_2O. The resulting tidal volume should be kept in the suggested ranges.

FRACTION OF INSPIRED OXYGEN In most cases, FIO_2 should be 100% when the patient is first intubated and placed on mechanical ventilation. Once proper tube placement is assured and the patient has stabilized, FIO_2 should be progressively reduced to the lowest concentration that maintains adequate oxygen saturation of hemoglobin, because high concentrations of oxygen produce pulmonary toxicity. Maintaining oxygen saturation of 90% or more is the usual goal. Occasionally, this goal is superseded by the need to protect the lung from excessive tidal volumes, pressures, or oxygen concentrations. In these circumstances, the target may be lowered to 85%, while optimizing the other factors involved in oxygen delivery (see chapter 1).

POSITIVE END-EXPIRATORY PRESSURE PEEP, as its name implies, maintains a set level of positive airway pressure during the expiratory phase of respiration. It differs from continuous positive airway pressure (CPAP) in that it is only applied during expiration, whereas CPAP is applied throughout the entire respiratory cycle.

The use of PEEP during mechanical ventilation has several potential benefits. In acute hypoxemic respiratory failure (type 1), PEEP increases mean alveolar pressure, promotes re-expansion of atelectatic areas, and may force fluid from the alveolar spaces into the interstitium. This allows previously closed or flooded alveoli to participate in gas exchange. In cardiogenic pulmonary edema, PEEP can reduce left ventricular preload and afterload, improving cardiac performance.

a.

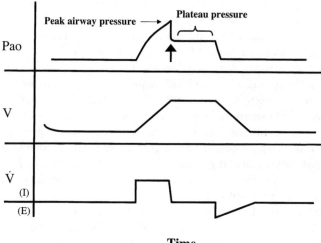

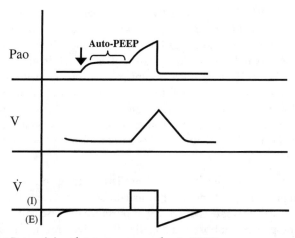

Time

FIGURE 4–4 Determining plateau pressure and auto-PEEP.
a. Method for determining plateau pressure. Graphs of airway pressure, volume, and flow versus time are shown during volume-targeted ventilation. An inspiratory pause is performed in relaxed patient by occluding airway at end-inspiration (thick arrow). Pressure drops from peak to plateau as flow stops and end-inspiratory volume is maintained. When airway occlusion is released, expiratory flow occurs and lung volume returns to FRC.
b. Method for estimating auto-PEEP. An expiratory pause is performed in a relaxed patient by occluding airway at end-expiration (thick arrow). Measured pressure rises as flow stops and P$_A$ equilibrates with airway pressure. The next breath from ventilator causes flow to resume, and airway pressure and lung volume rise. (Modified with permission from Aldrich TK, Prezant DJ. Indications for mechanical ventilation. In Tobin MJ, ed. Principles and practice of mechanical ventilation. *New York: McGraw-Hill, 1994:155–189.)*

In hypercapneic respiratory failure (type 2) resulting from airflow obstruction, patients often have insufficient time to exhale, resulting in dynamic hyperinflation. This results in an end-expiratory alveolar pressure that is above atmospheric pressure, or "auto-PEEP." This pressure can be estimated with an expiratory hold maneuver in the relaxed patient (Figure 4–4*b*). Triggering the ventilator in the presence of auto-PEEP requires a negative airway pressure that exceeds both trigger sensitivity and auto-PEEP. If the patient is unable to achieve this, inspiratory efforts are futile and merely increase the work of breathing. Applying PEEP can counteract this problem. In effect, a given amount of applied PEEP *subtracts* an equivalent portion of auto-PEEP from the total negative pressure required for ventilator triggering (Figure 4–5). Generally, PEEP is slowly increased until patient efforts consistently trigger the ventilator, up to a maximum of 85% of the estimated auto-PEEP.[10]

Disadvantages of PEEP include elevation in the mean airway pressure which, if excessive, can result in barotrauma. Elevation in the mean airway pressure can also impair cardiac output, especially in the setting of volume depletion.

TRIGGER SENSITIVITY Trigger sensitivity is the negative pressure that the patient must generate to initiate a ventilator-supported breath. It should be low enough to minimize the work of breathing but high enough to avoid oversensitivity and the delivery of breaths without true patient effort. In general, this pressure is −1 to −2 cm H_2O. A more recent adaptation, known as "flow-by," employs a baseline flow rate through the ventilator circuit; patient effort is detected when flow rate decreases. Some studies suggest that flow-by reduces the work of breathing in comparison to pressure-triggering.[11,12] In general, ventilator triggering occurs when the patient decreases baseline flow by 1 to 3 L/min.[2]

FLOW RATE This is often the "forgotten ventilator setting" on volume-targeted modes. Although the respiratory therapist usually sets flow rate without the need for a physician order, this rate is of critical importance because it affects the work of breathing and patient comfort and directly affects dynamic hyperinflation and auto-PEEP. On some ventilators, it is set directly, and on others (e.g., Siemens 900c), it is determined indirectly from the respiratory rate and I:E ratio. This is demonstrated in the following example:

$$
\begin{aligned}
\text{Respiratory rate} &= 10 \\
\therefore \text{Respiratory cycle time} &= 6 \text{ sec} \\
\text{I:E ratio} &= 1{:}2 \\
\therefore \text{Inspiratory time} &= 2 \text{ sec} \\
\therefore \text{Expiratory time} &= 4 \text{ sec} \\
\text{Tidal volume} &= 500 \text{ mL} \\
\text{Flow rate} &= \text{volume/inspiratory time} \\
&= 500 \text{ mL every 2 sec} \\
&= 250 \text{ mL/sec} \times 60 \text{ sec} = 15 \text{ L/min}
\end{aligned}
$$

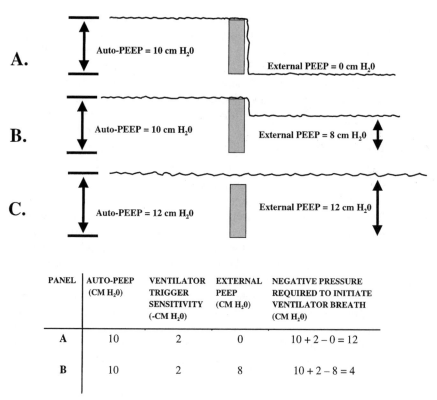

PANEL	AUTO-PEEP (CM H_2O)	VENTILATOR TRIGGER SENSITIVITY (-CM H_2O)	EXTERNAL PEEP (CM H_2O)	NEGATIVE PRESSURE REQUIRED TO INITIATE VENTILATOR BREATH (CM H_2O)
A	10	2	0	$10 + 2 - 0 = 12$
B	10	2	8	$10 + 2 - 8 = 4$

FIGURE 4–5 *Relationship between auto-PEEP and external PEEP in setting of expiratory air flow limitation, in analogy to water over dam. In panel a, water above dam is 10 cm high (auto-PEEP = 10 cm H_2O) and water below dam is at ground level (external PEEP = 0 cm H_2O). In panel b, water level above dam remains at 10 cm, but below dam, it has risen to 8 cm. This decreases the distance between water levels on either side of dam (the auto-PEEP–induced work needed to trigger ventilator), but it does not impair flow of water above dam (rate of expiratory air flow). The graph shows work required for ventilator triggering in the two examples, assuming trigger sensitivity of –2 cm H_2O. In panel c, the downstream water has now risen above dam, increasing upstream water level (excessive external PEEP, causing worsening dynamic hyperinflation and auto-PEEP). (Modified with permission from Tobin MJ, Lodato RF. PEEP, auto-PEEP, and waterfalls.* Chest *1989; 96(3):449–451.)*

When flow rate is set directly, inspiratory time is determined by inspiratory flow rate divided by tidal volume. In turn, inspiratory time and set respiratory rate determine I:E ratio.

Under most circumstances, flow rate is set between 40 and 100 L/min. An inspiratory flow rate that is set too low for patient demand (as might be expected in the example) causes the patient to "tug" on the ventilator, thus increasing the work of breathing. During volume-targeted ventilation, the prescribed flow rate cannot be exceeded. If patient demand for inspiratory flow exceeds the set rate, the patient's efforts will be ineffective, increasing the likelihood of patient distress. Moreover, slower flow rates lengthen inspiratory time, shorten expiratory time, and predispose the patient to dynamic hyperinflation and auto-PEEP. Conversely, an excessive inspiratory flow rate increases peak airway pressures and may cause patient discomfort and patient-ventilator asynchrony. In general, it is best to err on the side of high flow rates. In pressure-targeted ventilation, inspiratory flow rate is a function of inspiratory time, patient effort, and respiratory system mechanics (compliance and resistance). In these modes, it is possible for patients to alter flow rate on demand, potentially enhancing comfort.

RATIO OF INSPIRATORY TO EXPIRATORY TIME As with inspiratory flow rate, the respiratory therapist sets the I:E ratio without need for a physician order. However, the clinician must understand how alterations in this ratio can affect respiratory system mechanics and patient comfort. A typical I:E ratio is 1:2. In acute hypoxemic respiratory failure, this ratio may be increased (lengthened inspiratory time), increasing mean airway pressure and recruiting collapsed or fluid-filled alveoli, which results in improved oxygenation. In severe hypoxemia, the I:E ratio is sometimes completely reversed to 2:1, while vigilance is maintained for adverse effects on hemodynamics and lung integrity. A complete review of inverse ratio ventilation is beyond the scope of this chapter. In obstructive lung diseases, the inspiratory time may be reduced to allow more time for exhalation and reduce the risk for dynamic hyperinflation and auto-PEEP.

Mechanical Ventilation for Specific Conditions

ACUTE HYPOXEMIC RESPIRATORY FAILURE
Acute Respiratory Distress Syndrome

Volume- and pressure-targeted modes of mechanical ventilation are both reasonable in patients with ARDS. The advantages of pressure-targeted modes include complete control of peak airway pressures and an inspiratory flow pattern that decelerates as the lung inflates, minimizing peak airway pressures; the disadvantages include variability in tidal volume and minute ventilation. Volume-targeted modes, on the other hand, dictate minute ventilation at the expense of peak airway pressure variability. Ultimately, the mode chosen should be based on patient comfort, the clinical situation, and the clinician's experience.

In patients with ARDS, alveolar flooding and atelectasis cause shunt physiology (mixed venous blood flows through nonventilated areas of lung), resulting in oxygen-refractory hypoxemia. Shunt fraction can be reduced with PEEP by recruiting collapsed lung units and perhaps shifting intra-alveolar fluid to the interstitium. In so doing, PEEP reduces the FIO_2 required for adequate arterial oxygenation. However, potential hazards of PEEP necessitate careful titration, which may be performed according to two strategies:

1. The "best PEEP" approach, in which PEEP is adjusted upward to allow use of an FIO_2 of below 0.60 or below [4]
2. The "open lung approach," in which PEEP is adjusted to a level of 2 cm H_2O above the lower inflection point of the respiratory system compliance curve[13]

The latter can be difficult to determine as a result of the complexities of compliance measurements in unstable patients. In general, PEEP levels of 10 to 20 cm H_2O are commonly required. PEEP should also be adjusted to keep plateau pressure at 35 cm H_2O or lower in most circumstances.

Tidal volume is of critical importance in patients with ARDS. Although chest radiographs often suggest diffuse and homogenous lung injury, CT scanning has shown that lung involvement is instead patchy, with marked abnormalities in dependent regions and relatively normal parenchyma in nondependent regions.[14] This finding has promoted the concept of the "baby lung" in patients with ARDS, that is, large areas of the lungs cannot be ventilated and gas exchange only occurs in the less affected areas. In this situation, tidal volumes should be adjusted downward to minimize overinflation. Moreover, recent data suggests that overinflation of an injured lung not only perpetuates lung injury but it also causes systemic inflammation that may damage other organs.[8] Accordingly, tidal volumes of 5 to 8 mL/kg of ideal body weight are now standard, especially in light of a recent multicenter randomized trial[7] directly comparing tidal volumes of 6 mL/kg with 12 mL/kg. In the low tidal volume group, there was a significant increase in the number of ventilator-free days, and the trial was stopped early because of a 22% mortality reduction.[7]

A compensatory increase in respiratory rate is often necessary to achieve an adequate minute ventilation with such low tidal volumes, and therefore, rates from 15 to 35 breaths per minute are necessary. Clinicians must often tolerate a modest degree of respiratory acidosis despite higher respiratory rates, a strategy known as "permissive hypercapnea."[15] Usually this means accepting a PCO_2 of 50 to 60 Hg and a pH of 7.30. Occasionally, more extreme hypercapnea may be required, allowing the PCO_2 to climb to 70 to 80 mm Hg.

FIO_2 is kept at the lowest level that maintains adequate oxygenation. The goal is an FIO_2 of 0.6 or less to reduce risk of pulmonary oxygen toxicity, while maintaining the oxyhemoglobin saturation at 90% or more. Again, occasionally a slightly lower oxyhemoglobin saturation goal must be accepted.

Cardiogenic Pulmonary Edema

Ventilator strategies for patients with this condition are similar to those for patients with ARDS. However, the primary mechanism of alveolar fluid accumulation is elevated left ventricular end-diastolic pressure, causing hydrostatic edema, instead of inflammatory lung injury, causing pulmonary capillary leak. Therefore, the risk of ventilator-induced lung injury and systemic inflammation may be lower, reducing the need to severely restrict tidal volume. This is fortunate because permissive hypercapnea can adversely affect cardiac function and predispose to arrhythmias in patients with underlying heart disease.[15] The cardiovascular benefits of positive pressure ventilation are particularly relevant in this patient population. The various effects that mechanical ventilation may have on cardiac function are illustrated in Figure 4–6.

HYPERCAPNEIC RESPIRATORY FAILURE
Chronic Obstructive Pulmonary Disease

Ventilator strategies for chronic obstructive pulmonary disease (COPD) have the common goal of reducing the workload imposed on failing respiratory muscles. The work of breathing increases with auto-PEEP and dynamic hyperinflation, making ventilator triggering more difficult as the compliance of the respiratory system decreases. Allowing adequate exhalation time by shortening inspiratory

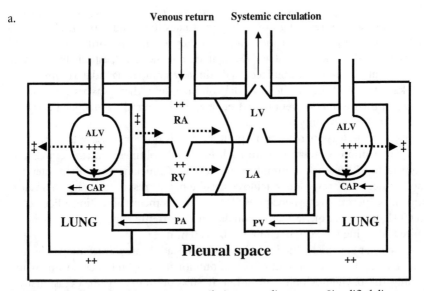

FIGURE 4–6 *Effects of positive pressure ventilation on cardiac output. Simplified diagrams of thorax. Blood flow (solid lines); pressure transmission (dotted lines). ALV, alveolus; RA, right atrium; RV, right ventricle; LA, left atrium; LV, left ventricle; PA, pulmonary artery; APC, pulmonary capillary; PV, pulmonary vein.*
a. Mechanisms for decreased cardiac output.[16] Positive pressure ventilation causes elevated alveolar pressure (+++), which is partially transmitted to the pleural space (++) and RA, causing reduction in venous return. LV preload is reduced, causing reduction in cardiac output. With lung distention, pulmonary vascular resistance may increase,[17] further increasing RA pressure and reducing venous return. Increased right-sided pressures can bow the interventricular septum to left, reducing left-sided chamber compliance, further reducing LV preload. Septal bowing can also increase afterload by causing LV outflow tract obstruction.

b.

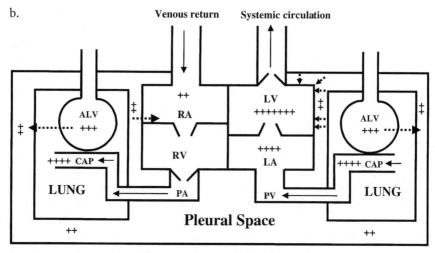

FIGURE 4–6 *(continued) Effects of positive pressure ventilation on cardiac output. Simplified diagrams of thorax. Blood flow (solid lines); pressure transmission (dotted lines). ALV, alveolus; RA, right atrium; RV, right ventricle; LA, left atrium; LV, left ventricle; PA, pulmonary artery; CAP, pulmonary capillary; PV, pulmonary vein.*
b. *Mechanisms for increased cardiac output.[18] Occurs in patients with impaired LV function and elevated LV filling pressures.[19] Patients typically have high LV afterload, which impairs cardiac output. Afterload is defined as transmural ventricular pressure required for ventricular systolic emptying. This pressure is estimated by subtracting pleural pressure (++) from ventricular systolic pressure (+++++). Higher pleural pressures reduce ventricular transmural pressure, or afterload. In addition, positive pleural pressures push on dilated ventricular wall, reducing its radius (small interrupted arrows). This reduces wall tension required to achieve same transmural pressure (or afterload), via LaPlace's relationship: $P = \frac{2T}{r}$, where P = transmural pressure, T = ventricular wall tension, and r = radius of ventricular wall. Preload reduction from decreased venous return does not impair LV cardiac output, because the left-sided filling pressures are high (++++).*

time, maximizing inspiratory flow rate, and reducing respiratory rate reduces the risk of these problems. Permissive hypercapnea is often a necessary by-product of such ventilator management. High flow rates combined with a high level of airway resistance result in elevated peak airway pressure, which is a poor indicator of barotrauma risk. Peak airway pressure can be markedly elevated while plateau pressure remains within acceptable limits, especially with COPD. The risk of barotrauma (e.g., pneumothorax, subcutaneous emphysema) is low if plateau pressure is kept at 35 cm H_2O or less.

Despite these interventions, some degree of dynamic hyperinflation and auto-PEEP are inevitable. Indeed, these conditions are often present even before intubation as a result of expiratory airflow limitation. As described above, judicious use of ventilator-applied PEEP can be helpful in reducing the work required for ventilator triggering.

Finally, efforts should be made to reduce oxygen consumption and carbon dioxide production by maximizing patient comfort through ventilator adjustments and judicious sedation. The work of breathing can remain elevated during mechanical ventilation. This is most easily detected by careful and repeated observation of the patient. Signs of increased work of breathing include patient distress, diaphoresis, accessory muscle use, paradoxical abdominal motion, hypertension, tachycardia, and rapid, shallow breathing.

Almost any mode of mechanical ventilation can be used to accomplish the goals described, so treatment should be individualized according to patient comfort and tolerance. Volume-targeted modes do have a safety advantage over pressure-targeted modes because they ensure adequate tidal volume. As described previously, pressure-targeted modes deliver the inspiratory pressure only for the defined inspiratory time. With high levels of inspiratory resistance, tidal volume declines, predisposing the patient to auto-PEEP, dynamic hyperinflation, and barotrauma. However, freedom to increase inspiratory flow rate with pressure-targeted modes may improve patient comfort. Again, individualizing the treatment to the patient is required.

Asthma

The ventilator strategies used for patients with asthma are similar to those described for patients with COPD. Inspiratory airway resistance is typically even higher in asthma patients, so peak airway pressures may become markedly elevated. But if plateau pressure remains at 35 cm H_2O or less, the risk of barotrauma remains low. Attempts to reduce peak airway pressure by decreasing inspiratory flow rate shorten expiratory time, promoting dynamic hyperinflation, auto-PEEP, and barotrauma. Permissive hypercapnea is frequently required in patients with status asthmaticus.

On occasion, therapeutic paralysis is necessary to eliminate the respiratory efforts that increase oxygen consumption and carbon dioxide production and can impair effective gas exchange in unstable patients. The use of neuromuscular blocking agents mandates concomitant use of intravenous sedation and analgesia to prevent patient wakefulness during paralysis. Risks of these drugs include prolonged neuromuscular blockade, myopathy, and increased incidence of the polyneuropathy of critical illness. All of these complications delay patient recovery, so use of these agents should be minimized.

Neuromuscular Disease

Patients with diseases of the CNS (e.g., massive stroke, cervical spine trauma, or drug overdose), peripheral nervous system (e.g., Guillain-Barré syndrome and amyotrophic lateral sclerosis), and muscle (e.g., myasthenia gravis and Eaton-Lambert syndrome) share the feature of hypoventilation with essentially normal lungs. Such patients are probably less vulnerable than others to lung injury, so they can receive ventilation with somewhat higher tidal volumes. Indeed, the primary problem in these patients is poor lung inflation, predisposing them to atelectasis and pneumonia. It is therefore acceptable to use tidal volumes from 8 to 12 mL/kg in this patient group. Many of these patients often prefer high inspiratory flow rates, on the order of 60 L/min. Small to moderate amounts of PEEP should be used to reduce the risk of atelectasis. The mode of ventilation varies depending on the clinical circumstances. Patients with intact mental status may prefer pressure-support ventilation alone, or SIMV with pressure support. Patients with an impaired central respiratory drive require a mode with sufficient mandatory ventilation to maintain adequate gas exchange, such as assist-control, pressure-control, or SIMV.

MIXED RESPIRATORY FAILURE Most patients in acute respiratory failure present with a combination of hypoxemic and hypercapneic physiology. These patients should be managed with ventilator settings that combine features of the strategies described above.

SPECIAL SITUATIONS
Restrictive Disease

These conditions cause mixed respiratory failure and include patients with interstitial lung fibrosis or severe kyphoscoliosis. These patients often require mechanical ventilation because of acute diseases (such as pneumonia) superimposed on chronic respiratory disease. Impaired oxygenation deteriorates further as acute air space filling is superimposed on chronic interstitial lung disease or atelectasis. Ventilation deteriorates as an additional workload is placed on respiratory muscles that are already compromised because of low compliance of the restricted lungs or chest wall. Moreover, in fibrotic lung disease, increases in dead space (i.e., lung that is ventilated but not perfused) accompany loss of the pulmonary capillary bed, thereby increasing the minute ventilation required to maintain a normal P_{CO_2}. The strategy in this group must include low tidal volumes of 5 to 8 mL/kg, as in patients with ARDS. However, PEEP can be particularly hazardous in this group. For patients with fibrotic lung disease, PEEP can increase the likelihood of barotrauma. Moreover, PEEP may increase physiologic dead space by compressing alveolar capillaries in ventilated lung units, creating West zone 1 regions (Figure 4–7). In the case of restrictive disease of the chest wall, much of the PEEP is transmitted to the pleural space. This, in turn, accentuates preload reduction to the left ventricle and predisposes patients to hemodynamic compromise (see Figure 4–6a).

Unilateral Lung Disease

Unilateral disease occurs with focal lung disease (as in lobar pneumonia) or with bronchopleural fistulas. In the former, PEEP should be kept at the lowest level that allows adequate oxygenation, because it can cause West zone 1 formation in

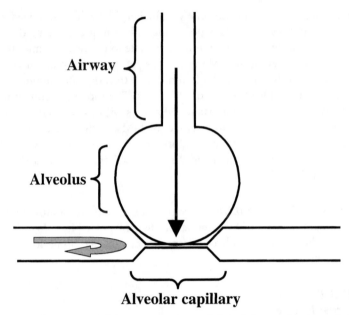

Airway

Alveolus

Alveolar capillary

FIGURE 4–7 West zone 1 conditions. Lung unit, consisting of airway, alveolus and alveolar capillary is shown. Positive airway pressure (black arrow) causes elevation in the alveolar pressure. If alveolar pressure is sufficiently elevated, it compresses the alveolar capillary, obstructing blood flow (curved arrow) and creating dead space. (Modified with permission from West JB. Blood flow and metabolism. In West JB, ed. Respiratory physiology: The essentials, *5th ed. Baltimore: Williams & Wilkins, 1995:41.)*

the unaffected lung, increasing dead space and shunting blood to the diseased areas.[20] So PEEP potentially *worsens* oxygenation in these patients. In the latter condition, PEEP should be minimized, because positive pressure maintains the air leak.[21] High inspiratory flow rates, low tidal volumes, and permissive hypercapnea are often used in both groups. If adequate ventilation cannot be achieved, independent-lung ventilation by means of a dual-lumen endotracheal tube may be attempted as a rescue maneuver.[2]

Increased Intracranial Pressure

Hypercapnea initiates a process of cerebral vasodilation, increased vascular hydrostatic pressure, and edema. It can thereby contribute to increased ICP in those with head injury or stroke. Although prophylactic hyperventilation is not recommended in these patients, hyperventilation to a P_{CO_2} of 25 to 30 mm Hg is reasonable if clinical evidence of increased ICP develops, until more definitive therapy can be instituted.[2] Once definitive therapies are in place, ventilator changes should be made gradually to allow the P_{CO_2} to normalize over 1 to 2 days.[2]

Complications

Many of the complications of mechanical ventilation have been alluded to in the preceding discussion. Dynamic hyperinflation and auto-PEEP have been discussed in detail. These complications are more common in patients with expiratory airflow obstruction but can occur in any patient if the respiratory system cannot return to FRC because of short expiratory time.

Another complication of over ventilation is respiratory alkalosis. This is potentially life-threatening because extreme alkalosis predisposes the patient to seizures, coma, ventricular arrhythmias, and hemodynamic collapse. Alkalosis of this severity is almost always an iatrogenic complication. To avoid this, a good rule of thumb is to set the ventilator rate a few breaths per minute below the patient's intrinsic rate. When the patient is not triggering the ventilator, periodic ABG samples should be drawn and analyzed to rule out unintended alkalosis.

A practical approach to complications manifested by high or low pressure is shown in Figures 4–8 and 4–9. A critical step in evaluating the deteriorating patient

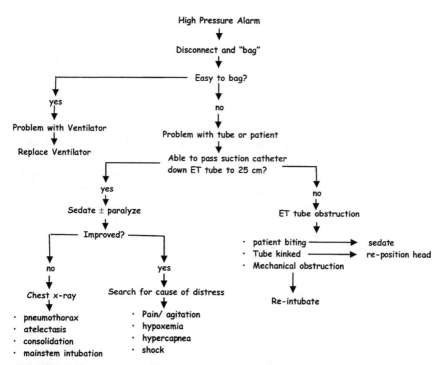

FIGURE 4–8 *High-pressure ventilator alarm. Algorithm for patient evaluation. (Adapted with permission from Schmidt GA, Hall JB. Management of the ventilated patient. In Hall JB, Schmidt GA, Wood LDH, eds.* Principles of critical care, *2nd ed. New York: McGraw-Hill, 1998; 517–535.)*

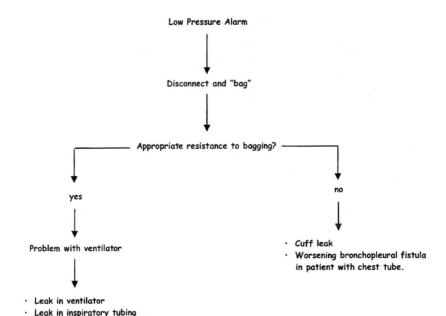

Low Pressure Alarm

Disconnect and "bag"

Appropriate resistance to bagging?

yes

no

Problem with ventilator

· Cuff leak
· Worsening bronchopleural fistula
  in patient with chest tube.

· Leak in ventilator
· Leak in inspiratory tubing
· Leak in Y-adaptor

FIGURE 4–9 *Low-pressure ventilator alarm. Algorithm for patient evaluation. (Adapted with permission from Schmidt GA, Hall JB. Management of the ventilated patient. In Hall JB, Schmidt GA, Wood LDH, eds.* Principles of critical care, *2nd ed. New York: McGraw-Hill, 1998; 517–535.)*

on mechanical ventilation is to separate problems with the patient and endotracheal tube from problems with the ventilator. This can be done by simply disconnecting the patient from the machine and ventilating by hand with a bag-valve-mask apparatus.[4] However, the patient should not be bagged too vigorously, because it may cause auto-PEEP and can result in catastrophic complications, including pneumothorax, hypotension, and cardiovascular collapse.[22] Tidal volumes of more than 1 L are commonly generated when "bagging" via an endotracheal tube with two hands,[23] so maintaining gentle ventilation at 15 to 20 breaths per minute (one breath every 4 to 5 seconds) is critical in avoiding complications.

Discontinuation of Mechanical Ventilation

Discontinuation is commonly referred to as "weaning," but it has been suggested that the term is misleading.[24] Weaning implies a gradual process of withdrawal from mechanical ventilation, during which the patient gradually regains the ability to breathe spontaneously. In most cases however, the capacity for spontaneous breathing is regained when the underlying illness that made mechanical ventilation necessary resolves sufficiently. This process has less to do with ventilator manipulation and more to do with accurate diagnosis and effective treatment of the underlying condition causing respiratory failure. Weaning also implies gradual withdrawal of a benevolent life-sustaining process,[4] when, in fact, mechanical ventilation should be considered a "necessary evil" to be removed at the earliest opportunity. Therefore, terms such as "discontinuation" and "liberation" probably are more appropriate. Nevertheless, the term "weaning" remains pervasive in the vernacular of the ICU.

Identifying the precise time when spontaneous breathing capacity returns is difficult, but attempting to do so is important because the risks accompanying mechanical ventilation increase with time. So, when the patient has medically stabilized, the patient should be assessed daily for the ability to breathe independently. From a mechanistic perspective, the ability to breathe independently after an episode of respiratory failure can be viewed as a restoration of the normal relationship between neuromuscular competence ("supply") and the load on the respiratory system ("demand"). Respiratory failure implies an imbalance in this relationship (Figure 4–10).

Other basic considerations in the decision to initiate the discontinuation process are oxygenation needs and cardiovascular function.[2] Spontaneous breathing trials should not generally be considered until the FIO_2 is 0.5 or less and the PEEP is 5 cm H20 or less. Patients with impaired cardiac function may benefit from the afterload- and preload-reducing effects of even small amounts of

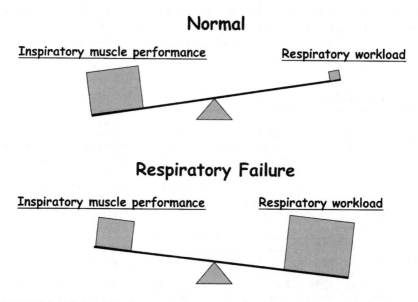

FIGURE 4–10 *Relationship between inspiratory muscle strength and respiratory workload. Normally, neuromuscular competence far exceeds imposed workload. In respiratory failure, neuromuscular competence is reduced or imposed workload is increased, or both. These conditions are commonly present in patients who are unable to tolerate discontinuation of mechanical ventilation. (Modified with permission from Aldrich TK, Prezant DJ. Indications for mechanical ventilation. In Tobin MJ, ed.* Principles and practice of mechanical ventilation. *New York: McGraw-Hill, 1994; 155–189.)*

PEEP. At extubation, PEEP removal may increase preload and afterload, causing pulmonary edema and recurrent respiratory failure. Cardiac performance should be medically optimized before attempting extubation in such patients.

Psychological factors are probably important, especially in patients subjected to prolonged mechanical ventilation. To date, the contribution of these factors to the discontinuation process is poorly understood. However, effective treatment of pain, anxiety, delirium, or depression probably does increase the likelihood of successful liberation from mechanical ventilation.

Once the decision has been made to initiate the process of discontinuation, one must assess the patient's readiness at the bedside. Various "weaning criteria" have been developed (Table 4–5). These indices are applied during a trial of spontaneous breathing, when the ventilator provides either no support (T-piece trial) or minimal support. The latter typically consists of 3 to 5 cm H_2O of PEEP and 5 of 10 cm H_2O of pressure support. Pressure support is provided to overcome the resistance of the endotracheal tube, which may result in an "unfair" resistive load. The exact amount of pressure support required to overcome tube resistance in any individual patient is difficult to predict, but it increases with decreasing size of the endotracheal tube.[25]

Independently, most of the criteria listed have a limited ability to predict successful discontinuation of mechanical ventilation. In clinical practice, these criteria are often used in combination. Like the data derived from different elements of a complete history and physical examination, the data obtained from these weaning criteria should be synthesized to arrive at a working theory: does the patient have the capacity to breathe spontaneously or not? The criteria are best used in this way.

TABLE 4–5 Weaning Parameters

Parameter	Threshold	Ability to discriminate pts. able to breath spontaneously
PImax (NIF)[a]	> 30 cm H_2O	good sensitivity,[b] poor specificity[c, 26]
VC[d]	> 10 mL/kg	poor sensitivity and specificity[27]
$\dot{V}_E$[e]	< 15 L/min	good sensitivity, poor specificity[26]
MVV[f]	≥ 2 × resting $\dot{V}_E$	poor sensitivity, good specificity[28]
Rapid shallow breathing index	< 105 breaths/min/L	very good sensitivity, low specificity[26]

[a]PImax, maximal inspiratory pressure; NIF, negative inspiratory force, synonym for PImax. PImax is determined by asking the patient to make a maximal inspiratory effort against an occluded airway from resting lung volume and then measuring the pressure generated at the mouth. Poor patient cooperation limits the reliability of this test. A one-way valve, allowing expiration but not inspiration, permits performance of the test in uncooperative patients.
[b]Sensitivity is the likelihood of meeting the threshold if the patient can breathe spontaneously.
[c]Specificity is the likelihood of not meeting the threshold if the patient cannot breathe spontaneously.
[d]VC, vital capacity. VC is obtained by asking the patient to inhale to total lung capacity and exhale forcefully to residual volume. The volume of gas exhaled is measured.
[e]$\dot{V}_E$, minute volume. $\dot{V}_E$ is the V_T times respiratory rate. It is usually measured while breathing at rest.
[f]MVV, maximum voluntary ventilation. MVV measures the peak ventilation (L/min) that the patient can achieve over 12–15 seconds, breathing as fast and deep as possible.

One of the most powerful predictive criteria is the rapid shallow breathing index.[26] This is calculated by dividing the respiratory rate (in breaths per minute) by the tidal volume (in liters) when the patient is breathing on a T-piece, typically after 1 minute has elapsed. The volume is measured with a simple spirometer briefly attached to the T-piece. An index of less than 105 breaths per minute per liter identifies most patients who are capable of spontaneous breathing (i.e., the test has high sensitivity), although it may underestimate the capability of women and patients with small endotracheal tubes.[29] The specificity of the index (i.e., the likelihood of an index greater than 105 breaths per minute per liter if the patient is incapable of spontaneous breathing) is poor, however. So while the rapid shallow breathing index is a good screening test for capturing patients who can breathe spontaneously, it should be followed by a more sustained trial to "weed out" patients with a false-positive screening test who are incapable of sustaining spontaneous respiration. Most commonly, the T-piece or pressure-support trial is continued for 30 to 120 minutes. Failure is evident if the patient develops discomfort, diaphoresis, acute respiratory acidosis, or vital sign abnormalities. The latter are defined as progressive tachypnea, tachycardia with a heart rate more than 20 beats/min above the baseline, or hypertension with systolic or diastolic blood pressure more than 20 mm Hg above baseline.[30] If such events occur, mechanical ventilation should be resumed, while further efforts are directed at treating the underlying cause of respiratory failure.[30] If the patient remains comfortable with stable vital signs and without acute respiratory acidosis, it is very likely that spontaneous breathing can be sustained. Extubation should be considered, presuming mental status and spontaneous secretion clearance are adequate.

These criteria for discontinuation of ventilation are not able to predict extubation failure resulting from upper airway obstruction, a complication that occurs in 1% to 5% of extubated patients.[4] Treatment for this emergent complication includes nebulized racemic epinephrine and high-dose intravenous corticosteroids to reduce airway edema. Heliox, a helium and oxygen gas mixture with a density lower than room air, can reduce turbulent flow and thereby reduce airflow resistance through the upper airway.[31] Noninvasive mechanical ventilation has also been suggested as a temporizing measure,[30] while medical therapy is being initiated. If such interventions are unsuccessful, a low threshold should exist for reintubation. In this situation, the likelihood of a difficult intubation is increased. Appropriate precautions should be taken and personnel with expertise in airway management should be immediately available.

NONINVASIVE MECHANICAL VENTILATION

Noninvasive mechanical ventilation (NIMV) is positive-pressure ventilation delivered by means of a cushioned facial or nasal mask that is maintained over the appropriate area with elastic straps. NIMV has the advantage of not requiring an endotracheal tube. Risks of the endotracheal tube (including upper airway injury and iatrogenic infection from bypassing the barrier defenses of the airway) are therefore obviated. Moreover, speaking and eating are possible with NIMV, providing potential advantages in quality of life.

Indications and Objectives

Indications and objectives of NIMV are similar to those of invasive mechanical ventilation. NIMV has benefits in both hypoxemic (type 1) and hypercapneic (type 2) respiratory failure. Application of NIMV requires an otherwise medically stable patient who is cooperative and can protect their airway. NIMV is not appropriate in patients with severely altered mental status, hemodynamic instability, excessive tracheobronchial secretions, or facial fractures. Proper patient selection is the key to success with NIMV.

There are advantages and disadvantages to both facial and nasal masks in the delivery of NIMV (Table 4–6). In general, facial masks are more effective in patients with acute respiratory failure, because they typically breathe through their mouth, which results in unacceptable leaks with a nasal mask.[32]

Modes

CONTINUOUS POSITIVE AIRWAY PRESSURE Continuous positive airway pressure (CPAP) mode involves the application of positive pressure to the airway throughout the respiratory cycle. Benefits result from:

1) Improved oxygenation via increased mean alveolar pressure in acute hypoxemic respiratory failure
2) Improved ventricular performance via increased pleural pressure in cardiac dysfunction
3) Reduced threshold workload in severe obstructive lung disease complicated by auto-PEEP
4) Reduced upper airway resistance in obstructive sleep apnea

TABLE 4–6 Advantages of Facial vs. Nasal Masks in Noninvasive Mechanical Ventilation

Facial Mask	Nasal Mask
• Less air leak in mouth-breathers	• Less dead space: 105 mL vs. 250 mL
	• Less claustrophobia
• More effective in acute respiratory failure	• Vomiting less hazardous
	• Oral intake possible with mask in place
	• Speaking easier with mask in place
	• Sputum expectoration easier

SOURCE: Adapted with permission from Meduri GU. Noninvasive positive-pressure ventilation in patients with acute respiratory failure. *Clin Chest Med* 1996; 17(3):535.

For details concerning the first three benefits, see the previous discussion of invasive mechanical ventilation.

BI-LEVEL POSITIVE AIRWAY PRESSURE Bi-level positive airway pressure (BiPAP) provides different inspiratory and expiratory pressures. The inspiratory assistance can be either time-cycled (pressure-control ventilation) or flow-cycled (pressure-support ventilation). The ventilator is triggered when the patient makes an inspiratory effort. The methods of patient triggering (either reduction in airway pressure or baseline airflow) are similar to those used in invasive ventilation. For details regarding mechanical ventilation modes, see the previous discussion of invasive mechanical ventilation. Because of the additional inspiratory support, BiPAP is probably superior to CPAP alone when respiratory muscle fatigue is present.[33]

Ventilator Settings

During CPAP, a single positive airway pressure is applied; during BiPAP, an expiratory positive airway pressure (EPAP) and an inspiratory positive airway pressure (IPAP) are chosen. These settings should be titrated to attain certain specified endpoints. Examples of initial settings, ranges, and endpoints are shown in Table 4–7.

TABLE 4–7 Suggesting Settings for Noninvasive Mechanical Ventilation

Parameter	Usual Range	Adjust to Maintain
CPAP or EPAP	0–15 cm H_2O (Start at low level and increase in 2–3 cm H_2O increments until objectives met.)	O_2 sat ≥ 90% FIO_2 ≤ 0.6 Patient comfort Peak mask pressure ≤ 30 cm H_2O (to avoid gastric overdistention) Minimal air leak
IPAP	8–20 cm H_2O (Start at low level and increase progressively to attain objectives.)	Respiratory rate ≤ 25/min Expiratory V_T > 7 mL/kg Patient comfort Peak mask pressure ≤ 30 cm H_2O (to avoid gastric overdistention) Minimal air leak

ABBREVIATIONS: CPAP, continuous positive airway pressure; EPAP, expiratory positive airway pressure; IPAP, inspiratory positive airway pressure; V_T, tidal volume. SOURCE: Adapted with permission from Meduri GU. Noninvasive positive-pressure ventilation in patients with acute respiratory failure. *Clin Chest Med* 1996; 17(3):537–542.

Complications

NIMV is characterized by a lower risk of complications than invasive mechanical ventilation.[33] The most common adverse events in patients undergoing NIMV are facial skin necrosis, gastric distention, and conjunctivitis.[33] Facial skin necrosis can be prevented by avoiding overzealous tightening of the straps and accepting a small air leak and by placement of a wound dressing over the bridge of the nose.[33] Gastric distention is less likely if peak mask pressure is kept below 30 cm H_2O.[33] Routine placement of nasogastric tubes for gastric decompression are not considered necessary.[33] Manipulation of the mask to direct air leakage inferiorly toward the mouth rather than superiorly toward the eyes reduces the risk of conjunctivitis.

Discontinuation of Noninvasive Mechanical Ventilation

The general criteria for initiating discontinuation of NIMV are identical to those for invasive mechanical ventilation. To summarize, the underlying process initiating respiratory failure should be sufficiently improved, the patient should be otherwise medically stable, and oxygenation should be adequate on an FIO_2 of 0.5 or less and 5 cm H_2O or less of expiratory pressure (CPAP or EPAP). When these criteria are fulfilled, spontaneous breathing trials should be initiated. These are easier to accomplish with NIMV, since the mask can be simply removed and replaced as needed. This results in a true assessment of the patient's ability to breathe spontaneously. The confounding effects of the endotracheal tube and ventilator circuit on respiratory mechanics are avoided, as are the risks of reintubation if the trial fails. If a patient has difficulty, the time without ventilator support can be progressively increased on a daily basis or the level of support can be progressively reduced.[33]

CONCLUSION

Respiratory failure is common in critical illness, and mechanical ventilation is necessary in most patients. Careful monitoring of physical examination findings, pulse oximetry, ABG analysis, airway pressures, and tidal volume are necessary to avoid potential ventilator-induced harm to the patient. When used carefully, mechanical ventilation is a life-saving intervention that bridges the period of acute illness, providing support until the patient regains the ability to breathe spontaneously.

REFERENCES

1. Aldrich TK, Prezant DJ. Indications for mechanical ventilation. In Tobin MJ, ed. *Principles and practice of mechanical ventilation.* New York: McGraw-Hill, 1994: 155–189.

2. Slutsky AS. ACCP consensus conference: Mechanical ventilation. *Chest* 1993; 104(6): 1833–1859.

3. Marini, JJ, Smith TC, Lamb VJ. External work output and force generation during synchronized intermittent mechanical ventilation: Effect of machine assistance on breathing effort. *Am Rev Respir Dis* 1988; 138:1169–1179.

4. Schmidt GA, Hall JB. Management of the ventilated patient. In Hall JB, Schmidt GA, Wood LDH, eds. *Principles of critical care*, 2nd ed. New York: McGraw-Hill, 1998; 517–535.

5. Tobin MJ, ed. *Principles and practice of mechanical ventilation.* New York: McGraw-Hill, 1994.

6. Apostolakos MJ, Levy PC, Papadakos PJ. New modes of mechanical ventilation. *Clin Pulmon Med* 1995; 2(2):121–128.

7. The Acute Respiratory Distress Syndrome Network. Ventilation with lower tidal volumes as compared with traditional tidal volume for acute lung injury and the acute respiratory distress syndrome. *N Engl J Med* 2000; 342:1301–1308.

8. Ranieri VM, Suter PM, Tortorella C, et al. Effect of mechanical ventilation on inflammatory mediators in patients with acute respiratory distress syndrome: A randomized controlled trial. *JAMA* 1999; 282(1):54–61.

9. Hudson LD. Progress in understanding ventilator-induced lung injury. *JAMA* 1999; 282(1):77–78.

10. Ranieri VM, Giuliani R, Cinnella G, et al. Physiologic effects of positive end-expiratory pressure in patients with chronic obstructive pulmonary disease during acute ventilatory failure and controlled mechanical ventilation. *Am Rev Respir Dis* 1993; 147:5–13.

11. Polese G, Massara A, Poggi R, et al. Flow-triggering reduces inspiratory effort during weaning from mechanical ventilation. *Intens Care Med* 1995; 31:682–686.

12. Goulet R, Hess DR, Kacmarek RM. Pressure vs flow triggering during pressure support ventilation. *Chest* 1997; 111:1649–1653.

13. Amato MB, Barbas CS, Medeiros DM, et al. Effect of a protective-ventilation strategy on mortality in the acute respiratory distress syndrome. *N Engl J Med* 1998; 338:347–354.

14. Gattinoni L, Pesenti A, Torresin A, et al. Adult respiratory distress syndrome: Profiles by computed tomography. *J Thorac Imag* 1986; 1(3):25–30.

15. Tuxen DV. Permissive hypercapneic ventilation. *Am J Respir Crit Care Med* 1994; 150:870–874.

16. Johnston WE, Vinten-Johansen J, Santamore WP, et al. Mechanism of reduced cardiac output during positive end-expiratory pressure in the dog. *Am Rev Respir Dis* 1989; 140:1257–1264.

17. West JB, ed. *Respiratory physiology: The essentials*, 5th ed. Baltimore: Williams & Wilkins, 1995.

18. Pinsky MR, Summer WR, Wise RA, et al. Augmentation of cardiac function by elevation of intrathoracic pressure. *J Appl Physiol: Respir Env Exer Physiol* 1983; 54(4): 950–955.

19. Bradley TD, Holloway RM, McLaughlin PR, et al. Cardiac output response to continuous positive airway pressure in congestive heart failure. *Am Rev Respir Dis* 1992; 145:377–382.

20. Mink SN, Light RB, Cooligan T, Wood LDH. Effect of PEEP on gas exchange and pulmonary perfusion in canine lobar pneumonia. *J Appl Physiol* 1981; 50(3):517–523.

21. Dennis JW, Eigen H, Ballantine TVN, et al. The relationship between peak inspiratory pressure and PEEP on the volume of air lost through a bronchopleural fistula. *J Ped Surg* 1980; 15(6):971–976.
22. Rogers PL, Schlichtig R, Miro A, et al. Auto-PEEP during CPR: An "occult" cause of electromechanical dissociation? *Chest* 1991; 99:492–493.
23. Manoranjan CS, Harrison RR, Keenan RL, et al. Bag-valve-mask ventilation; two rescuers are better than one, preliminary report. *Crit Care Med* 1985; 13(2):122–123.
24. Hall JB, Wood LDH. Liberation of the patient from mechanical ventilation. *JAMA* 1987; 257:1621–1628.
25. Fiastro JF, Habib MP, Quan SF. Pressure support compensation for inspiratory work due to endotracheal tubes and demand continuous positive airway pressure. *Chest* 1988; 93:499–505.
26. Yang LK, Tobin MJ. A prospective study of indexes predicting the outcome of trials of weaning from mechanical ventilation. *N Engl J Med* 1991; 234(21):1445–1450.
27. Tahvanainen J, Salmenpera M, Nikki P. Extubation criteria after weaning from intermittent mandatory ventilation and continuous positive airway pressure. *Crit Care Med* 1983;11:702–707.
28. Sahn SA, Lakshminarayan S. Bedside criteria for discontinuation of mechanical ventilation. *Chest* 1973;63: 1002–1005.
29. Epstein SK, Ciubotaru RL. Influence of gender and endotracheal tube size on preextubation breathing pattern. *Am J Respir Crit Care Med* 1996; 154:1647–1652.
30. Manthous CA, Schmidt GA, Hall JB. Liberation from mechanical ventilation: A decade of progress. *Chest* 1998; 114:886–901.
31. Boorstein JM, Boorstein SM, Humphries GN, et al. Using helium-oxygen mixtures in the emergency management of upper airway obstruction. *Ann Emerg Med* 1989; 18:688–690.
32. Carrey Z, Gottfried SB, Levy RD. Ventilatory muscle support in respiratory failure with nasal positive-pressure ventilation. *Chest* 1990; 97:150–158.
33. Meduri GU. Noninvasive positive-pressure ventilation in patients with acute respiratory failure. *Clin Chest Med* 1996; 17(3):513–553.

CHAPTER 5

Approach to Renal Failure

ANDREW B. LEIBOWITZ

"The dumbest kidney is smarter than the smartest doctor."

THOMAS IBERTI, MD

INTRODUCTION

Acute renal failure is a common diagnosis in the ICU that increases morbidity and mortality in any patient group. Diagnosis and management of acute renal failure in the critically ill patient should be a subject with which the ICU physician is intimately familiar and should rarely require outside consultation.

HOW IS RENAL DYSFUNCTION DEFINED AND QUANTIFIED?

The adequacy of renal function is assessed by quantification of urinary output, laboratory determination of the blood urea nitrogen (BUN) and creatinine (Cr) levels, and calculation of the creatinine clearance (CrCl) either by estimation or direct measurement. Further, measurement of the urine osmolarity (Uosm), urine sodium (UNa) concentration, and calculation of the fractional excretion of sodium (FeNa) may be helpful.

Urinary Output

Urinary output in a critically ill patient should be measured hourly and quantified every "shift" (6 to 8 hours) and daily. This requires placement of a Foley catheter in most patients. Despite the importance of early recognition of renal dysfunction and failure, in this author's opinion, far too much effort is expended on maintaining some "magical" minimum urinary output in all patients (usually more than 30 mL/hr or 0.5 mL/kg per hour). A reduction in urinary output is most often a sign of an underlying process that requires elucidation, not a disease itself. For example, oliguria in the presence of hypotension and hypovolemia is renal success, not renal failure; restoration of the blood pressure and circulating intravascular volume in this circumstance is of paramount importance, while an increase in the urinary output is simply a sign that the effort is a success.

Traditionally, oliguria is defined as urinary output of less than 400 mL/day, although many physicians loosely refer to patients producing less than 0.5 mL/kg per hour or 30 mL/hr as being oliguric. Anuria is defined as urinary output of less than 50 mL/day. The presence of anuria should always raise the suspicion that the Foley catheter is not properly functioning and mandates that the bladder be irrigated and free return of fluid be observed to rule out a mechanical problem.

Blood Urea Nitrogen and Creatinine

BUN is the breakdown product of protein. Measurement of the BUN level is commonly performed daily on all ICU patients. The BUN level directly varies with protein intake and increases in the presence of gastrointestinal bleeding and corticosteroid administration. A reduction in BUN level may be seen in patients with starvation and malnutrition, muscle wasting, and liver disease. Although most patients with acute renal failure have a rising BUN level, these concomitant conditions may lead to a "false" rise or fall, and thus an overestimation or underestimation of the change. Thus, interpretation of the BUN level should rely more on its change over time than its absolute value and should always take into consideration these concomitant conditions and other measures of renal function. In the absence of these contributing conditions, the BUN level typically rises 10 to 15 mg/dL per day in patients with acute renal failure.

Creatinine is the breakdown product of muscle. Measurement of the creatinine level, like the BUN level, is commonly performed daily on all ICU patients. Its absolute value and change over time is a much more reliable indicator of underlying renal function than the BUN level. In acute renal failure, the creatinine level rises by 1 to 2 mg/dL per day. In rhabdomyolysis, the rise in serum creatinine level may be greater. Indeed, a rise in the creatinine of more than 2 mg/dL per day should clue the physician into the possibility of rhabdomyolysis and the need to determine the creatinine kinase (CK) concentration.

Creatinine Clearance

Creatinine clearance is actually what we should be interested in and only infer from the above measurements. Two normal kidneys usually clear approximately 120 mL of creatinine per minute, and it is not until creatinine clearance falls below 10 mL/min in chronic renal failure that dialysis is required. A crude estimation of the creatinine clearance is given by the following equation:

$$\text{CrCl (mL/min)} = \frac{(140 - \text{age}) \times \text{weight (kg)}}{72 \times \text{serum Cr (mg/dL)}}$$

This equation is simply the ratio of the expected amount of muscle breakdown (which is directly related to young age and large size) to the presence of this breakdown product present in the serum multiplied by a "fudge factor." Females typically have less muscle mass than their same-age male counterparts, and so this value should be multiplied by 0.85 for female patients. However, in rapidly failing kidneys of critically ill patients, this formula usually overestimates the creatinine clearance. Therefore, more direct determination of creatinine clearance may be necessary.

Creatinine clearance may be more accurately determined by collecting all the urine produced over a time interval. This is usually 24 hours in a chronically ill patient, but for the sake of convenience in an ICU patient with a Foley catheter placed, a 4- or 6-hour collection is actually more practical. The following equation is used:

$$\text{CrCl(mL/min)} = \frac{\text{Urine [Cr] (mg/dL)} \times \text{volume (mL/min)}}{\text{Plasma [Cr] (mg/dL)}}$$

Urine Sodium

When perfusion of the kidney is reduced, sodium reabsorption increases and excretion decreases. Typically, a urinary sodium concentration of less than 20 mEq/L results. Perfusion of the kidney may be reduced from hypovolemia, secondary to dehydration or hemorrhage, or from decreased forward flow, as may be seen in patients with severe heart failure. In ICU patients suffering from severe hypoperfusion a urinary sodium concentration of less than 10 mEq/L may be seen, but such values should always raise the suspicion that the patient may have an hepatorenal syndrome.

Sodium reabsorption in a kidney with an acute injury (e.g., acute tubular necrosis) is impaired and an increase in sodium excretion results. Typically a urinary sodium level of greater than 20 mEq/L, or even greater than 40 mEq/L, results. Often, a combination of factors may occur (e.g., hypovolemia in addition to chronic renal failure) making interpretation of the urinary sodium level particularly difficult, hence the fractional excretion of sodium measurement has evolved.

Fractional Excretion of Sodium

The fractional excretion of sodium is helpful in determining whether the rise in creatinine level is a prerenal or renal problem. The fractional excretion of sodium is calculated as follows:

$$FeNa = \frac{Urine\ [Na]/plasma\ [Na]}{Urine\ [Cr]/plasma\ [Cr]} \times 100$$

A fractional excretion of sodium measurement of less than 1% is evidence that the problem is prerenal (e.g., hypovolemia, severe heart failure), and a fractional excretion of sodium measurement of more than 2% is evidence that the problem is renal (e.g., acute tubular necrosis).

CAUSES

The cause of renal failure may be classified as prerenal, renal, or postrenal.

Prerenal

Hypoperfusion of any origin causes the kidney to concentrate urine, the urinary output to fall, and the BUN and creatinine levels to rise. The BUN level usually, but not always, rises out of proportion to the creatinine level, and a ratio of more than 20:1 is achieved. Prerenal "failure" is therefore most accurately and commonly not a failure at all but a normal response on the part of the kidney to an abnormal perfusion. Common causes include hypovolemia, CHF, and extreme vasodilatation. Genuine renal injury probably does not result from these causes, unless there is a superimposed insult (e.g., exposure to a nephrotoxin). The rise in the BUN and creatinine levels is rapidly and completely reversible by restoration of effective circulating intravascular volume, maximization of cardiac function, and treatment of abnormal vasodilatation.

Renal

Renal failure occurring within the kidney itself is the most common cause of acute renal failure and the need for dialysis in critically ill patients. Acute tubular necrosis is commonly (but semantically incorrectly) used as a "waste-basket" term to generally describe all renal injuries that progress to acute renal failure. Traditional medical teaching usually divides intrarenal renal failure into 3 categories:

1. Tubular failure, including genuine acute tubular necrosis
2. Interstitial nephritis
3. Glomerulonephritis and vasculitis

It is probably more helpful in critically ill patients to classify de novo intrarenal failure into two relatively large and intentionally vague groups. The first group would contain iatrogenic and avoidable causes that are usually a complication of therapy, or failure to make an expeditious diagnosis and implement appropriate intervention. Examples of this first group include: 1) intrarenal injuries secondary to administration of therapeutic agents (particularly the aminoglycoside antibiotics and amphotericin), or diagnostic agents (i.e., radiographic contrast agents) with known nephrotoxic potential; 2) myoglobinuria secondary to rhabdomyolysis; or hemoglobinuria secondary to massive hemolysis and 3) interstitial nephritis, which is a frequently unrecognized allergic reaction seen with a wide variety of drugs, including penicillin, furosemide, and NSAIDs. The second group would include origins in which intrarenal failure is part and parcel of the process, causing acute intrarenal failure in a fashion that is well recognized but poorly understood; examples of this second group include massive transfusion, multisystem trauma, severe pancreatitis, liver failure, ARDS, shock, and sepsis.

Postrenal

Renal failure with a postrenal cause can occur when there is obstruction to urinary flow anywhere distal to the renal pelvis. Obstruction is always the leading diagnosis when there is anuria. Normally, both ureters (one, if there is only one kidney) or the urethra must become obstructed to cause acute postrenal failure. However, unilateral ureteral obstruction and partial urethral obstruction may complicate ongoing intrarenal processes in critically ill patients. Clinical suspicion of these pathologies should remain high in patients with pelvic and retroperitoneal disease. A Foley catheter should always be placed in the bladder to exclude the possibility of a distal obstruction. Mechanical obstruction of the Foley catheter and obstruction of the Foley's holes by debris and clots should always be considered in patients with an indwelling Foley catheter and acute changes in urinary output. Abdominal ultrasound, which can be performed at the patient's bedside, is the diagnostic test of choice. If an obstruction distal to the bladder is discovered and released, hematuria and postobstructive diuresis may result.

DIAGNOSTIC CONSIDERATIONS

The patient's history of exposure to harmful substances, particularly nephrotoxins, ongoing disease processes (such as liver failure), and periods of hypotension should be noted.

Physical Examination

Physical examination of the critically ill patient with acute renal failure is relatively simple but often unrewarding. Attention should be paid to the vital signs and orthostatic hypotension[7]. Estimation of the central venous pressure (CVP) by examination of the jugular venous pressure and assessment of blood volume status by noting peripheral edema are two often highly touted techniques that are probably relatively useless in a critically ill patient. A careful review of daily fluid intake and output and changes in body weight might be helpful adjuncts in determining volume status.

Urinalysis

Urinalysis and microscopic examination may be diagnostic. Certainly the presence of blood suggests that embolic phenomena should be considered, and a large number of casts suggests that there is acute tubular necrosis, but "dirty" results on urinalysis are a common finding in critically ill patients.

Ultrasonography

Abdominal ultrasonography is the diagnostic test of choice when considering the diagnosis of postrenal failure. In the presence of obstruction to urinary flow, the proximal ureter dilates, resulting in hydronephrosis. Ultrasound is also helpful in determination of kidney size, which in patients with unclear histories may give a clue as to the cause of underlying chronic renal disease. Small kidneys usually signify long-standing hypertension; large kidneys may result from diabetes or amyloidosis.

Nuclear Studies

Nuclear imaging of the kidney should be considered when there is concern about abnormal blood flow, which is commonly the concern in patients with a suspected embolus to the kidneys or vascular compromise (e.g., status posttransplant, renal artery stenosis).

ACUTE MANAGEMENT ISSUES

Use of Diuretics and Dopamine

Diuretics and "renal-dose" (low-dose) dopamine are frequently administered in hope of either: 1) converting anuric or oliguric renal failure to nonoliguric renal failure, because patients with de novo nonoliguric renal failure have better outcomes than patients with oliguric renal failure; or 2) amelioration of the renal injury with subsequent decreased intensity or duration of dialysis.

Unfortunately, although nonoliguric patients may be more easily managed than oliguric patients, diuretics and dopamine have largely been disproven to favorably influence patient outcome. These agents are frequently administered anyway, under the assumption that the potential benefit outweighs the risk. Furosemide can cause interstitial nephritis and hearing loss, and even low-dose dopamine may cause undesirable tachycardia, arrythmias, and myocardial ischemia.

Other Measures

There are a variety of "soft" interventions that may ameliorate renal injury and certainly will delay the need for dialysis and reduce the intensity of dialysis required. First, restore circulating intravascular volume and maintain a mean arterial blood pressure of more than 50 mm Hg, which is the lower limit for renal autoregulation. Successfully accomplishing this may require measurement of the CVP, pulmonary artery catheterization, or echocardiography. Second, on first recognition of worsening renal function, immediately eliminate or appropriately reduce the dose of nephrotoxic therapies (e.g., change amphotericin to fluconazole if possible; reduce the dose of gentamicin and vancomycin). Third, if the blood pressure is normal and hypovolemia is not an issue, aggressively reduce maintenance-level intravenous fluid administration to avoid fluid overload. Fourth, reduce the administration of acid (commonly administered in the form of 0.9% sodium chloride solution, which has a pH of 5.0), potassium, magnesium, and phosphate in maintenance fluids in intravenous and enteral feeds. Fifth, feed the patient—starved patients with renal failure clearly have worse outcomes than fed patients. Also, try to maximize enteral nutrition and discontinue intravenous nutrition when possible, in view of preliminary evidence that, in critically ill patients in general and with renal failure in particular, morbidity and mortality may be improved with the administration of enteral compared with parenteral nutrition.

DIALYSIS

Dialysis may be emergent or elective. Emergency dialysis should rarely be required in a hospitalized patient, because the need for dialysis should be anticipated and early intervention initiated. Severe acidosis, hyperkalemia, uremia (e.g., change in mentation, pleuritis, pericarditis, bleeding), and volume overload are the classic indications for emergency dialysis. Elective dialysis is usually initiated in anticipation of one or more of these issues arising. Many ICU physicians advocate early dialysis, but there is no evidence that it improves outcome. Usually, daily observance of the BUN and creatinine levels and estimation of the creatinine clearance is performed, and dialysis is begun when the BUN level exceeds 100 mg/dL, or the creatinine clearance is less than 15 mL/min; however, these values are completely arbitrary. Opinion regarding the optimal time to start dialysis varies markedly from physician to physician, institution to institution, and country to country.

There are four contemporary modes of dialysis to be considered: peritoneal dialysis (PD), hemodialysis (HD), continuous arteriovenous hemofiltration (CAVH), and continuous venovenous hemofiltration (CVVH).

Peritoneal

PD is generally impractical in most ICU patients because of the high incidence of previous intra-abdominal surgery and ongoing intra-abdominal pathology. In addition, patients with respiratory insufficiency and failure often cannot tolerate fluid in the peritoneum. Therefore, except in the most rudimentary of ICUs, PD is rarely used.

Continuous Arteriovenous Hemofiltration

CAVH was the continuous method of choice before the development of CVVH. Its reliance on an adequate pressure head, lack of external apparatus to control flow and provide warning alarms, and need to insert a large-bore catheter into an artery, with the potential for resultant bleeding, thrombosis, clot, and pseudo-aneurysm formation, have generally led to its abandonment. Nonetheless, in certain patients in institutions where CVVH is not available, CAVH is a method that warrants consideration.

Continuous Venovenous Hemofiltration

CVVH has been rapidly emerging as the dialysis mode of choice. It can be combined with continuous arteriovenous hemodialysis (CAVHD). The slow method of solute and fluid removal results in an extremely hemodynamically stable milieu. In additon, CVVH can remove large quantities of cytokines, which may reduce the incidence and ameliorate the progression of multisystem organ failure. New CVVH machines have incorporated a pump, air detector, and pressure monitor, which makes CVVH far safer than CAVH was. Management of CVVH usually requires one-to-one nursing and frequent (i.e., every 4 to 6 hours) electrolyte level measurement. However, removal of large quantities of fluid, sometimes as much as 10 L per day, is possible, often shortening the time that mechanical ventilation is required and reducing the stay in the ICU.

Intermittent Hemodialysis

Intermittent HD is frequently used in critically ill patients, but, especially in patients with hypotension, it is fraught with imminent danger. It is virtually impossible to adequately perform hemodialysis on a hypotensive patient with an intermittent method. It may be necessary to administer vasopressors at the time of HD to maintain a near-normal blood pressure, and the resultant cardiac effect (i.e., tachycardia and possible myocardial ischemia) and peripheral vasoconstrictive effects are theoretically injurious.

HD has been declining in popularity in ICUs because of its association with hypotension and the inability to remove significant quantities of fluid, given HD's relatively short (i.e., 3 to 4 hours) duration.

Although there is an emerging consensus among ICU physicians that CVVH is the preferred method of dialysis in critically ill patients, many institutions still rely primarily on HD for a variety of bureaucratic, logistical, and political reasons.

PRESCRIBING COMMON DRUGS IN RENAL FAILURE

All medication prescribed for patients who have renal failure should be reviewed and an adjustment made for the reduction of organ function and the effects of dialysis. Failure to do this results in potential drug toxicity and possibly even promulgation of the underlying renal failure. Drugs most commonly administered to critically ill patients that will require adjustment include penicillins, carbipenems, cephalosporins, vancomycin, aminoglycosides, amphotericin, digoxin, and some muscle relaxants. Opioids and benzodiazepines are for the most part metabolized by the liver, but many have active metabolites eliminated by the kidney and thus a reduction in dose is often necessary.

LONG-TERM OUTCOME

Renal failure definitely has an attributable mortality in the critically ill patient. However, most renal failure that occurs in the critically ill patient is potentially reversible, and 90% of critically ill patients who have renal failure during the ICU stay do not become dialysis-dependent for life if they survive their illness.

Renal failure often occurs as part of the spectrum of multiorgan failure, in which case, prognosis may be poor if two or more other organs have failed.

ACID-BASE ABNORMALITIES

Determination of the critically ill patient's acid-base status is, simply, critical. It has been estimated that 90% of all critically ill patients have an acid-base abnormality, yet upwards of 40% of physicians cannot accurately interpret ABG analysis results.

Basics

All critically ill patients need an ABG analysis to adequately access their acid-base status. An ABG analysis gives an estimate of the serum bicarbonate concentration that may be misleading, and therefore a direct serum bicarbonate measurement should be made. One of the cardinal rules of acid-base interpretation is that the body's natural tendency is to correct acid-base abnormalities by compensating, using metabolic and respiratory means, but never overcompensating (Table 5–1).

The anion gap (AG) often is explained at length, although its utility in the ICU is often limited. The anion gap is calculated as follows:

TABLE 5–1 Rapid Interpretation of Acid Base Abnormalities

Primary Disorder	Primary Change		Compensatory Change	Common Causes in the ICU
Metabolic Acidosis	↓ HCO_3	↓pH	↓$Paco_2$	Lactic acidosis, renal failure, exogenous poisons
Metabolic Alkalosis	↑ HCO_3	↑pH	↑$Paco_2$	Excessive diuresis, nasogastric drainage, corticosteroid use
Respiratory Acidosis	↑ $Paco_2$	↓pH	↑HCO_3	Acute respiratory failure (e.g., COPD, Guillian-Barré)
Respiratory Alkalosis	↓ $Paco_2$	↑pH	↓HCO_3	Hyperventilation, sepsis syndrome

ABBREVIATIONS: HCO_3, bicarbonate; COPD, chronic obstructive pulmonary disease.

$$AG = \text{Measured cations} - \text{measured anions}$$
$$= (Na + K) - (Cl + HCO_3)$$
$$\text{Normal } AG = \text{less than 12} \qquad mEq/L$$

Calculation of the anion gap is commonly used to help determine the cause of metabolic acidosis. Practically, it is assumed that:

1. There are commonly occurring negatively charged anions that we do not routinely measure (e.g., phosphate, sulfate, proteins, other endogenous acids).
2. The difference between the measured cations and measured anions is equal to the sum of these unmeasured anions.
3. The difference should not exceed 12.

If it does exceed 12, the implication is that there is another unmeasured anion (e.g., lactate, a common endogenous acid; salicylate, an exogenous acid) or an unusually large amount of naturally occurring acids (e.g., sulfates, phosphates, and other organic acids) have accumulated because of renal failure or other metabolic disturbance. Unfortunately, the anion gap often is misleading as a factor in the interpretation of acidosis in critically ill patients. Resuscitation of critically ill patients dilutes the serum bicarbonate or raises the serum chloride, especially if sodium chloride solutions are used for resuscitation. This, in turn, lowers the anion gap. Therefore, measurement of the lactate level in critically ill patients is essential, because it is a common cause of metabolic acidosis that often is not suspected if the anion gap is used as the sole means of measurement. In fact, in many ICUs, an "arterial panel" includes the lactate level as a routine measurement.

Essentially, only four distinct acid-base abnormalities exist. All other abnormalities are derived from a combination of these four abnormalities.

Acidosis

Acidosis exists when the pH is less than 7.35. It is classified into metabolic and respiratory types.

METABOLIC A pH of less than 7.35 along with a $Paco_2$ of less than 45 mm Hg signifies that metabolic acidosis exists. Metabolic acidosis is the result of acid addition or base loss. Common acids that may be added to the circulation are lactate, hydrochloride (from sodium chloride), diabetic ketoacids, poisons (e.g., salicylic acid, methanol, and paraldehyde), and uremic toxins. Common sources of base loss include diarrhea and renal tubular acidosis. Over time, the respiratory system compensates for metabolic acidosis by hyperventilating and reducing the $Paco_2$ in the blood. The $Paco_2$ falls by 1.2 mm Hg for every fall in the HCO_3 of mEq/L. However, the $Paco_2$ can rarely be lowered by more than 10 to 15 mm Hg, and patients who are on mechanical ventilation or who have incipient respiratory failure may be unable to compensate in this manner. When the pH is less than 7.20, consideration should be given to administration of exogenous intravenous bicarbonate, especially in cases of base loss and ARF. The administration of exogenous bicarbonate for lactic acidosis and diabetic ketoacidosis is probably not indicated, and may indeed be harmful.

RESPIRATORY A pH of less than 7.35 along with a $Paco_2$ of more than 45 mm Hg signifies respiratory acidosis. Common causes include any pathologic process that reduces minute ventilation (e.g., COPD exacerbation, weakness secondary to underlying neurologic illness) or increased dead space ventilation, thus reducing carbon dioxide elimination. An acute rise in the $Paco_2$ of 10 mm Hg causes the pH to fall by .08. This is one of the most important rules of acid-base interpretation. Conversely, an acute fall in the $Paco_2$ of 10 mm Hg causes the pH to rise by 0.8. Chronic carbon dioxide retention signals the kidney to retain bicarbonate, and the pH falls from its baseline (presumably about 7.40) by .03 per 10 mm Hg rise in the $Paco_2$. A pH decrease of more than .08 per 10 mm Hg rise in the $Paco_2$ implies that, in addition to respiratory acidosis, there is accompanying metabolic acidosis. This is a very common situation in critically ill patients.

Acute respiratory acidosis almost always requires respiratory intervention, such as chest physiotherapy, inhaled beta-agonists (in the case of asthma), or medications to treat neuromuscular weakness (such as pyridostigmine in the case of myasthenia gravis), but often mechanical ventilation is also required. Bicarbonate administration does not improve the situation, because for bicarbonate to buffer the acid in the blood, it must be broken down into carbon dioxide, which then must be expired.

Alkalosis

Alkalosis exists when the pH is greater than 7.45. Alkalosis can be classified into metabolic and respiratory types.

METABOLIC A pH of more than 7.45 and a $Paco_2$ of more than 40 mm Hg signify metabolic alkalosis. Common causes include loss of acid (e.g., vomiting, nasogastric drainage), addition of base (e.g., administration of sodium bicarbonate or bicarbonate precursors, such as acetate and citrate), and change of tubular transport characteristics (corticosteroid administration). Aggressive diuresis is a common cause of metabolic alkalosis in critically ill patients. Classically, metabolic alkalosis is divided into chloride-responsive and chloride-unresponsive types on the basis of the urinary chloride. If the urinary chloride concentration is < 15 mEq/L the most common causes are gastric losses, prior diuretic administration, and adaptation to chronic hyperventilation. If the urinary chloride is > 20 mEq/L the most common causes are steroid excess (exogenous or endogenous), administration of bicarbonate or bicarbonate precursors, diuretic administration, and severe hypokalemia. Treatment should be tailored to reverse the underlying cause, usually administration of potassium chloride and on occasion administration of acetazolamide. Acetazolamide is a carbonic anhydrase inhibitor which will promote bicarbonate excretion by the kidney. On occasion, infusion of an acid, such as ammonium chloride or, even more rarely, hydrochloric acid, may be required; however, this author suggests that renal consultation be obtained when infusion of acids is under consideration. Central line access is necessary to infuse hydrochloric acid.

RESPIRATORY A pH of more than 7.45 with a $PaCO_2$ of less than 35 mm Hg signifies respiratory alkalosis. The most common cause of respiratory alkalosis in the ICU patient is sepsis, which causes an unexplained primary hyperventilation. Frequently, critically ill patients are mechanically hyperventilated without reason. Obviously, any cause of hyperventilation causes a fall in the $PaCO_2$ level and a rise in the pH. On rare occasions, severe respiratory alkalosis may cause seizures and muscular spasm. Usually, however, respiratory alkalosis is benign.

APPROACH TO MANAGEMENT OF HYPONATREMIA AND HYPERNATREMIA

Hyponatremia

Hyponatremia is defined as a serum sodium level of less than 135 mmol/L. Hyponatremia is a common finding in hospitalized patients and is even more common in ICU patients, perhaps because of the interplay between fluid administration, diuretic administration, and abnormal antidiuretic hormone (ADH) secretion. Typically, hyponatremia is divided into states of low, normal, and high extravascular volume.

Unless the sodium level has fallen to less than 120 mmol/L, there is usually no medical urgency to correct it. Most patients are best managed with simple fluid restriction. When the sodium has fallen to less than 120 mmol/L, especially if the fall has been rapid, there is a significant risk that the patient will develop neurologic symptoms, including confusion, coma, and possibly seizures. Generally, administration of hypertonic saline is required in this circumstance. Hypertonic saline solution comes in 3% and 5% strengths. Obviously, fluid overload as a result of hypertonic fluid administration can occur and, thus, meticulous calculation of the sodium deficit, accurate administration, and frequent (i.e., at least hourly for the first 2 to 3 hours) measurement of the serum sodium concentration is mandated. The other major risk factor in the correction of low serum sodium levels is central pontine myelolysis (CPM), which results from the too-rapid correction of hyponatremia.

Few subjects have stirred as much debate as the proper rate of sodium solution infusion in the severely hyponatremic patient. In general, if the patient is not actively having seizures, correcting the sodium level at a rate of less than

1 mmol/L per hour appears to be safe. If the patient is having seizures, however, more rapid correction, perhaps as rapid as 2 mmol/L per hour, or in some authors' opinions, even 3 mmol/L per hour, may be indicated. Obviously, the risk of hyponatremia and seizure needs to be weighed against the risk of developing CPM. Notably, however, there is rarely any need to correct the sodium level above 120 mmol/L, so aggressive efforts to raise the sodium level further should stop, which limits the potential for CPM. Alcoholic patients and those with cirrhosis are particularly prone to CPM and slower correction may be indicated.

To estimate the amount of sodium required to raise the serum sodium level to a given degree, the following formula is used:

Serum Na deficit = Body weight (kg) × 0.70 × (desired Na level − current Na level)

For example, a 60-kg patient with a sodium level of 112 mmol/L requires 336 mmol of sodium to raise the serum sodium level to 120 mmol/L (i.e., 60 × 0.70 × [120 − 112]). Hypertonic saline 3% solution contains 513 mmol/L of sodium; thus, approximately 600 mL should be administered. If the patient is not actively having seizures, this author suggests infusing this volume over at least 8 hours and checking the serum sodium level hourly to insure a correction rate of 1 mmol/hr maximum. If the patient is actively having seizures, an infusion of this volume can be given over 4 to 6 hours, attempting to keep the rate of correction perhaps as rapid as 2 mmol/hr and not exceed a serum sodium level of 120 mmol/L.

Hypernatremia

Hypernatremia is defined as a serum sodium level of more than 145 mmol/L, which either results from the loss of fluid with a sodium level of less than 145 mmol/L or gain of a fluid with a sodium level of more than 145 mmol/L (e.g., normal saline contains 154 mmol/L of sodium). Manifestations of hypernatremia include altered mentation, lethargy and weakness. Severe hypernatremia may cause seizures. A serum sodium level of less than 150 mmol/L rarely requires active intervention. Most textbooks divide their sections on the diagnosis and management of hypernatremia based on whether the patient has low, normal, or high effective circulating intravascular volume. However, for the sake of simplicity, in the absence of recent hypertonic fluid administration, hypernatremia in the critically ill patient almost always represents free water depletion. Free water depletion in critically ill patients commonly results from nasogastric suctioning, diarrhea, administration of hypertonic enteral feeding without free water addition, diabetes insipidus (nephrogenic or central), osmotic diuresis (e.g., mannitol or glucose), overzealous diuretic administration, and, although less often recognized, underresuscitation of the septic patient. In the absence of hypotension or a markedly low extracellular volume, as may be assessed by the presence of tachycardia, orthostatic hypotension, or measurement of filling pressures with a central venous catheter or PAC, administration of free water is the most appropriate intervention. Free water may be administered enterally or, as dextrose 5% in water (D5W), be given intravenously. For the hyperglycemic patient, in whom administration of D5W may present a management difficulty, 0.45% sodium chloride solution is a reasonable alternative; however, it may contain more sodium than is present in the fluid being lost, and correction of the hypernatremia may, in that circumstance, be impossible. Attempted normalization of the serum sodium level should take place over 24 to 48 hours, and the sodium level should fall by no more than 0.5 mmol/hr to avoid cerebral edema, which may in turn cause seizures and neurologic damage.

The free-water deficit is calculated as follows:

$$\text{Free-water deficit} = \text{Body weight (kg)} \times 0.70 \times$$
$$(\text{current Na} - \text{desired Na})/(\text{desired Na})$$

So, for example, an average-sized adult patient with a serum sodium level of more than 150 mmol/L usually has a fluid deficit of at least 3 L (i.e., $60 \times 0.7 \times [150 - 140/140]$). To correct such a patient's level down to 140 mmol/L, 3 L of free water, in addition to necesssary maintenance fluid, would need to be administered. A frequent ICU error is to forget about ongoing losses of free water, which lead to an uncorrectable serum sodium level. Careful attention must be paid to urinary output, fluid lost through drains, third spacing, and evaporation.

SUMMARY

Acute renal failure is a common problem seen in all intensive care units. The critical care physician should be facile in diagnosing the etiology of the renal failure as well as with management. CVVH is fast becoming the usual practice for renal replacement therapy in ICUs because of its ability to maintain a hemodynamically stable milieu in critically ill patients.

SUGGESTED READINGS

Bellomo R, Tipping P, Boyce N. Continuous venovenous hemofiltration with dialysis removes cytokines from the circulation of septic patients. *Crit Care Med* 1993; 21(4): 522–526.

Better OS, Stein JH. Early management of shock and prophylaxis of acute renal failure in traumatic rhabdomyolysis. *N Engl J Med* 1990;22(12):825–829.

Brivet FG, Kleinknecht DJ, Loirat P, et al. Acute renal failure in intensive care units—causes, outcome, and prognostic factors of hospital mortality; a prospective, multicenter study (French Study Group on Acute Renal Failure). *Crit Care Med* 1996 Feb; 24(2):192–198.

Cottee DB, Saul WP. Is renal dose dopamine protective or therapeutic? No. *Crit Care Clin* 1996;12(3):687–695.

Davenport A, Will EJ, Davidson AM. Improved cardiovascular stability during continuous modes of renal replacement therapy in critically ill patients with acute hepatic and renal failure. *Crit Care Med* 1993;21(3):328–338.

Forni LG, Hilton PJ. Continuous hemofiltration in the treatment of acute renal failure. *N Engl J Med* 1997; 1(18):1303–1309.

Jochimsen F, Schafer JH, Maurer A, et al. Impairment of renal function in medical intensive care: Predictability of acute renal failure. *Crit Care Med* 1990;18(5):480–485.

Kellum JA. Use of diuretics in the acute care setting. *Kidney Int Suppl* 1998;66:S67–70.

Klahr S, Miller SB. Acute oliguria. *N Engl J Med* 1998; 338(10):671–675.

Murray P. Hall J. Renal replacement therapy for acute renal failure. *Am J Respir Crit Care Med* 2000; 162:777–781.

Spurney RF, Fulkerson WJ, Schwab SJ. Acute renal failure in critically ill patients: Prognosis for recovery of kidney function after prolonged dialysis support. *Crit Care Med* 1991;19(1):8–11.

Sterns RH. Hypernatremia in the intensive care unit: Instant quality—just add water. *Crit Care Med* 1999;26(6):1041–1042.

Thadhani R, Pascual M, Bonventre JV. Acute renal failure. *N Engl J Med* 1996;334(22):1448–1460.

Approach to Infectious Disease

DOUGLAS SALVADOR

ROBERT F. BETTS

INTRODUCTION

Infection is one of the most common diagnoses in the ICU, whether it is the reason for admission or acquired during the hospital stay. Nosocomial infections have been shown to increase mortality, prolong stay, and increase cost. Successful prevention, diagnosis, and treatment of infections in the ICU requires the clinician to be familiar with the expected rates of infection, risk factors for infection, the clinical parameters that define an infection, and the treatment options for each type of infection.

In the United States, data on nosocomial infections has been maintained since 1970 by the National Nosocomial Infections Surveillance System (NNIS).[1,2] They have a convenient website that releases up-to-date surveillance data from around the country. The most common sites of infection are listed in Table 6–1.

Infections contracted in the ICU in part depend on the presence of certain common risk factors.[3] These include:

1. Increased length of stay (more than 48 hours)
2. Use of mechanical ventilation
3. Diagnosis of trauma
4. Use of central venous catheter
5. Use of pulmonary artery catheter
6. Use of urinary catheter
7. Prophylaxis for stress ulcer

The infection control practices of health care workers in the ICU are of utmost importance, especially handwashing and maintenance of asepsis in inserting and maintaining devices. Many of these factors act to break down the host's defenses. The use of invasive instruments is common in this setting (Table 6–2) and is directly related to the incidence of infection.[3]

This chapter begins with a discussion of fever and its causes to outline a directed, logical approach to evaluation of the febrile critically ill patient. The re-

TABLE 6–1 CDC Surveillance of Nosocomial Infections in ICUs: Distribution for Reported Cases, 1992–1997

Site of Infection	Percentage of Cases	Rate of Infection
Urinary tract	35%	6.5 per 1,000 catheter days
Pneumonia (lung)	24%	11.7 per 1,000 ventilator days
Primary bloodstream	17%	5.0 per 1,000 catheter days
GI tract	4%	
Surgical site	4%	
Cardiovascular	4%	
ENT	2%	

TABLE 6–2 Percentage of ICU Patients on Whom Invasive Instruments
Are Used in ICUs

Instrument	ICU Patients (%)
Urinary catheter	75.3
Central venous catheter	63.9
Mechanical ventilation	63.0
Arterial catheter	44.2
Pulmonary artery catheter	12.8
Wound drain	30.6

mainder of the chapter is aimed at diagnosis and treatment of common ICU infections. Standard disease definitions are offered and their limitations examined
to help foster accurate diagnosis in this notoriously difficult setting. Practical
methods for use of antimicrobial agents are provided. In addition, the chapter
addresses the new challenges brought on by immunocompromised patients and
antimicrobial resistance.

FEVER

Fever is defined as a rise of the body temperature above the normal variation.
Fever develops because of a reset of the hypothalamic temperature set-point,
which may be caused by endogenous or exogenous pyrogens, chiefly through
prostaglandin E_2 (PGE_2). This must be distinguished from hyperthermia, which is
an elevation of the core temperature when the hypothalamic set-point is nor-
mothermic. Excessive heat production or diminished heat dissipation causes hyperthermia (Table 6–3).

TABLE 6–3 Causes of Hyperthermia

Mechanism	Cause
Excessive production	Exertion
	Malignant hyperthermia of anesthesia
	Neuroleptic malignant syndrome
	Pheochromocytoma
	Salicylate intoxication
	Thyrotoxicosis
Diminished dissipation	Heat stroke
	Occlusive dressings
	Dehydration
	Autonomic dysfunction
	Anticholinergic drugs

The magnitude of temperature elevation that defines a fever, which takes into account a 1°C circadian variation with the peak in late afternoon and trough in early morning, is 38.3°C or above. Body temperature is usually about 0.5°C lower in elders. Temperature may be measured orally, rectally, or in the auditory canal. The site depends on patient position, intubation, instrumentation, and other factors. Axillary temperatures do not correlate well with core temperature and should not be used.

Fever is common in patients in the ICU; it has myriad causes and often results in ordering of costly laboratory and radiologic studies, which carry their own adverse side effects. We advocate a directed evaluation of the patient with fever, which should take into account noninfectious and the common infectious causes. Fever in the ICU population is most commonly secondary to infection.[4] Because of this, the evaluation of the febrile patient should be directed at excluding infection. All of the noninfectious causes should be considered when the initial evaluation does not reveal an infectious one (Table 6–4).

Approach

A directed approach to the febrile patient is summarized in Table 6–5. The history and physical examination may suggest an explanation for fever, leading to appropriate diagnostic measures and treatment. Every patient with new fever should be completely evaluated with X-ray studies and laboratory testing for electrolyte levels and CBC count with differential, if this has not been done recently. From this evaluation, some information may suggest the need for immediate response or careful follow-up without therapeutic intervention. An example of the former is that a new infiltrate seen on chest radiographs and a deteriorating oxygen saturation level may suggest pneumonia, while a low serum bicarbonate level with the presence of anion gap may indicate lactic acidosis and sepsis. Other findings are important but often do not require immediate action. Although a normal WBC count does not exclude serious infection, a WBC count of less than 4,000/μL, especially in older patients, can be a sign of serious infec-

TABLE 6–4 Noninfectious Causes of Fever

Drug fever
Endotoxin release from colonization
Neurologic causes: stroke, seizure, hemorrhage
Ischemic colitis
Transfusion reaction
Myocardial infarction
Procedure-related causes
Thrombosis
Acute respiratory distress syndrome (ARDS)
Malignant tumor

TABLE 6–5 Evaluation of Patients with New Fever

- Review of patient history, including:
  - Comorbidities
  - New medications prescribed
  - Blood products administered
  - Recent procedures
- Thorough physical examination, including special attention to:
- All wounds and sites of intravascular catheters
  - Skin rashes that indicate a drug reaction
  - Flank discoloration (indicates retroperitoneal hemorrhage)
  - Lesions suggestive of disseminated candidiasis (fundoscopic examination)
- The following tests *must* be ordered:
  - Serum electrolyte levels
  - Complete blood cell (CBC) count, with differential
  - Examination of respiratory secretions
  - Urinary microscopy
  - Urine Gram's stain
  - Quantitative urine culture
  - Blood cultures
  - Chest radiograph (for mechanically ventilated patients)
- The following tests should be ordered *only* if suggested by findings or if fever is persistent and unexplained:
  - Diarrheal stool sample for *Clostridium difficile*
  - Gram's stain of any purulent discharge from vascular catheter site
  - Computed tomographic (CT) scan of sinuses
  - CT scan of abdomen
  - ECG tracing and myocardial enzyme levels
  - Ventilation/Perfusion nucleotide scan or lower extremity ultrasonograhy

tion. The presence of immature forms of polymorphonuclear leukocytes totalling more than 10% of total blood cells is also suggestive of sepsis caused by infection. A high WBC count also raises concern. There are relatively few infections that cause the leukocyte count to rise above 30,000/µL. In this case, disseminated candidiasis, *Clostridium difficile* colitis, and beta-hemolytic streptococci should be suspected. The absolute value of the WBC count, by itself, does not mean that therapeutic intervention is required, but appropriate diagnostic measures should be initiated. Some findings lead to further laboratory testing, which may include liver enzyme levels, ABG analysis, and specific imaging studies. Other findings often do not require immediate action.

Since the goal is to exclude infectious causes, samples must be obtained for microbiologic examination. Samples for Gram's stain of respiratory secretions, urine, purulent wound drainage, or catheter sites should be collected. Samples for cultures of urine, respiratory secretions, and blood should be sent. The intricacies of culture sampling in the respiratory tract are discussed in the section on pneumonia. However, the decision to treat should be based on the evaluation of the patient, not solely on what grows in culture. The obvious exception is positive results from a blood culture for a recognized pathogen. Once the evaluation dictates that treatment is necessary, the appropriate antibiotic agent can be deduced from a Gram's stain of the specimen or culture and results of susceptibility testing, if they are available. If not, treatment must be empiric.

Samples for blood cultures should be obtained at the first sign of fever. There is much confusion surrounding the number and sites at which to draw blood samples. In the first 24 hours, there is little additional diagnostic value to taking more than three blood samples for culture. Regardless of whether the patient has a vascular catheter placed, two blood samples should be obtained from separate peripheral sites, and these samples should be spaced 10 minutes apart, if possible. If two samples for culture cannot be obtained in a patient with vascular access, obtain one culture from the most recent vascular catheter. This decreases the likelihood that the culture result will be a false-positive because of colonization, which increases with the length of time that the access device is used. Paired cultures of peripheral site and vascular catheter samples are performed, using quantitative culture methods, to aid in diagnosis of catheter-related bloodstream infection. This should only be done when there is suspicion of catheter-related bloodstream infection, which is discussed later.

After the first 24 hours, blood cultures should be obtained only if bacteremia or fungemia is suspected. In general, more than one pair of blood cultures per day is unhelpful. Blood cultures are not required for each occurrence of temperature elevation.

There are several ways to increase the accuracy of blood cultures; the most critical is taking a sample that is large enough. A sample of at least 15 mL improves sensitivity. In addition, the skin should be cleaned with an iodine preparation that is allowed to dry, and the injection port of the culture bottles should be wiped clean with alcohol to decrease contamination.

For patients on mechanical ventilators, a new fever warrants a chest radiograph. In the ICU, it is not feasible to do posteroanterior and lateral chest films. The anteroposterior portable chest radiograph should be taken in the upright position, during deep inspiration, if possible.

Although the initial history and physical examination are used to guide evaluation of fever, based on the most likely causes in a particular patient, quite often this information leads to further testing to determine the cause of a fever. A postoperative patient or patient with known coronary artery disease (CAD) may need an ECG and measurement of cardiac enzyme levels. Ventilation-perfusion scanning or lower extremity Doppler imaging may be performed in patients at risk for deep venous thrombosis (DVT) and pulmonary embolism. CT scan of the abdomen is useful for diagnosis of an intra-abdominal abscess and hemorrhage. Hemorrhage may be suspected as the cause of fever in a patient who has undergone femoral artery catheterization or abdominal surgery, in which splenic laceration is a possible complication. Abscess may be a complication of gastrointestinal (GI) or biliary surgery or may occur as a result of trauma.

In a patient who continues to have a fever after an initial evaluation with negative results, one approach is to stop all antibiotic therapy. After all, in many cases, the therapy is not working.

Antipyretics

In general, antipyretics are not indicated. Host defenses may be improved at higher body temperatures, and observation of temperature trends can help guide diagnosis and treatment. Patient comfort is often used as a reason for antipyresis but an abrupt drop in temperature can cause diaphoresis and discomfort. There is no question that body temperatures above 42°C impair immune function and that antipyresis should be used at this threshold. Extremely high fevers may cause delirium, and any fever in the patient with tenuous cardiac function can be detrimental.

Hyperthermia should always be treated by cooling the patient. This is not a problem which the hypothalamic set-point affects, so antipyretics are useless. The patient must be physically cooled externally.

Treatment

The most difficult decision an intensivist must make is when to treat. Because it is so difficult to make definitive diagnoses of many infectious diseases in the ICU and because most of the patients are critically ill, the impulse is to initiate antibiotic therapy with little data and no clinical evidence of unstable physiology. There is undoubtedly a part in each of us that says: "Go ahead, give antibiotics, it can't hurt—and if there is infection and you don't, the patient will suffer." However, if antibiotics are used unnecessarily, the patient will also suffer. *C. difficile* colitis, disseminated yeast infection, and colonization with resistant organisms predisposing the patient to difficult-to-treat infections later are just some of the possibilities.

Some febrile patients develop hemodynamic deterioration. There are objective findings to look for in an "unstable patient" (Table 6–6). Such a patient should re-

TABLE 6–6 **Findings in the Febrile ICU Patient that Suggest Use of Empiric Antibiotics**

- Hemodynamic instability
  - Abrupt drop in blood pressure
  - Difficulty in keeping blood pressure normal
  - Required use of vasopressor agents without obvious cardiogenic or hemorrhagic explanation
- Respiratory failure
  - Increases in ventilatory requirements (unexplained by patient status) in a febrile patient
- Decline in mental status in a previously alert patient that cannot be explained by administration of sedative agents or presence of a noninfectious illness (e.g., CHF, hepatic encephalopathy)
- All of the five clinical criteria for ventilator associated pneumonia

ceive empiric antibiotics. However, there are many patients in the ICU who become febrile, have no such worrisome objective signs, and overall, are stable or improving. The reflex response to a febrile episode should not be initiation of antibiotic therapy. Instead, realize that most patients are in the ICU for several days at least. Because they are "captives" and can be closely evaluated and because unnecessary antibiotics may lead to later problems, we advocate delaying antibiotic therapy for patients without definitive objective findings. Patients may harbor organisms, such as coagulase-negative staphylococcal bacteremia, that lead to fever but do not cause invasive disease or compromise physiology. Endotoxin released from gram-negative bacteria that are colonizing bladder catheters or endotracheal tubes may leak into the bloodstream, leading to fever but not significant decline of status.

Furthermore, many of the causes of fever in the ICU are noninfectious. For example, in the patient with chemical pneumonitis, the body temperature will return to normal without intervention. The stable patient with fever should be monitored carefully: the fever often disappears without intervention. However, some patients require empiric antibiotic therapy.

Antibiotic therapy in the ICU is initiated empirically or against a specific identified pathogen. Every effort should be made to obtain specimens that allow identification of the responsible pathogen, so that the therapeutic regimen can be adjusted to treat that organism with narrow coverage. This is often not possible, forcing the use of empiric therapy.

Empiric therapy is guided by knowledge of the most common organisms that cause an infection. This is influenced by site of infection, host factors, and local flora. Intimate knowledge of the resistance patterns in your ICU is essential to making rational choices about empiric therapy. For example, in many major centers across the United States the prevalence of oxacillin-resistant *Staphylococcus aureus* is high, necessitating the use of vancomycin empirically for line sepsis and nosocomial pneumonia.

When a diagnosis of infection is made, antibiotic therapy should be started promptly. Before instituting therapy, it is imperative that appropriate cultures of all relevant fluids be obtained. Antibiotic therapy should be started empirically in an unstable patient, and it is imperative that treatment be effective. If a specific site of infection is identified, for example, a ventilator associated pneumonia(VAP), and samples are available for Gram's stain, the results may help focus therapy. If not, initial empiric therapy must cover resistant gram-negative rods and methicillin-resistant *S. aureus* (MRSA), if those organisms are prevalent in your ICU. All too often, the clinician identifies a site of infection (e.g., VAP) in a critically ill unstable patient and initiates ampicillin sodium and sulbactam sodium therapy, which is ineffective against many causes of VAP infection.

The next key step in the process is to reconsider the choice of antibiotics when the culture results return. If, for example, the initial diagnosis was VAP infection, for which gentamicin and piperacillin/tazobactam were initiated, but the blood and urine cultures return positive for *Escherichia coli*, the spectrum should be narrowed, even though the patient has responded to the initial choice. Culture data should be reviewed daily until it is finalized, because new information may help further narrow antibiotic coverage.

Specific considerations regarding the most common infections in the ICU are laid out in each respective section of the chapter. Empiric therapeutic regimens appear in Table 6–7. With many new antibiotics undergoing clinical trials, the

TABLE 6–7 Choices for Empiric Antibiotic Therapy

Infectious Disease	Agent(s)	Alternative Agents
Ventilator-Related Pneumonia		
Predominantly gram-positive	Vancomycin	
Predominantly gram-negative	Aminoglycoside + piperacillin	Combination of two: aminoglycoside, antipseudomonal cephalosporin, antipseudomonal fluoroquinolone, piperacillin, piperacillin-tazobactam, aztreonam; or imipenem alone
Gram's stain not available	Aminoglycoside + piperacillin + vancomycin	Combinations above + vancomycin
Sinusitis		
Gram-positive	Vancomycin	
Gram-negative	Aminoglycoside + piperacillin	Combination of two: aminoglycoside, antipseudomonal cephalosporin, antipseudomonal fluoroquinolone, piperacillin, piperacillin-tazobactam, aztreonam; or imipenem alone.
Uncertain and severe	Aminoglycoside + piperacillin + vancomycin	Above combination + vancomycin
Catheter-Related Sepsis[a]	Vancomycin + aminoglycoside +/- fluconazole	Vancomycin + cefepime or aztreonam, or imipenem +/- fluconazole
Urinary tract infection[b]		
Gram-positive chains	Ampicillin	Vancomycin
Gram-positive clusters	Vancomycin	
Gram-negative	Aminoglycoside	Fluoroquinolone, third-generation cephalosporin, or cefepime
Fungal	Fluconazole	Amphotericin B bladder wash or systemic therapy

[a]For severe catheter-related sepsis, add antifungal until culture results are available. Catheter should be removed and tip should be cultured.
[b]If catheter remains, treat only if hemodynamically unstable.

empiric regimen of choice may change in the near future. In general, newer drugs should be substituted only if they show a clear advantage (i.e., in efficacy, width of spectrum, or decreased cost) over an accepted regimen.

PNEUMONIA

Pneumonia is the second most common nosocomial infection in the ICU, with an incidence of 11.7 infections per 1,000 days the patient is on a ventilator. Various estimates of prevalence of nosocomial pneumonia in the ICU range from 10% to 50%.[5,6] The significance of the problem lies in these outcomes: increased mortality, increased multiple organ dysfunction, increased duration of mechanical ventilation, longer ICU stay, and increased cost of care. The clinician who wants to decrease the burden of this problem must understand the pathogenesis and risk factors for nosocomial pneumonia and the diagnostic dilemma it poses. Only then can steps to prevent infection and initiate appropriate therapy be taken.

Pathogenesis and Risk Factors

Bacteria invade the lower respiratory tract primarily from aspiration of oropharyngeal fluids, ventilator-tube condensation, or gastric contents.[7] Bacteria, much less frequently, may also be inhaled in aerosols or spread to the lungs via the bloodstream. Nearly half of healthy adults aspirate during sleep. Critically ill patients are even more prone to aspiration.[8]

The risk factors for development of pneumonia are related to host factors, factors that enhance colonization, and factors that favor aspiration and time on the ventilator (Table 6–8).

Prevention

Prevention of ventilator-related pneumonia is aimed at modifying the known risk factors.

TABLE 6–8 Risk Factors for Pneumonia in ICUs

Category of Risk	Risk Factors
Host	Age, immunosuppression, severity of illness
Colonization	Antibiotic exposure, use of antacids
Aspiration	Supine position, nasogastric tube, reintubation, large gastric volumes, witnessed aspiration, paralytic agents, patient transport, neurologic impairment
Duration of ventilation	Risk increases by up to 1% per day

CROSS CONTAMINATION Health care workers frequently transmit microorganisms to patients on hands that have been transiently colonized. Although it is universally known that frequent handwashing can reduce the transmission of microorganisms, compliance with this simple technique remains a challenge. Routine use of gloves has therefore been recommended to reduce cross contamination. All health care workers in the ICU, including physicians, should wear gloves when they visit individual patients, and then remove gloves and wash hands before seeing others. Recently, use of antiseptic impregnated towelettes dispensed outside each patient's room has decreased cross contamination.

ASPIRATION Aspiration is more common in patients who:

1. Have a depressed level of consciousness (caused by disease or medication)
2. Have endotracheal, tracheostomy, or enteral tubes in place
3. Are receiving enteral feeding

Since some of these risks are necessary to patient comfort and nutrition status, attempts must be made to reduce the risk.

Regurgitation is less likely if the patient is semirecumbent, with the head of the bed partially elevated. When using enteral feeding, the residual volume of the stomach should be regularly monitored and feeding should be withheld if the volumes are large. There do not appear to be differences when bolus feeding is used as opposed to continuous or jejunal tube feeding as opposed to gastric. Remove all tubes as soon as they are no longer essential.

COLONIZATION It is common practice in critically ill and intubated patients to use antacids and histamine (H$_2$) blockers to prevent stress ulcer bleeding. Use of these agents has been associated with gastric bacterial overgrowth. A recent meta-analysis of trials comparing the rate of pneumonia in critically ill patients receiving H$_2$-blockers to those receiving no prophylaxis showed a trend towards higher rates of pneumonia for those receiving H$_2$-blockers.[9] Sucralfate, a cytoprotective agent, has been studied as an alternative to H$_2$-blockers, because it has little effect on gastric pH and may have bactericidal properties. The Canadian Critical Care Trials Group performed the best study to date that compares sucralfate and ranitidine in 1200 patients requiring mechanical ventilation in the ICU.[10] They used strict criteria for the diagnosis of pneumonia and found no significant difference in the incidence of pneumonia between the two groups. Therefore, there is no basis for the use of sucralfate for prophylaxis of ventilator-associated pneumonia.

Selective decontamination of the GI tract has been evaluated as prophylaxis for pneumonia. A paste of a combination of nonabsorbable antibiotics is applied to the oropharynx and allowed to flow down the gastric tube. Recent meta-analyses of studies, which unfortunately have nonuniform diagnostic criteria for pneumonia and relatively short follow-up periods, of selective decontamination have shown a trend toward decreased pneumonia with selective decontamination but do not show any mortality benefit. Selective decontamination is expensive, and a tendency toward development of resistant organisms has not been studied. Based on current information, selective decontamination cannot be recommended.

Diagnosis

The diagnosis of nosocomial pneumonia, specifically ventilator-related pneumonia, is notoriously difficult. The differential diagnosis is extensive (Table 6–9).

Fever, cough, sputum production, and pulmonary infiltrate—the hallmarks of the diagnosis of pneumonia in an ambulatory population—are present in a large number of critically ill patients who do not have pneumonia. In one study of patients who had been intubated for more than 48 hours and had fever, new or progressive pulmonary infiltrates, leukocytosis, or purulent tracheal aspirate, only 42% had pneumonia.[11] Clinical judgment was tested against quantitative bacterial counts by bronchoscopy using protected specimen brush (PSB) in another study. Clinicians predicted the presence or absence of pneumonia accurately 62% of the time.[12] Logistic regression analysis of 16 parameters from the same study group revealed no parameter or combination of parameters that could predict nosocomial pneumonia. Therefore, no intensivist should feel confident in his or her ability to make a diagnosis of pneumonia in the ICU on clinical grounds.

This raises the alternative possibility of using microbiologic methods for diagnosis. As a comparator, in the ambulatory population, Gram's stain of expectorated sputum has a sensitivity of 50% to 60% and a specificity of more than 80% for a causative organism in pneumonia, and sputum culture yields a pathogen in

TABLE 6–9 **Possible Diagnoses for Fever and Pulmonary Infiltrates**

One of the following:

Atelectasis
Acute respiratory distress syndrome (ARDS)
Congestive heart failure (CHF)
Pulmonary fibroproliferation
Pulmonary hemorrhage
Peritonitis
Pulmonary embolism

Plus any of the following may cause fever where one of the former is responsible for an infiltrate:

Catheter-related infection
Drug fever
Clostridium difficile colitis
Sinusitis
Urinary tract infection

30% to 40% of cases.[13] This contrasts with the ICU environment, where colonization of respiratory secretions is common. This can obscure the interpretation of microbiologic data.

The more rigorous approach requires bronchoscopic sampling of respiratory secretions (Table 6–10).[14] However, the cost and expertise required prohibits its widespread use. The diagnostic difficulty, combined with the fact that every patient in the ICU is critically ill and mortality in patients with nosocomial pneumonia is high, leads to the often-practiced approach in which every patient with fever and possible pneumonia is treated with empiric antibiotic therapy immediately. This exposes the patient to the risks of using intravenous antibiotics, the most serious of which is subsequent colonization with a more resistant bacterial strain, which will prove more difficult to treat if a true pneumonia develops later. Risks also include allergic response, induction of fever, and adverse effects. Huge medical costs of treament accrue.

The most reasonable approach to limit the unnecessary use of antibiotics is to insist on all five clinical criteria before initiation of therapy (Table 6–11). Pneumonia should be suspected in patients with fever, leukocytosis, purulent respiratory secretions, new or progressive infiltrate on chest radiograph, and deterioration of gas exchange. When there is a clinical suspicion of pneumonia, other studies should be obtained to confirm the diagnosis (Table 6–12). In patients with new

TABLE 6–10 Criteria for Confirming or Ruling Out Pneumonia

Confirmed Pneumonia

1. Evidence on CT scan of abscess with positive results on analysis of needle aspirate
2. Histopathologic evidence from analysis of lung-tissue postmortem or open-lung biopsy specimen

Probable Pneumonia

1. Positive results on blood cultures that are unrelated to another source and are obtained within 48 hours before or after the identical organism is isolated from respiratory sample
2. Positive results on pleural fluid culture with identical organism isolated from respiratory sample
3. Positive quantitative culture of secretion samples from the lower respiratory tract, which have been obtained by one of the following methods: protected specimen brush (PSB), bronchoalveolar lavage (BAL), protected bronchoalveolar lavage(PBAL)

Pneumonia Ruled Out

1. Absence of histologic evidence of pneumonia on postmortem
2. Definite alternative cause of symptoms with no bacterial growth indicated on results of culture of reliable respiratory specimen
3. Cytologic evidence for a disease process other than pneumonia (e.g., malignant tumor) with no bacterial growth indicated on results of culture of reliable respiratory specimen

TABLE 6–11 Criteria for Clinical Suspicion of Pneumonia

1. Fever
2. Leukocytosis
3. Radiographic appearance of new or progressive pulmonary infiltrates
4. Purulent tracheobronchial secretions (more than 25 leukocytes and less than 10 squamous cells per low-power field)
5. Deterioration of gas exchange

NOTE: All criteria must be present.

fever and pleural effusion that is unexplained, pleural fluid sampling should be done, because it can quickly confirm the diagnosis of pneumonia.

ENDOTRACHEAL ASPIRATION Endotracheal sampling is usually done by the nursing staff, using a sterile-trap system. A flexible tube is advanced through the endotracheal tube as far as is easily accomplished. Suction is applied with or without the addition of several milliliters of sterile saline solution. The specimen is collected in a sterile trap, which has been connected in a series with the suction tubing. This sample may be stained and cultured for bacteria. There is no accepted role for endotracheal aspiration in the diagnosis of pneumonia because it is difficult to separate colonization from true pneumonia on the basis of the upper airway sample.

BRONCHOSCOPIC TECHNIQUES[15] Flexible bronchoscopes are used to obtain samples with bronchoalveolar lavage (BAL) and PSB techniques. Standard preparatory technique and monitoring methods are used for each.

Quantitative Bronchoalveolar Lavage

The flexible bronchoscope is advanced into the bronchial tree and "wedged" in a segment corresponding to infiltrate on chest radiograph, if a specific infiltrate is identified. In the absence of a focal infiltrate, any dependent lung segment is

TABLE 6–12 Studies for Patients in Whom Pneumonia Is Clinically Suspected

1. Blood chemistry panel and complete blood cell (CBC) count
2. Blood cultures for suspected organisms
3. Arterial blood gas (ABG) sample analysis
4. Microbiologic specimens obtained by:
   Deep tracheal suctioning
   Bronchoscopic protected specimen brush (PSB)
   Bronchoalveolar lavage (BAL)
   Pleural fluid sample analysis to obtain: pH, Gram's stain, culture, protein level, CBC count, acid-fast bacteria (AFB) smear and culture, cytology

used. Once the bronchoscope is wedged, 120 mL of sterile saline is infused into the lung segment. Through another port in the bronchoscope, suction is used to aspirate fluid. This fluid can be stained and examined for the presence of organisms and can be cultured. A threshold of 10^4 CFU/mL is considered a definitive diagnosis of pneumonia. This corresponds to a bacterial concentration of 10^5 to 10^6 in the original respiratory secretions.

Protected Specimen Brush Technique

Alternatively, the bronchoscopist can use a double catheter, inside of which is a brush protected by a biodegradable plug. When the outer cannula is positioned at the segmental opening, an inner cannula is advanced. The plug is ejected and a brush is advanced into the airway. The brush is rotated gently and pulled back into the inner cannula. The inner cannula is pulled into the outer one, and the entire bronchoscope is removed. In this way, the brush is not exposed to organisms that may be colonizing the upper airway. The brush is clipped into 1 mL of sterile fluid and agitated vigorously. This fluid is then cultured. The threshold for a diagnosis of pneumonia is 10^3 CFU/mL, which corresponds to a concentration of 10^5 to 10^6 bacteria in the original respiratory secretions.

PSB and BAL are well-accepted ways of confirming the diagnosis of VAP infection. An additional advantage is that bronchoscopy can aid in diagnosing other causes of fever and pulmonary infiltrates. The morbidity and mortality of bronchoscopy in the hands of an experienced endoscopist are low. The major complications are pneumothorax, hemorrhage, and anesthetic complications.

Each of the bronchoscopic methods of sampling the respiratory secretions has been studied extensively (Table 6–13).[16–24] There is still uncertainty in the diagnosis, partially because many of these studies used clinical criteria, or the method being tested as the gold standard, for the diagnosis. More recent studies used postmortem histologic tests to make a diagnosis of pneumonia.

TABLE 6–13 Accuracy of Microbiologic Samples in Testing for VAP Infection

Type of Sample	Positive Result	Sensitivity	Specificity
Endotracheal	10^6 CFU/mL	55%	85%
aspirate	10^5 CFU/mL	63%	75%
	Gram's stain	38%	40%
BAL	10^4 CFU/mL[a]	47–91%	78–100%
	5% intracellular organisms	44–91%	47–100%
PSB	10^5 CFU/mL	57–82%	77–88%
BAL + PSB	See above	91%	78%

[a]Of retrieved fluid.
ABBREVIATIONS: CFU, colony-forming units; BAL, bronchoalveolar lavage; PSB, protected specimen brush.

Causes

Many nosocomial pneumonias are polymicrobial. Aerobic bacteria are by far the most commonly isolated organisms. Of these, the major cause is *S. aureus*, followed closely by individual gram-negative bacilli, including *Pseudomonas* species, *Klebsiella* species, and *Acinetobacter baumanii*. The relative contribution of anaerobic bacteria and viruses is not known, because most hospitals do not routinely culture for these. Fungi are thought to cause a small percentage of pneumonias.

Because therapy is often initiated before the results of microbiologic testing are available, knowledge of the common pathogens and their resistance patterns in your locale is essential (Table 6–14).[15,26] The prevalence of methicillin-resistant *S. aureus* is highly variable. In some ICUs, it may account for more than half of the *S. aureus* isolates, while in others it may be rare.

Therapy

As noted above, the diagnosis of ventilator-related pneumonia is difficult; however, meeting each of the five criteria is highly specific for pneumonia, although the sensitivity is low. If all of the criteria are not met, a watchful, waiting approach may help to distinguish patients who are actually infected from those with noninfectious causes of pulmonary infiltration. If the intensivist does not have access to bronchoscopic testing, endotracheal aspiration will be the most accessible sample to test. Results must be interpreted with caution. If a predominant organism is found on Gram's stain, therapy may be directed towards either gram-negative or gram-positive organisms.

If all of the clinical criteria are met, empiric antibiotic therapy may be started after microbiologic specimens are collected and appropriate Gram's stain studies

TABLE 6–14 Common Pathogens in Ventilator Related Pneumonia

Causative Pathogen	NNIS[1] 1986–1998 N = 1635	Luna et al[25] 1997 N = 65	Kollef et al[26] 1998 N = 70
Staphylococcus aureus	21%	26%	30%
Pseudomonas aeruginosa	14%	11%	29%
Enterobacter spp.	9%	5%	6%
Klebsiella pneumoniae	8%	14%	1.5%
Candida albicans	6%	3%	3%
Escherichia coli	4%	2%	1.5%
Serratia marcescens	4%	0%	6%
Acinetobacter spp.	3%	26%	4%
Hemophilus influenzae	3%	1%	1.5%
Other	16%	15%	7%

have been done. The antibiotics selected for empiric therapy should have a sufficient spectrum to be active against the organisms identified on Gram's stain, taking into account the resistance pattern in your local ICU. Several recent studies investigated the effect that bronchoscopic sampling has on empiric therapy for ventilator-related pneumonia.[17,25–27] Each confirmed the importance of an adequate initial choice of antibiotics. Mortality was higher in groups in which the initial antibiotic choice was not active against the resident flora of the ICU and was subsequently changed, in comparison to groups in which the initial antibiotic choice covered the causative agent.

Therefore, when the Gram stain shows pure gram-negative rods, the empiric regimen should cover the most resistant bacteria present in the specific unit where the patient is housed. Third-generation cephalosporins without antipseudomonal activity and antipseudomonal monotherapy may represent inadequate regimens.[28,29] Gram's stain evidence of gram-positive bacteria should prompt the use of vancomycin. In the absence of a Gram's stain or when both morphologic types are present, an inclusive regimen should be initiated. Once susceptibility results return, the coverage can be narrowed appropriately. Seven days of intravenous and/or oral antibiotic therapy is adequate for treatment of nosocomial pneumonia. Treatment may be extended to 10 or 14 days for slow clinical resolution.

CATHETER-RELATED BLOODSTREAM INFECTION

Catheter-related bloodstream infection is one of the most serious complications for patients in the ICU. It is less common than nosocomial urinary tract infection, but certainly more costly in terms of morbidity, mortality, and expenditure. The incidence is approximately 5 infections per 1,000 catheter days and, at any given time in ICUs across the United States, more than half of the patients have an indwelling central venous catheter or PAC.

Risks

Biofilms form around the catheter where it passes through the subcutaneous tissue, even in the absence of bacteria. Organisms colonize catheters most commonly by embedding in the biofilm. Rarely, colonization leads to infection. There is a correlation between the virulence of the organism and its burden and likelihood of infection. There are many risk factors for the development of infection.[30] These include:

1. Nonsterile conditions at placement
2. Poor catheter maintenance technique
3. Long duration of catheter use
4. Type of catheter

5. Patient's immune status
6. Use of catheter for total parenteral nutrition (TPN)
7. Number of organisms colonizing catheter surface

Organisms that cause infection originate from one of three places. For catheters that have been in place less than 10 days, the most common site is the skin insertion. The organisms migrate from the skin or gloves of health care providers along the external surface of the catheter to colonize the tip. Catheters that have been in place longer than 10 days are more likely to be colonized from the hub. In either instance, colonizing organisms may generate from the hands of health care providers. The third and, by far the least, likely source of catheter contamination is hematogenous spread.

Prevention[31]

Central venous catheters are essential to the care of some patients in the ICU. Aside from limiting their use, many precautions can be taken to reduce the risk of catheter related bloodstream infection. These include:

1. Use of sterile technique during insertion and maintenance
2. Cutaneous antisepsis (with chlorhexidine or mupirocin)
3. Use of an antimicrobial-coated or silver-impregnated catheter
4. Use of an antimicrobial lock or flush
5. Use of a tunneled catheter
6. Use of an antiseptic hub

CATHETER TYPE The highest risk for infection is with temporary, noncuffed central venous catheters, typically placed in ICU patients by physicians. The incidence of infection ranges up to 10 per 1,000 catheter days.[4] The risk is much lower for surgically or radiographically placed tunneled devices: about 2 infections per 1,000 catheter days. Because of urgency, convenience, or cost, most lines in the ICU are not the tunneled type. Whenever feasible, a tunneled catheter should be placed when central access is anticipated to be necessary for more than 14 days. In this case, the benefits likely outweigh the added cost. An alternative with lower risk for infection is a peripherally inserted central venous catheter.

Antimicrobial-impregnated catheters have been used to prevent catheter-related infection. A recent meta-analysis of studies comparing catheters impregnated with clorhexidine and silver sulfadiazine with conventional nonimpregnated catheters showed a significant decrease in catheter colonization and bloodstream infection.[32] Newer catheters may further reduce the risk. These catheters were compared with catheters impregnated with minocycline and rifampin, which were one-third as likely to be colonized and one-half as likely to lead to bloodstream infection.[33] Because of the higher cost of antimicrobial-impregnated catheters, the decision to use one must be made after considering the cost of the catheter with the baseline rate of infection. The higher the rate of infection in your area, the more likely it will be cost effective to use the impregnated catheters.

INSERTION AND MAINTENANCE Strict adherence to aseptic technique when placing a catheter has been shown to produce a sixfold reduction in the rate of bacteremia.[31] During insertion of a central venous line, careful handwashing; sterile gloves, mask, gown, and cap; and large sterile drapes create the aseptic environment. Manipulation of the catheter is also shown to increase the risk of sepsis. Since the site of access for most infections is the skin insertion site, this area should be protected. Firm anchorage to the skin prevents the catheter from sliding in and out and allowing the entrance of organisms from outside. The use of antimicrobial ointments has been shown to reduce the number of bacteremias, but the incidence of fungemia rises. The risk of developing antimicrobial resistance is thought to be low with these ointments, but the level of risk is unknown.

The site of catheter insertion also affects the risk of infection. Subclavian catheters pose the least risk for infection, followed by jugular and then femoral sites. The risk of infection must be weighed against the risk of mechanical complication (e.g., pneumothorax, subclavian artery puncture, hemothorax, thrombosis) when choosing a site of insertion.

Routine replacement of central venous catheters has been advocated to prevent infection. Routine replacement without clinical indication (signs of infection) has not been shown to decrease the risk. The risk accrued daily from the presence of a catheter remains constant with either a new or an old catheter. While many hospitals have guidelines for the replacement of central venous catheters, the clinician should feel comfortable extending their life in the absence of signs of infection.

Diagnosis

As part of the workup of the febrile patient, all catheter sites should be inspected and palpated for tenderness, warmth, swelling, or purulent discharge. Any purulent discharge should be gram-stained and cultured. Sometimes, infection derives from organisms that colonize the lumen of the catheter, and the catheter appears normal. The diagnosis of catheter-related bloodstream infection requires paired positive blood cultures (Table 6–15). One sample set must be a quantitative culture drawn from the line and the other drawn from a peripheral site. An alternative method is to remove the line and culture the tip, correlating this to a positive peripheral blood culture result. There are several culture methods in practice for the culture of blood and intravascular devices (Table 6–16).

When only one blood culture sample is obtained, a positive result may indicate either true infection or contamination. However, if two or three other samples test negative, usually the positive result is a contaminant. Organisms colonizing the lumen of the catheter may be released into the bloodstream peri-

TABLE 6–15 Definitions of Catheter-Related Infections

Catheter-related bloodstream infection: Isolation of the same organism from (1) a semi-quantitative or quantitative culture of a catheter segment and (2) a peripherally drawn blood sample of a patient with accompanying clinical symptoms of bloodstream infection and no other apparent source of infection

Catheter colonization: Growth of more than 15 colony-forming units (CFUs) by semiquantitative culture or more than 10^3 CFU/LPF by quantitative culture from a catheter segment in the absence of clinical symptoms

Local catheter-related infection: Evidence of catheter colonization plus erythema, warmth, swelling, or tenderness at catheter insertion site and negative results on blood culture analysis

---

odically from injections and flushing. This may cause transient bacteremia, which may be the cause of fever, but does not reflect infection. This is especially true for coagulase-negative staphylococci. In stable patients without clinical signs of bacteremia in whom the organisms isolated are coagulase-negative staphylococci, we would advocate reserving treatment for a situation in which all of multiple blood cultures show positive results.

Clinical findings that may point to infection include: bacteremia or fungemia in a patient at low risk for sepsis, local signs of infection, onset of fever with catheter already in place, and multiple blood culture results containing organisms that may otherwise be considered contaminants (e.g., coagulase-negative staphylococci, *Corynebacterium jeikeium*, *Bacillus* species, *Candida* species, or *Malassezia* species). Remember that a single positive blood culture result from a catheter may indicate either infection or colonization. If a catheter is left in place

TABLE 6–16 Microbiologic Methods for Evaluation of Catheter-Related Infections

---

Semiquantitative culture: A segment of catheter that has been removed is rolled along the surface of an agar plate. After overnight incubation, the number of colony forming units (CFU) is counted and a result of more than 15 CFU is considered a potential source of infection.

Quantitative culture: Catheter segment is sonicated in broth or flushed with and immersed in broth. The broth is quantitatively cultured. A value of $>10^3$ CFU is a cutoff for consideration as a potential source of infection.

Quantitative blood culture: If the catheter is not removed, quantitative blood culture samples taken from the catheter and periphery can aid in the diagnosis. In catheter-related bloodstream infection, there is usually a fivefold to tenfold increase in the number of colony-forming units in the sample from the catheter. The increase is in comparison to the peripheral sample. Often the catheter sample results are positive, even when the peripheral culture results are negative.

NOTE: These methods are helpful when results of peripheral blood cultures are positive for the same organism as the catheter cultures. By themselves, positive catheter cultures are not a reason to treat and may represent colonization.

long enough, it will become colonized with bacteria and produce a positive culture result, even in the absence of true infection.

Cause

The pathogenesis of catheter-related bloodstream infection implicates migrating organisms from patient skin or the hands of health care workers. The causative agents should come as no surprise (Table 6–17). They are predominantly skin flora, coagulase-negative staphylococci, and *S. aureus*. The remainder are aerobic gram-negative organisms or *Candida* species that colonize many of the patients in ICUs.

Therapy

If Gram's stain or culture results are available at the time of diagnosis, then narrow coverage may be selected. Broader empiric therapy is used when a patient is at risk for bacteremia and is clinically unstable. This requires broad-spectrum antibacterial coverage. It should include vancomycin wherever the prevalence of MRSA is high and also coverage for *Pseudomonas* species, where this organism is common.

Coagulase-negative staphlyococci are often the cause when positive blood culture results and fever are present. In the stable patient with a single positive blood culture result, consider withholding therapy and watchful waiting. If there are multiple positive culture results, vancomycin is the drug of choice because almost all of these organisms are resistant to penicillins. The infected catheter need not always be removed. This infection should be treated for 7 days.[30]

Catheter-related bloodstream infection by *S. aureus* is a very serious disease. Once it has been documented, the catheter should be removed. Complications

TABLE 6–17 Causes of Catheter-Related Bloodstream Infections

Organism	NNIS[1] N = 1159
Coagulase-negative staphylococci	37%
Staphylococcus aureus	24%
Enterococcus spp.	10%
Escherichia coli	3%
Enterobacter spp.	3%
Candida albicans	2%
Klebsiella pneumoniae	2%
Pseudomonas aeruginosa	2%
Serratia marcescens	2%
Candida glabrata	2%
Other *Candida* spp.	2%
Other	11%

include endocarditis, septic thrombosis, osteomyelitis, and abscesses. If there are no complications and the patient responds to antibiotic therapy in the first 3 days, a course of 2 weeks may be used. If the catheter is removed and defervescence is prompt, subsequent culture results are negative, and transesophageal echocardiogram results are negative, 1 week of therapy may be sufficient. By contrast, if these good prognostic features are not present, therapy should be continued for a minimum of 4 weeks.

The gram-negative bloodstream infections may be managed similarly. A 7-day course of antibiotic therapy is generally adequate. The catheter should be removed, especially in the presence of *Pseudomonas, Stenotrophomonas,* and *Acinetobacter* species.

URINARY TRACT INFECTION

Urinary tract infections (UTI) are the most common nosocomial infection, according to the NNIS.[1] The incidence is 6.5 infections per 1,000 catheter days. In one surveillance study, 75% of patients in the ICU had indwelling urinary catheters. The definition of UTI used by the Centers for Disease Control and Prevention (CDC) does not take into account asymptomatic bacteriuria: these numbers may be artificially high. As many as 50% of these "infections" may be asymptomatic. The difficulty lies in deciding when bacteria or yeast in the urine constitutes an infection that requires intervention. We discuss the diagnosis and indications for treatment and outline proven methods of prevention.

Risks

Most organisms causing UTI ascend to the bladder through the urethra. Most of these organisms can be found as colonizers of the rectum or vagina. Urinary catheterization facilitates this migration in several ways. Insertion of the catheter may inoculate bacteria into the bladder. The catheter, once inserted, can serve as a path through the urethra. Growth in the urine collection bag may spread up the lumen of the catheter. Catheters may mechanically break down the uroepithelial barrier to adhesion, which has been shown to retard antibacterial polymorphonuclear leukocyte formation. Finally, catheters may not completely empty the bladder, leaving standing urine. The factors that affect colonization are listed in Table 6–18.[34]

The urinary tract is only very rarely infected hematogenously. This occurs most commonly with *S. aureus* bacteremia and candidal fungemia.

Prevention

The most important aspect of prevention of UTI is more stringent criteria for catheterization. However, many patients in the ICU require urinary catheteriza-

TABLE 6–18 Risk Factors for Nosocomial Urinary Tract Infection

1. Duration of catheterization
2. Absence of use of a urinometer
3. Microbial colonization of the drainage bag
4. Patient with diabetes mellitus
5. Absence of antibiotic use
6. Female patient
7. Abnormal serum creatinine level at placement
8. Indication other than surgery or urinary output measurement
9. Errors in catheter care

tion; therefore, prevention is aimed at preventing bacteria from getting to the bladder. Observing aseptic technique during insertion of the catheter is critical. The closed catheter system can be maintained by obtaining urine specimens through the urine port after cleaning with alcohol. Even with the utmost care, it is simply a matter of time before bacteriuria occurs. Once this happens, there are no good ways to prevent the complications.

The most important aspect of prevention of UTI is preventing the catheterization. Each day the clinician should review the need for catheterization and promptly remove all unnecessary catheters.

Several researchers have tried using silver-impregnated catheters to reduce the risk of infection. A recent meta-analysis attempted to clarify whether silver-coated catheters were less likely to lead to bacteriuria than standard urinary catheters.[35] There was a significant decrease in the incidence of bacteriuria with silver-alloy catheters. The studies did not use symptomatic infection, bacteremia, or death as outcomes. The cost for silver-alloy catheters is about double that of standard catheters. There is no clear advantage to the use of the silver-alloy catheter in large populations.

Diagnosis

The CDC divides UTIs into symptomatic UTI and asymptomatic bacteriuria (Table 6–19).[36] Determination of prevalence of infection is made by lumping together asymptomatic bacteriuria with symptomatic UTI. The most common causative organisms are listed in Table 6–20. When organisms initially colonize the catheterized bladder, fever may develop from endotoxin release even in the absence of invasive infection.

Organisms in catheterized bladders change spontaneously without treatment. Those that invade the bloodstream most often do so immediately after they appear in the bladder. Most times, organisms in the bladder do not invade the bloodstream; they release endotoxin without becoming invasive (i.e, colonization). Endotoxin may cause fever in the absence of signs of unstable physiology. Unnecessary treatment of organisms colonizing the catheterized bladder leads to

TABLE 6–19 **Definition of Nosocomial Urinary Tract Infection**

Symptomatic Urinary Tract Infection

Fever (higher than 38°C), urgency or frequency of urination, dysuria, or suprapubic tenderness, plus one of the following:
1. Urine culture results showing ≥ 105 CFU/mL containing no more than two species of organisms
2. Any of the following: (a) positive dipstick results for leukocyte esterase and/or nitrate, (b) pyuria (> 10 WBC/mL^3 or > 3 WBC/mL^3 of uncentrifuged urine), (c) organisms seen on Gram's stain of urine, (d) two urine cultures with repeated isolation of the same pathogen with > 102 CFU/mL urine, or (e) urine culture with < 105 CFUs/mL of a single pathogen in patient being treated with appropriate antimicrobials

Asymptomatic Bacteriuria

One of the following:
1. An indwelling urinary catheter is present within 7 days before urine is cultured *and* patient has no fever, urgency or frequency of urination, dysuria, or suprapubic tenderness *and* urine culture results show more than 105 organisms per milliliter of urine with no more than two species of organisms
2. No indwelling urinary catheter within 7 days before the first of two urine cultures show more than 105 organisms per milliliter of urine with the same organism and with no more than two species of organisms *and* patient has no fever, urgency or frequency of urination, dysuria, or suprapubic tenderness

greater resistance. When a catheter is removed, organisms in the bladder pose a greater threat (can be thought of as an undrained abscess).

Therapy

Asymptomatic bacteriuria or fungus in the urine need not be treated as long as the catheter remains in place. Exceptions include:

1. Bacteria that cause a high incidence of bacteremia that originates as bacteriuria in a particular hospital (i.e. *Serratia marcescens*)
2. Therapy that is designed to control a cluster of infections by the same organism
3. High-risk patients, such as pregnant women, organ transplant recipients, and granulocytopenic patients
4. Patients who must undergo urologic surgery

Patients in the ICU often are unable to complain of symptoms. The task of the clinician then becomes to rule out alternative sources of fever and to judge whether the fever is likely to be caused by bacteriuria or fungus in the urine and whether or not treatment is indicated. If the patient is stable with fever, the fever often will disappear.

TABLE 6–20 Causative Organisms in Nosocomial Urinary Tract Infection

Organism	NNIS[1] N = 2321
Escherichia coli	28%
Enterococcus spp.	14%
Candida albicans	10%
Psuedomonas aeruginosa	7%
Klebsiella pneumoniae	6%
Enterobacter spp.	4%
Proteus mirabilis	4%
Staphylococcus aureus	3%
Candida glabrata	3%
Other *Candida* spp.	4%
Other fungi	5%
Other	12%

When a decision is made to treat, usually because of unstable physiology, the choice of drug should be guided by results of Gram's stain. For gram-positive infections in areas with a low prevalence of MRSA, ampicillin and sulbactam is a good first choice. If the prevalence of MRSA is high, vancomycin should be used. For gram-negative infections a third-generation cephalosporin or aminoglycoside, or both, may be used. Candidal infection can be managed with amphotericin B bladder washings for 3 days or with fluconazole. A 7-day course is adequate for most nosocomial UTIs; almost all are the result of a bladder catheter,[37] which should be removed or changed.

DISSEMINATED CANDIDIASIS

Disseminated candidiasis is rapidly increasing in incidence. It is primarily a nosocomial disease that is found in the ICU more often than other parts of the hospital. The NNIS data for 1986 to 1990 indicate that *Candida* species were the fourth most commonly isolated pathogen in patients with nosocomial bloodstream infection, accounting for 10.2%.[38]

Pathogenesis and Risks

In critically ill patients, the risk factors predisposing to candidiasis are common and include:

1. Treatment with antibiotics
2. Immunosuppression (especially neutropenia)
3. Abdominal surgery or other disruption of the GI tract

4. Isolation of *Candida* species from other sites
5. Placement of central venous catheters

In addition, host defenses are compromised. It is especially true in neutropenic patients (e.g., those with acute leukemia) and those where the skin barrier is interrupted (e.g. patients with catheters, burn patients). The normal flora is altered by the use of antibacterial agents; this may allow for overgrowth of *Candida* species. There is increased risk for development of candidemia with previous use of antibiotics.[39] There was an exponential increase in risk for each antibiotic class used. Researchers in a study of candidemia in patients with acute leukemia found colonization of the stool to be a marker for dissemination.[38]

Diagnosis

The diagnosis is suspected in patients with new fever and risk factors. Patients with disseminated candidal infection may present with fever of unclear cause or fulminant sepsis. The most common way the diagnosis is made is by positive blood culture results. But if blood cultures are relied on, the diagnosis is often missed. The sensitivity of blood culture techniques is approximately 50%.[40] The diagnosis can also occasionally be confirmed by characteristic fundoscopic findings or skin biopsy. Candidal endopthalmitis may appear as white exudates in the chorioretina that extend into the vitreous matter, which presents as a red eye. Skin lesions of disseminated disease are usually small nodules (0.5 to 1.0 cm) that are single or multiple and pink or red in color and are often found on the upper torso. Punch biopsy reveals fungi on histologic examination.

Presumptive diagnosis is often made on the basis of colonization of urine, stool, oral secretions, or respiratory secretions, which may be the precursor to disseminated disease. However, most patients with colonization at multiple sites do not progress to disseminated disease. The presumptive diagnosis should only be made in patients at high risk, who have colonization of multiple sites and also have objective signs of infection that cannot otherwise be explained.

Therapy

The initiation of antifungal therapy for disseminated candidiasis may be in response to a positive blood culture result or positive histologic result or may be an empiric response for certain high-risk patients. Disseminated candidal infection may be treated with amphotericin B or fluconazole; the superiority of one over the other has not been established, with the exception of *Candidal* strains that exhibit fluconazole resistance (i.e., *C. krusei* and *C. glabrata*). Recently, more "non albicans" species of *Candida* have been isolated in invasive disease (Table 6–21).[41,42] In a study of nonneutropenic patients with candidemia, there was no significant difference in the rates of successful treatment with fluconazole or amphotericin B.[43] There was less toxicity with fluconazole. Two other recent studies, one in nonneu-

TABLE 6–21 Species of Candida Implicated in Disseminated Disease

	NEOMS[41] 1993–95 N = 408	Nolla-Sallas et al[42] 1991–92 N = 46
C. albicans	56%	60%
C. parapsilosis	20%	17%
C. glabrata	11%	2%
C. tropicalis	7%	8%
C. krusei	3%	2%
Other	3%	11%

tropenic patients[44] and the other in a more heterogeneous population[45] had similar results. However, in the past, these patients were treated with line removal without antifungal therapy, making assessments of this kind frought with difficulty.

SINUSITIS

Sinusitis is relatively less common than other infections in the ICU. Pinning down the incidence is problematic because many studies include cases in which the diagnosis is made by radiographic criteria alone. Nevertheless, it is a serious problem with which all intensivists should be familiar.

Risks

The only factor that has been shown to increase the risk of sinusitis is nasotracheal intubation.[46] Sinusitis occurs when the drainage of the sinuses through their ostia in the nasal canal is impaired or blocked. A nasotracheal tube may cause trauma and inflammation to the area around the ostia or simply act as a barrier to drainage. Other factors that have been proposed, but not proven to increase the risk of sinusitis are nasogastric tubes, high-dose corticosteroids, facial fractures, and unconsciousness.

Diagnosis

The diagnosis of acute sinusitis in the outpatient setting is usually made clinically (Table 6–22).[47] It is even more difficult in the critically ill patient. Symptoms may not be elicited from intubated patients, and purulent nasal discharge is only present in 25% of proven cases of sinusitis. Therefore, if sinusitis is suspected, the workup should include CT scan of the sinuses.

A CT scan that shows evidence of sinusitis *must* be followed by microbiologic sampling.[4] Sterile sinus puncture is the sampling method of choice. It involves disinfection of the nasal mucosa (with povidone iodine) and puncture and aspiration of the sinus. Since the sinuses should be sterile and the nasal mucosa is

TABLE 6–22 Diagnosis of Acute Sinusitis in Outpatients

Diagnosis requires two major criteria or one major and two minor criteria, lasting for more than 7 days.

Major criteria

Cough
Purulent nasal discharge

Minor criteria

Periorbital edema
Headache
Facial pain
Tooth pain
Earache
Sore throat
Halitosis
Wheezing
Fever

colonized with bacteria, if the disinfection is done properly, this method is definitive for the diagnosis.

Cause

The organisms that cause sinusitis are common colonizers of the oropharynx in the ICU patient. Two-thirds of cases are caused by *Pseudomonas aeruginosa* and other aerobic gram-negative bacteria; nearly one-third are caused by gram-positive bacteria, most common of which is *S. aureus*. Fungi cause a small percentage of cases.

Therapy

Sinusitis can be thought of as a closed-space infection. Antibiotic therapy is only an adjunct to drainage for this infection. Drainage may be accomplished by the aspiration done for diagnosis or may require aspiration of multiple sinuses, most often accompanied by irrigation. There is a high failure rate with drainage alone,[46] which is why we recommend antibiotics as well. Because the diagnosis requires sinus puncture, there should always be Gram's stain data to help guide therapy.

Predominantly gram-negative sinusitis should be treated with double coverage for *Pseudomonas* species until culture data becomes available. For gram-positive sinusitis, vancomycin should be started, pending culture data.

There may be treatment failures with drainage and antibiotic therapy. If symptoms do not abate after 7 days, it may be necessary to insert a drainage catheter in the infected sinus.

DIARRHEA

Many patients in the ICU have diarrhea, and most patients develop fever at some point in the ICU stay. The challenge is discovering which cases of fever are caused by the diarrhea. There is only one common cause of diarrhea in the ICU that should also cause fever: *C. difficile*.[4]

Differential diagnosis for diarrhea should include consideration of the potential contribution of enteral feedings and medications, such as promotility agents, erythromycin, clindamycin, quinine, theophylline, alprazolam, chemotherapeutic agents, valproic acid, gemfibrozil, and many others. The differential diagnosis of infectious diarrhea includes *Salmonella, Shigella, Aeromonas,* and *Yersinia* species; *Campylobacter jejuni; E. coli* 0157:H7; *Entamoeba histolytica;* and several viruses. These are community-acquired infections and should not be considered in a patient unless they are admitted to the hospital with diarrhea. The list expands to include: *Cyclospora, Strongyloides, Salmonella,* and *Microsporidium* species; cytomegalovirus (CMV); and *Mycobacterium avium* complex for patients with a travel history or HIV infection. Only patients with these risk factors should have an evaluation for one of these relatively rare causes of diarrhea.

Clostridial Infection

The major risk factor for developing *C. difficile* diarrhea is previous antibiotic use. Any antibiotic may be the offending agent. The most commonly implicated are cephalosporins, penicillins, and clindamycin. Anyone who develops diarrhea and fever within 3 weeks of antibiotic therapy should be evaluated. The spore of the organism may also be spread from patient to patient in the ICU on the hands of health care workers.

The clinical spectrum of disease varies from asymptomatic to toxic megacolon, requiring urgent surgical intervention. Patients may have leukocytosis. In fact, it is one of few infections that causes WBC counts of more than 30,000/μL.

The workup for diarrhea in the ICU should include:

1. Send stool for *C. difficile* evaluation
2. If the first evaluation is negative, send a second sample for evaluation
3. For severe illness or in an unstable patient, consider empiric treatment while awaiting test results
4. For patients with HIV infection, send stool to be evaluated for ova and parasites, leukocytes, acid-fast bacilli (AFB), bacterial culture

For patients with diarrhea and fever with no obvious cause, evaluation should be performed. The tests are relatively rapid and empiric therapy is discouraged because of the risk of promoting resistant organisms. A diarrheal stool sample should be sent for enzyme immunoassay for toxin. If the first sample results are negative for toxin, then a second sample should be sent for evaluation more than

12 hours after the first. The sensitivity of two samples in making the diagnosis has been shown to be 84%, compared with 72% for a single sample.[48] False-negative results are uncommon, and empiric therapy for a patient with two negative results should be reserved for unstable ill patients.

The standard test for *C. difficile* is the enzyme immunoassay for detecting toxin. It is less sensitive than the gold standard, which is tissue culture assay, but it is less expensive and much faster to perform. *C. difficile* cultures are not useful.

The diagnosis may also be made by visualization of pseudomembranes by flexible sigmoidoscopy or colonoscopy. Pseudomembranes are more common with more severe disease. These procedures carry the risk of perforation of infected bowel. There is little role for these procedures in the workup. Stool studies are fast, reliable, and cheaper.

Therapy

When the diagnosis is made by one of the above methods, therapy should be initiated for *C. difficile*. There are some false-negative test results with the *C. difficile* enzyme immunoassay. For patients with no other source of fever and previous antibiotic exposure, empiric therapy may be started. It should, in general, be avoided, because of the risk of selecting for resistant organisms.

Treatment may be given for 7 to 14 days; the duration should be guided by clinical response in body temperature and severity of diarrhea. Relapse may occur in up to 20% of treated patients.

Recommended treatment regimens are metronidazole, 500 mg orally, three times daily; metronidazole, 500 mg intravenously, three times daily[49]; and vancomycin, 125 mg orally, four times daily. For relapse, the recommended regimen is metronidazole plus rifampin, 300 mg orally, twice daily for 10 days.

IMMUNOCOMPROMISED PATIENTS

The approach to the febrile immunocompromised patient in the ICU is different from the one outlined for the normal host. Immunocompromise results in two changes. First, it alters the presentations of common infections, and second, it permits a wider spectrum of infectious agents, requiring more aggressive diagnostic and treatment strategies. Infectious diseases in compromised patients may progress more quickly and be more severe. This section refines the approach to febrile patients in the ICU as it relates to three specific immunocompromised states: neutropenia, HIV infection, and organ transplantation.

Neutropenia

Neutropenia may result from drug therapy, radiation, malignant tumors, HIV infection, or immune disease. Of all febrile neutropenic patients, 50% to 60% have infection, of which approximately one-third are bacteremias.[50] The epidemiology of bacteremias in the neutropenic host is similar to that of nosocomial bacteremia in others. The most common are gram-positive infections with coagulase-negative staphylococci, *Streptococcus viridans*, or *S. aureus*. Aerobic gram-negative infections including *E. coli* and *Klebsiella* and *Pseudomonas* species are next in frequency. Fungi may cause infection in patients receiving broad-spectrum antibiotics or occasionally be a primary cause of neutropenic fever.

Clinical signs of infection are less pronounced in the neutropenic patient. Patients have localized complaints without findings to support those complaints. A careful search for subtle signs of inflammation at common sites of infection should direct diagnostic testing. Mouth, perineum, skin, catheter sites, and lungs should all be examined and suspicious sites sampled for culture. In cases of pneumonia, there may not be a visible infiltrate or sputum production. If the clinician is suspicious, sputum may be induced or CT scanning and bronchoscopy used early to aid diagnosis.[51] Blood samples for culture should be obtained from venous catheters and peripheral sites, and at least one should be quantitative. Any catheter with signs of entry site inflammation should be removed and the tip quantitatively cultured. Patients with diarrhea should be evaluated for *C. difficile* toxin. If this test result is negative and the patient has been hospitalized for less than 72 hours, stool should be cultured for bacteria, viruses, and protozoa. Neutropenic patients are at risk for diarrhea from *Salmonella, Shigella, Campylobacter, Yersinia,* and *Cryptosporidium* species and CMV and rotavirus.

Infections may be rapidly fatal in the neutropenic patient. Therefore, all febrile neutropenic patients in the ICU should be treated promptly with broad-spectrum intravenous antibiotics. The Infectious Disease Society of America recommends one of three regimens[50]:

1. Aminoglycoside plus an antipseudomonal beta-lactam agent (e.g., piperacillin, ticarcillin)
2. Ceftazidime, imipenem, or cefepime monotherapy
3. Vancomycin plus ceftazidime

The empiric use of vancomycin should be reserved for patients in whom catheter-related bloodstream infection or nosocomial pneumonia is suspected and who are in ICUs where methicillin-resistant *S. aureus* is common. Vancomycin should be discontinued if blood culture results are negative.

HIV Infection

Concerns about the management of the HIV-infected patient have led to many debates on the appropriate use of intensive care resources. With the advent of highly active antiretroviral therapy, this is no longer a debate. Although overall mortality of HIV-infected patients receiving care in the ICU has been high, two recent series show that short-term mortality is related mainly to the severity of acute illness, whereas long-term mortality depended primarily on the natural history of the HIV infection.[52,53] Survival rates were excellent for patients who were discharged from the ICU. The three most common diagnoses were respiratory failure, neurologic disorders, and sepsis.

RESPIRATORY FAILURE Studies of series of HIV-infected patients admitted to the ICU with respiratory failure reveal an even split between *Pneumocystis carinii* pneumonia (PCP) and bacterial pneumonia as the cause.[53,54] If the patient has been compliant with trimethoprim-sulfamethoxasole therapy or if the CD4 count is greater than 350/μL, PCP is much less likely. Other infectious agents cause a much smaller percentage of these cases. All HIV-infected patients in the ICU who are in respiratory distress should have a chest x-ray study, CBC count, ABG analysis, Gram's stain of sputum, sputum culture, CD4 count, lactate dehydrogenase (LDH) level measurement, and blood cultures. Management should be directed by the x-ray findings and prophylaxis history (Table 6–23).[55] This approach assumes that a patient is ill enough to require ICU admission and is different from the approach to the general medical patient with the same complaints.

The decision to start empiric antibiotic therapy must be made with the clinical status of the patient and the previously mentioned factors in mind. The same clinical criteria used to decide whether or not to treat patients suspected of having ventilator-acquired pneumonia hold for the HIV patient with respiratory distress. The major difference is the expanded differential diagnosis of the cause, which can be stratified by CD4 count.[56] When the CD4 count is above 500/μL, the infectious causes are essentially the same as for patients without HIV disease. Community-acquired pneumonia, bronchitis, and common noninfectious causes of respiratory distress should be considered. At CD4 counts of 200 to 500/μL, pulmonary tuberculosis becomes more likely, but bacterial infections are most common. At CD4 counts below 200/μL, the differential expands to include PCP and toxoplasmosis for those not on prophylaxis and histoplasmosis, coccidioidomycosis, miliary tuberculosis, and less commonly, CMV and *M. avium* complex for those who are. It is the patients with low CD4 counts for whom early bronchoscopy to make a microbiologic diagnosis is essential.

PCP is the most feared cause of respiratory distress in the HIV-infected patient. Empiric therapy is often started, especially if the patient is sufficiently ill to require intensive care and has not been receiving trimethoprim-sulfamethoxazole (TMP/SMX). Factors that lead to suspicion of PCP are: indolent clinical course, hypoxemia, elevated LDH level, and a CD4 count of less than 200/μL. Of the patients with PCP admitted to the ICU in one series, the average room-air PaO_2 was 41 mm Hg.[54] Elevated LDH levels are sensitive, but not at all specific, for PCP. Patients who are at risk should be started on empiric therapy. In the case of the ICU patient, the PO_2 will almost always be less than 70 mm Hg and therapy should include corticosteroids. Attempts at making the diagnosis should be carried out as quickly as possible, because other causes aggravated by unopposed corticosteroids may, in fact, be present. The most accurate technique for

TABLE 6–23 Work up for Fever and Respiratory Distress in HIV-Infected Patients

Radiographic Evidence	Work up Required	Common Pathogens Found
Normal	Induced sputum sample for PCP/AFB x 3	*Pneumocystis carinii, Mycobacterium tuberculosis, Cryptococcus* spp., *M. avium*
Interstitial infiltrate		*P. carinii,* miliary tuberculosis, histoplasmosis, coccidioidomycosis, cytomegalovirus, *Toxoplasma gondii*
$PaO_2 > 70$ mm Hg	Induced sputum sample for PCP/AFB x 3 Bronchoscopy, if sputum is negative	
$PaO_2 = 50$–70 mm Hg	Induced sputum sample for PCP x 1 Bronchoscopy	
$PaO_2 < 50$ mm Hg	Empiric treatment for PCP Immediate bronchoscopy	
Pulmonary lobar consolidation	Gram's stain, culture, *Legionella* DFA Sputum sample for AFB, fungi, cytology Consider bronchoscopy	Bacteria, cryptococcosis, Kaposi's sarcoma, *Legionella* spp., nocardiosis, *M. tuberculosis*
Pleural effusion	Thoracentesis for pH, cell counts, protein Gram's stain, bacterial culture AFB stain and culture, cytology Sputum sample for AFB x 3 Pleural biopsy, if above test results are negative	Bacteria (*S. aureus, S. pneumoniae, Pseudomonas aeruginosa*), *M. tuberculosis,* cryptococcosis, Kaposi's sarcoma, heart failure, hypoalbuminemia, aspergillosis

ABBREVIATIONS: PCP, *Pneumocystis carinii* pneumonia; AFB, acid-fast bacteria; DFA, direct fluorescent antibody staining.

the diagnosis is bronchoscopy with BAL. This should be done whenever PCP is suspected in the severely ill patient, unless tracheal aspiration in an intubated patient yields a diagnosis.

First-line therapy for PCP is TMP/SMX, at a dose of 15 mg/kg per day of trimethoprim in three to four divided doses initially, tapered to 10 mg/kg per day if there is improvement, and especially if there appears to be toxicity. Duration of treatment is 21 days. Alternative regimens include pentamidine, 3 or 4 mg/kg per day intravenously; clindamycin, 600 mg every 8 hours intravenously, plus primaquine, 30 mg/day orally; or atovaquone suspension, 750 mg with meals twice daily—each lasting for 21 days.[55] In mild to moderate disease, the latter compares favorably with pentamidine.

NEUROLOGIC DISORDERS The most common diagnosis for patients with HIV infection admitted to the ICU with a neurologic disorder was toxoplasmic encephalitis followed by cryptococcosis, cerebral tuberculosis, bacterial meningitis, and nocardiosis.[57] Low CD4 counts widen the differential possibilities. Patients admitted to the ICU with fever and neurologic findings should have a CT scan and, if there is no mass lesion, lumbar puncture to rule out CNS infection. CSF tests should include cell counts, protein and glucose levels, VDRL, bacterial culture, fungal culture, viral culture, AFB culture, cryptococcal antigen, and cytology. Levels of serum cryptococcal antigen and toxoplasma serology should be tested as well. If a diagnosis can be made from this evaluation, appropriate treatment should be initiated. Additional steps include further imaging of the brain (e.g., MRI with contrast dye) or brain biopsy, depending on the findings of the imaging study.

A diagnosis of cryptococcal meningitis is made using serum cryptococcal antigen tests and confirmed by lumbar puncture with culture or tests for CSF antigen. Treatment is with amphotericin B, 0.7 mg/kg per day intravenously, with or without flucytosine, 100 mg/kg per day orally, for 10 to 14 days, followed by fluconazole, 400 mg orally twice daily for 2 days, then 400 mg orally every day for 8 to 10 weeks. An alternative regimen is fluconazole, 400 mg/day orally for 6 to 10 weeks. Regardless of initial therapy, maintenance therapy with fluconazole, 200 mg/day, is required for life.

Toxoplasmic encephalitis is usually diagnosed by finding multiple ring-enhancing lesions on CT scan or MRI in a patient with positive toxoplasma serology. Response to empiric therapy of pyrimethamine, 100 to 200 mg loading dose, then 50 to 100 mg/day orally; sulfadiazine, 4 to 8 g/day orally; and folinic acid, 10 mg/day orally, confirms the diagnosis. Corticosteroids should be avoided, if at all possible, because lymphoma responds to corticosteroids and confuses the clinician. The treatment is for 6 weeks or more, with maintenance therapy required for life.

SEPSIS The same algorithm outlined for catheter-related bloodstream infections can be used for HIV-infected patients with the sepsis syndrome. If another source is obvious, empiric antibiotics should be directed at the likely pathogens, based on that source of sepsis. If no source is obvious, broad-spectrum antibacterials are used. In a recent survey of nosocomial infections, HIV-infected patients with CD4 counts of more than 200/μL were at higher risk for acquiring bloodstream infection than the NNIS population.[57] Patients with CD4 counts of less than 200/μL were felt to be protected by TMP/SMX prophylaxis for PCP. The risk of acquiring other nosocomial infections was not greater in the HIV-infected population.

Organ Transplantation

Organ transplant recipients are immunosuppressed for a variety of reasons.[58] These include use of immunosuppressive drugs to minimize rejection of the transplant, broken mucocutaneous barriers (e.g., from catheters), infection with immunomodulating viruses (i.e., CMV, Epstein-Barré virus, hepatitis B and C viruses, HIV), and metabolic derangements. In general, the approach to infection in the organ transplant recipient is similar to that already outlined for immunocompetent patients. Pulmonary infection is known to be the most common infection encountered in this group. The risk should be stratified by time from transplantation. In the first month after transplant, the vast majority of infections are nosocomial bacterial infections of the lungs or candidal and bacterial wound, urinary tract, or vascular catheter infections. The approach to each has already been outlined. In the period from 1 to 6 months after transplant, the doses of immunosuppressive drugs are higher than in ensuing months and many of the immunomodulatory viruses reactivate endogenously or from the transplanted organ. When CMV is transplanted with the solid organ into the previously nonimmune host, it reactivates in that organ and causes clinical disease in the recipient. In concert with this reactivation, opportunistic pathogens emerge including *Listeria monocytogenes, Nocardia asteroides, Mycobacterium tuberculosis, Pneumocystis carinii, Asperillus fumigatus, Cryptococcus neoformans,* and far less commonly than in AIDS, *Toxoplasma gondii.*

In the recipient of a bone marrow allograft, CMV reactivates and replicates in pulmonary macrophages. The engrafted marrow recognizes pulmonary macrophages, which are supporting replication of CMV, as being more foreign and hence CMV pneumonitis parallels graft versus host disease.

Once the recipient has survived 6 months past the transplant date, the risk of infection is similar to the general population with the exception of those undergoing recurrent or chronic rejection. This puts them back into the 1- to 6-month risk group.

ANTIMICROBIAL RESISTANCE

Drug-resistant organisms are isolated more commonly from patients in the ICU than from general hospital or community patients.[59] Bacteria with resistance to antibiotics are prevalent in the ICU because of the use of broad-spectrum antibiotics. When a patient is treated with an antibiotic, their normal flora is suppressed, allowing the nosocomial organisms, which are transferred between patients on the hands of personnel or on devices, to take over the mucosal surfaces. These nosocomial organisms survive in the ICU because of their antibiotic resistance. In addition, via genetic transfer, they can donate resistance genes to organisms from another strain. Furthermore, these nosocomial organisms adhere, via a biofilm, to the tubes and catheters that are inserted into the patients. If a specific patient has not received antibiotics, he or she is less likely to be colonized by resistant organisms because the presence of normal flora excludes the nosocomial organisms. Physicians caring for patients in the ICU should be familiar with risks of infection with resistant organisms and preventative measures. The best ways to curb the spread of resistance are observing good infection control practices (chiefly wearing gloves and washing hands between patient encounters) and limiting the use of and appropriate selection of antibiotic agents. The Society for Healthcare Epidemiology of America and Infectious Diseases Society of America have published guidelines for the prevention of antimicrobial resistance.[60]

To treat infections caused by resistant organisms, it is first essential that a physician be familiar with local rates of resistance. If MRSA has not yet become a significant problem in a given hospital, vancomycin should not be a part of the empiric therapy for nosocomial infections in the ICU. The following national rates may be useful, but do not substitute for local data.

Methicillin-Resistant Staphylococcus aureus

S. aureus is a major cause of nosocomial infections in the ICU, especially VAP and catheter-related bloodstream infection. *S. aureus* resistance to methicillin is mediated through an altered penicillin-binding protein (mec A). Among the resistant bacterial species, it is the most virulent pathogen. In a 1997 surveillance study of more than 5,000 isolates causing bloodstream infection from multiple centers in the United States and Canada, methicillin resistance was found in 26.2% of U.S. isolates.[61] It was present in 46.7% of isolates from the ICU collected by the NNIS in 1998.[62] The characteristics of patients at highest risk for infection with MRSA are that they are older people, have recently been hospitalized, have severe underlying disease, have recently used antibiotic agents, and are on mechanical ventilation for pneumonia.[63]

Vancomycin is the treatment of choice in MRSA infection. Newer agents such as quinupristin-dalfopristin (Synercid) or linezolid are likely to prove clinically useful in the future. Vancomycin should be used as part of empiric therapy in patients at high risk for MRSA infection in hospitals where the prevalence is high.

Vancomycin-Resistant Enterococci

Vancomycin-resistant enterococcus (VRE) was first reported in the mid-1980s. Since then, the prevalence of VRE has steadily increased. The NNIS Antimicrobial Resistance Surveillance Report found that in the first 11 months of 1998, 23.9% of enterococcal isolates from the ICU were vancomycin-resistant.[62] Increasing vancomycin use has led to increasing resistance. Risk factors for infection with VRE include proximity to patients infected with VRE, hospitalization in an ICU, immunocompromised status, and exposure to antibiotics, including vancomycin, cephalosporins, metronidazole, and clindamycin.[64] Barrier isolation and the use of devoted medical instruments, such as individual glass thermometers and stethoscopes, is indicated. Most importantly, extremely careful hand-washing after patient contact is required.

Resistance is conferred through an alternate set of genes that encode for enzymes that synthesize new cell-wall precursors. These cell-wall precursors end in D-alanine-lactate, instead of the usual D-alanine-alanine, which is the binding site of vancomycin.

The importance of VRE infection is debated. In general, enterococci are not virulent organisms. They chiefly cause UTI and abdominal wound-related bacteremia. Some strains are susceptible to tetracyclines, chloramphenicol, rifampin, or ciprofloxacin, and several of these used in combination are sometimes effective. There are several drugs that show promise for activity against VRE. These include quinupristin/dalfopristin (Synercid), oxazolidinones, and everninomycin. The greatest risk with VRE is that it will confer its resistance, which can be found in genes on a transposon or on chromosomes, to other species of bacteria.

Drug-Resistant Streptococci

Drug-resistant *S. pneumoniae* (DRSP) is a fairly recent entity in the United States. In 1989 the rate of penicillin-resistance overall was 3.8%.[65] Virtually all of this was intermediate resistance; minimum inhibitory concentration (MIC) is 0.12 to 1 μg/mL. By 1992 the combined intermediate-level and high-level resistance (MIC, > 1 μg/mL) rose to 17.8%. A 30-center surveillance study found 24.6% resistance, with a full one-third being high-level in 1994.[66] The most recent prevalence study, conducted with more than 1600 isolates from the U.S. and Canada in 1997, revealed an overall penicillin-resistance rate of 43.8%, with 27.8% intermediate and 16.0% high-level.[67] In this study, 18.1% of the organisms were resistant to amoxicillin; 4%, to cefotaxime; 11.7% to 14.3%, to macrolides; and 19.8% to TMP/SMX. The rate of increase is alarming.

Penicillin resistance is mediated by alterations in the penicillin-binding proteins. There is some cross-resistance with all beta-lactam antibiotics. The rise in penicillin resistance has been observed to coincide with a rise in resistance to other classes of antibiotics and multiply resistant strains. This is probably caused by selective pressure of antimicrobial use for a relatively few strains of resistant *S. pneumoniae*.

Risks for DRSP infection have been identified from several population studies. Risk factors include age, recent antimicrobial therapy, coexisting illness or underlying disease, HIV infection, immunodeficient status, recent or current hospitalization, and being institutionalized. Patients in the ICU have some of these factors. The clinical relevance of intermediate and high-level resistance to *S. pneumoniae* is unclear. When empirically treating infections like community-acquired pneumonia in the ICU, awareness of local rates of drug resistance is imperative. In outcome studies, penicillin is effective in cases in which the pneumococci have intermediate resistance and in cases where the pneumococci are highly sensitive. If high-level penicillin resistance is suspected based on local patterns and individual risk factors, vancomycin may be used empirically until susceptibility test results are obtained.

Antibiotic-Resistant Gram-Negative Bacteria

Gram-negative organisms, which seldom cause disease in the community, are major colonizers in ICU patients and, given the right set of circumstances, cause disease in this group. Examples of this include *Pseudomonas aeruginosa* and *Acinetobacter baumanii*. When these organisms first appear as colonizers in the ICU, they are generally susceptible to the aminoglycoside antibiotics, piperacillin, ceftazidime, and imipenem-cilastatin. However, as these patients are given antibiotics to suppress the colonization, greater resistance ensues. In some instances, these organisms become resistant to all available antibiotics. If the clinician uses antibiotics to curb these organisms only when true infection occurs, evolution to complete resistance is slowed.

Klebsiella species are one of the better examples of acquisition of genes that allow emergence of resistance. *Enterobacter* species transfer resistance genes to the members of the *Klebsiella* tribe, which become resistant to all the beta-lactam antibiotics. Controlling the use of these antibiotics often eliminates the organisms from the ICU.

Stenotrophomonas maltophilia is a nonfermenting gram-negative bacterium, which is highly antibiotic-resistant and rarely causes infection in the community or in normal hosts. It has become an important organism in the ICU largely because it is resistant to imipenem-cilastatin and aminoglycosides. It causes ventilator-related pneumonia, bacteremia, and UTI. It is sensitive to high doses of TMP/SMX, ticarcillin-clavulanate, and unpredictably, to certain beta-lactam agents. In vitro susceptibility test results do not predict in vivo success.

ANTIBIOTICS

Penicillins

The penicillin class of antibiotics contains many different drugs that are useful in the treatment of infections in the ICU.[68] They share a mechanism, which is inhibition of synthesis of the bacterial cell wall and activation of the endogenous autolytic system of bacteria. The class shares its adverse effect profile. Most common is allergic or hypersensitivity reaction, occurring in 3% to 10% of the general population. These reactions can range from rash to anaphylaxis and include drug fever and interstitial nephritis. Less commonly psuedomembranous colitis, hepatotoxicity, seizures, and hypokalemia may occur. Most penicillins are not metabolized, are excreted by the kidneys, and require dose adjustment in renal failure (except for oxacillin, nafcillin, and ureidopenicillins).

AMINOPENICILLINS (AMPICILLIN, AMOXICILLIN, BACAMPICILLIN) The aminopenicillin (ampicillin, amoxicillin, bacampicillin) group is notable for its activity against gram-negative bacteria. There is activity against *S. pneumoniae* (but with growing resistance), *Hemophilus influenzae*, enterococci, and gram-negative bacteria, such as *E. coli* and *Proteus* and *Listeria* species. Absent from the spectrum is activity against *S. aureus* and *Klebsiella, Serratia, Enterobacter,* and *Pseudomonas* species. UTI with susceptible organisms may be treated with ampicillin.

PENICILLINASE-RESISTANT PENICILLINS (OXACILLIN, NAFCILLIN) The penicillinase-resistant penicillins (oxacillin, nafcillin) have a narrow spectrum of activity for gram-positive organisms. They are the treatment of choice for infections with *Staphylococcus* species. There is no activity against gram-negative bacteria. There is spreading resistance in *S. aureus*, a major ICU pathogen. In susceptible strains, this class is an excellent choice for the treatment of bloodstream infection, sinusitis, and pneumonia.

UREIDOPENICILLINS (PIPERACILLIN, MEZLOCILLIN, AZLOCILLIN) Ureidopenicillins (piperacillin, mezlocillin, azlocillin) have activity against most major gram-negative ICU pathogens, including *E. coli* and *Klebsiella, Serratia, Proteus,* and *Pseudomonas* species. They retain activity against streptococci and enterococci, but not beta-lactamase–producing *S. aureus* or *H. influenzae*. There is additional coverage against many anaerobic bacteria. Piperacillin is an excellent choice in the empiric treatment of gram-negative pneumonia or sinusitis, in combination with an aminoglycoside.

AMPICILLIN-SULBACTAM The spectrum of this drug, while broad, lacks coverage for many *E. coli* and for *Pseudomonas* and *Serratia* species. It should not be used empirically in critically ill patients with suspected bacteremia or pneumonia.

PIPERACILLIN-TAZOBACTAM Tazobactam adds to the activity of piperacillin by including methicillin-sensitive *S. aureus*, *E. coli,* and most *Klebsiella* species, which are resistant to piperacillin, and many anaerobic bacteria. This is an excellent drug for empiric coverage of sepsis from an unknown source or as a second-line agent in pneumonia, sepsis, or UTI.

Cephalosporins

The cephalosporin class of antibiotics is among the most used in the ICU.[69] The mechanism of action is the same as penicillin, i.e., binding to penicillin-binding proteins in the cytoplasmic membrane of bacteria and interfering with cell-wall synthesis. They also activate the autolytic system of bacteria. The drugs are generally well-tolerated, even though the known adverse effects are numerous. One to three percent of patients have a hypersensitivity or allergic reaction to the drug.

Anaphylaxis is rare. *C. difficile* colitis may be seen after cephalosporin use. Uncommon effects include eosinophilia, thrombocytopenia, nausea, vomiting, and hypoprothrombinemia and thrombophlebitis with intravenous administration. Cephalosporins are generally excreted in the urine and should be dose-adjusted in renal failure. The spectrum is given here for representative members of each generation that are commonly used in the ICU. No member of the class is a reliable agent against anaerobic infections.

FIRST-GENERATION (CEFAZOLIN) Cefazolin has a very narrow spectrum of antibacterial activity. It is active against MRSA and also *E. coli, Klebsiella pneumoniae*, and *Proteus mirabilis*. It may be used for the treatment of bacteremia, pneumonia, or sinusitis with proven-sensitive *S. aureus*.

SECOND-GENERATION (CEFUROXIME) Cefuroxime has better activity than cefazolin against *E. coli, Klebsiella* species, and *P. mirabilis*. It has less activity against *S. aureus*, but adds coverage for *S. pneumoniae*. Again, many of the common ICU pathogens are not covered. In general, there is little use for this drug in the ICU setting.

THIRD-GENERATION (CEFTRIAXONE, CEFTAZIDIME) Ceftriaxone has activity against *S. pneumoniae, Klebsiella, E. coli, P. mirabilis*, and *H. influenzae*. It is active against the typical bacteria that cause community-acquired pneumonia in the ICU. Many physicians use a macrolide with ceftriaxone to include the "atypicals" in the spectrum. A fluoroquinolone may be substituted for the macrolide. Ceftriaxone's lack of pseudomonal coverage prevents its empiric use for infections acquired in the ICU.

Ceftazidime has activity similar to that of ceftriaxone against *Hemophilus* or *Moraxella* species and adds pseudomonal coverage. However, it lacks effective activity against *S. pneumoniae* or anaerobes, so it should not be used for community-acquired pneumonia. It may be used empirically in combination with another anti-pseudomonal drug for gram-negative sinusitis, gram-negative ventilator-associated pneumonia, sepsis of unknown cause, and neutropenic fever.

FOURTH-GENERATION (CEFEPIME) Cefepime is the other cephalosporin with activity against *Pseudomonas* species. It has enhanced activity against *S. pneumoniae*. Its uses are similar to ceftazidime. It may be used as monotherapy for neutropenic fevers, if catheter-related bloodstream infection is not suspected.

Vancomycin

Vancomycin has very important use in the ICU, but it is often overused. Because of its virtually universal activity against gram-positive organisms, it is a mainstay of empiric therapy in the ICU. Its overuse, however, leads to the selection of resistant organisms. The mechanism of action is inhibition of cell-wall synthesis. Vancomycin binds to a peptide precursor of the cell wall, preventing the synthesis of peptidoglycan.[70]

Vancomycin is cleared from the body almost entirely through glomerular filtration. A dose adjustment is required in patients with renal failure, and peritoneal dialysis and hemodialysis do not clear the drug. The major reason to monitor drug levels is to assure, in the critically ill patient, that sufficient levels are maintained. Peak-and-trough drug concentrations should be measured for patients with renal failure, those concomitantly on aminoglycosides, and critically ill patients far above or below their ideal body weight.[71]

Gram-positive aerobic and anaerobic organisms are covered by vancomycin, including MRSA and *Corynebacterium, Bacillus,* and *Clostridium* species. It is most useful in the ICU for the treatment of serious infections with bacteria that are resistant to all other drugs, such as some strains of *S. aureus,* enterococci, coagulase-negative staphylococci, and *Corynebacterium* species. Because *S. aureus* is such a prevalent pathogen in the ICU, vancomycin is used empirically in hospitals with a high incidence of MRSA. However, in spite of its spectrum, it is not as effective against MSSA as oxacillin or cefazolin. Furthermore, it is not as effective against penicillin-sensitive bacteria as any of the penicillins, so its use should be restricted to those gram-positive organisms that are resistant to other antibiotics.

The "red man syndrome" is pruritis, erythema, angioedema, and hypotension, caused by nonimmunologic release of histamine. The incidence is decreased by slow infusion of vancomycin (over 60 minutes). It is unclear whether vancomycin causes ototoxicity and nephrotoxicity or simply potentiates the ability of other drugs to do this. Uncommon adverse effects include drug fever, rash, agranulocytosis with high cumulative doses, and thrombophlebitis related to the infusion.

Aminoglycosides

The aminoglycosides remain an important drug in the ICU because of its broad gram-negative coverage and the need to empirically treat for *Pseudomonas* species infection with two drugs. They are bacteriocidal by binding to the 30S subunit of ribosomes, preventing protein synthesis. This requires energy-dependent transport of the drug across the outer bacterial membrane.[72]

Most of the drug is excreted by glomerular filtration. Dose must therefore be adjusted in patients with renal failure. Approximately half of the serum level of aminoglycosides is cleared effectively with hemodialysis. Therefore, aminoglycosides should be administered after dialysis sessions. In traditional administration every 8 hours, toxicity has been associated with high trough concentrations in the blood. However, this may reflect the fact that renal tissue has become saturated and serum levels increase just before the creatinine level begins to rise, rather than just high trough concentrations "cause" renal failure. The concentration of aminoglycoside in the blood is altered by many variables, including age, sepsis, ascites, burns, fluid status, and renal function.[73] Most patients in the ICU have at least one of these confounding factors, and the volume of distribution is likely to change with the course of illness. This is why we advocate the use of traditional dosing with regular monitoring of concentration of the drug in the blood in the ICU. The use of once-daily dosing regimen has the potential for increasing toxicity, even though in a general medical population the toxicity has been proven equal to traditional dosing.

Aminoglycosides are effective against most gram-negative anaerobes, including *Klebsiella*, *Pseudomonas*, *Acinetobacter*, and *Serratia* species. There is activity against coagulase-negative staphylococci. Aminoglycosides may be used synergistically with beta-lactam antibiotics against enterococci, group A and B streptococci, and *S. viridans*. Aminoglycosides are a mainstay in the empiric treatment of ICU-related infections, such as ventilator-associated pneumonia, sinusitis, sepsis of unknown cause, and gram-negative UTI.

The most common side effects of treatment are nephrotoxicity, ototoxicity, and neuromuscular blockade. Nephrotoxicity is a result of binding to receptors on the proximal tubular cells; it usually manifests 4 to 7 days after initiation of drug therapy and is almost always reversible after discontinuation of therapy. Nephrotoxicity usually produces a nonoliguric decrease in creatinine clearance and is potentiatied by volume depletion, age, and co-administration of vancomycin, amphotericin B, or furosemide.[74] Ototoxicity and vestibular toxicity result from accumulation of drug or metabolite in hair cells of the organ of Corti or ampullar cristae. Risks include loud ambient noise, duration of therapy, high trough concentrations in the blood, and concomitant administration of vancomycin or loop diuretics. Neuromuscular blockade is associated with rapid increase of drug concentration. With administration of aminoglycoside over at least 30 minutes, this adverse effect is rare.

Fluoroquinolones

The development of new agents in the fluoroquinolone class has increased the importance of this drug class in the treatment of infections in the ICU. There is potential for misuse, however, which may lead to the emergence of resistance. Quinolones bind to topoisomerase II (an enzyme found only in bacteria), which inhibits the supercoiling of DNA.

There are multiple excretion pathways for the quinolones. The doses are generally not adjusted for hepatic failure, and those agents that are predominantly renally excreted are only dose-adjusted for severe renal impairment (ofloxacin, lomefloxacin). None of the agents is effectively cleared with hemodialysis.[75]

The fluoroquinolones are generally safe, with few side effects. Some patients experience nausea, vomiting, diarrhea, headache, or dizziness. Arthropathy has been found in dog models, and this is the reason that fluoroquinolones are not approved for use in children. Arthropathy is a rare finding in adults. Hepatotoxicity has also occurred in treatment with quinolone agents.

CIPROFLOXACIN Ciprofloxacin has excellent activity against the Enterobacteriacea, including *Pseudomonas* species. It is not an effective agent for community-acquired pneumonia, because of the lack of activity against *S. pneumoniae*. In the

ICU, it is well-suited to treatment of gram-negative UTI, gram-negative sinusitis, or as part of an empiric regimen for VAP-related infection.

Imipenem

Imipenem is a beta-lactam antibiotic with an extended spectrum of activity. It is useful in the treatment of life-threatening infections in the ICU. The mechanism of bacterial killing is attachment to penicillin-binding proteins. Its molecular size allows entry into the periplasmic space of gram-negative bacteria, and its structure gives it resistance to most beta-lactamases.[76]

The drug is renally cleared and dose must be adjusted for severe renal impairment. Additional doses must be given after hemodialysis. The most common adverse effects are nausea, vomiting, and diarrhea. There is a spectrum of possible allergic reactions, as there are with other beta-lactam antibiotics. There is a risk of seizure that is greater with higher dosing and in patients with underlying neurologic disease.

Before the introduction of newer generation fluoroquinolones, imipenem was the antibiotic with the broadest spectrum available, because of its affinity for multiple penicillin-binding proteins found in different species of bacteria. Anaerobic organisms are very susceptible, with the exception of C. difficile. Imipenem is ineffective against MRSA and Enterococcus faecium. It has excellent activity against the important gram-negative pathogens in the ICU, including Pseudomonas species, although resistance quickly develops if the agent is not used in combination with another antipseudomonal drug.

Imipenem is generally reserved as an alternative drug in severe infections. Its value is greatest for infections in which first-line therapy has failed or against bacteria that are resistant to other agents. It may be used as an alternative in the empiric treatment of neutropenic fever, VAP infection, sinusitis, and sepsis of unknown cause.

Aztreonam

Aztreonam is a monobactam antibiotic with an affinity for the penicillin-binding protein 3, found exclusively in gram-negative bacteria, which accounts for the drug's spectrum of activity. It is useful as an alternative to aminoglycosides.

Aztreonam is a very safe drug. The most common side effects are local reactions, rash, diarrhea, nausea, and vomiting.[77] It is active against most gram-negative ICU pathogens, including Pseudomonas species, but with the exception of Acinetobacter species.

Fluconazole

Fluconazole is a useful antifungal agent in the ICU. The mechanism of action is interference with synthesis and permeability of fungal cell membranes.[78] The enzymatic conversion of lanosterol to ergosterol, a major component of most fungal membranes, is inhibited. The most common use in critical care is treatment of candidiasis. There may be treatment failures against C. krusei or C. glabrata.

Fluconazole has excellent bioavailability when taken orally and should only be used intravenously when there is impairment of gut absorption. Most of the drug is excreted by the kidneys, and dose adjustment is required in patients with renal failure. Fluconazole is safe and well-tolerated. Most commonly, patients experience GI distress. There may be headache or mild elevation of transaminase level. Fluconazole increases the plasma concentration of theophylline, warfarin, cyclosporine, phenytoin, zidovudine, and oral hypoglycemics when used in combination.

Amphotericin B

Amphotericin B has traditionally been the first-line agent for most serious fungal infection, despite its considerable toxicity. It binds to ergosterol in the cell membranes of fungi, which alters permeability, allowing cellular contents to leak out and resulting in cell death. Virtually all fungi that cause disease are susceptible to amphotericin B.

Toxicity occurs acutely with infusion or chronically with cumulative doses. The acute reactions include fever, chills, rigors, malaise, nausea, vomiting, headache, hypertension, and hypotension. Premedication with 400 to 600 mg of ibuprofen or with aspirin, acetaminophen, diphenhydramine, meperidine, or hydrocortisone may relieve these effects in some patients. Nephrotoxicity is the most serious chronic effect. The mechanism is not well understood. Between 20% and 30% of patients receiving the drug experience a rise in serum creatinine level. Renal failure is almost always reversible with discontinuation of the drug. There is a protective effect of sodium administration before infusion of amphotericin B. Most patients receiving the drug require supplementation of potassium and magnesium. Other chronic effects include anemia, CNS disturbances (including delirium), depression, tremors, vomiting, and blurred vision.[79]

The half-life of amphotericin B is extremely long, and serum concentrations are not altered significantly in hepatic or renal failure. Clearance is unchanged with dialysis. The liposomal or lipid complex form is usually substituted in patients with renal failure. However, experience indicates that creatinine levels often peak at 3.0 g/dL, even when standard amphotericin B therapy is maintained, and renal failure usually reverses when therapy is discontinued.

Three alternate formulations of amphotericin B are currently available for use: amphotericin B lipid complex (ABLC), amphotericin B cholesteryl sulfate complex (ABCD), and liposomal amphotericin B. Each has proven less nephrotoxic compared with amphotericin B deoxycholate. Because of the enormous difference in cost compared with amphotericin B deoxycholate, the alternate formulations are generally reserved for patients with renal insufficiency before treatment, patients in whom acute renal failure develops while receiving amphotericin B deoxycholate, and patients in whom treatment fails with the traditional agent.

Amphotericin B, in any of its forms, remains the first-line therapy for life-threatening fungal infection. It is used for invasive aspergillosis, disseminated candidiasis with fluconazole-resistant strains, empiric treatment of patients with fever and neutropenia, and cryptococcosis. A summary of commonly used antimicrobials and their dosages is provided in Table 6–24.[80]

SUMMARY

Infectious diseases cause much morbidity and mortality in the intensive care unit. Intimate knowledge of your local antibiotic resistance patterns as well as familiarity with the diagnostic considerations discussed in this chapter are essential

TABLE 6–24 Intravenous Dosages for Commonly Used Antimicrobials

Drug	Normal Adult Dose	Renal Failure Parameter	Renal Failure Dose
Penicillins			
Ampicillin	1 g q4–6h[a]	Cr Cl: 10–50	q6–12h
	1.5 g q4h[b]	< 10	q12–24h
		HD	Supplement post-HD
Nafcillin	1 g q4h[c]		No change
	1.5–2 g q4h[b]		
Piperacillin	3–4 g q4–6h	Cr Cl: 20–40	3–4 g q8h
		< 20	3–4 g q12h
		HD	2 g q8h with 1 g post-HD
Ampicillin-sulbactam	1.5–3 g q6h	Cr Cl: 30–50	1.5–3 g q6–8h
		15–29	1.5–3 g q12h
		5–14	1.5–3 g q24h
Piperacillin-tazobactam	3.375 g q6h	Cr Cl: 20–40	2.25 g q6h
	4.5 g q6h[d]	< 20	2.25 g q8h
		HD	2.25 g q8h plus 0.75 g post-HD
Cephalosporins			
Cefazolin	0.5–1 g q8h	Cr Cl: 10–49	0.5–1 g q12h
		< 10	0.5–1 g q24–48h
Cefuroxime	0.75–1.5 g q8h	Cr Cl: 10–29	0.75–1.5 g q12h
		< 10	0.75 g 24h
		HD	May use supplemental dose post-HD
Ceftriaxone	1–2 g q12h	HD	500 mg q24h (not meningitis)
Cefepime	1–2 g q12h	Cr Cl: 30–60	1–2 g q24h
		11–29	0.5–1 g q24h
		< 10	0.25–0.5 g q24h
		HD	Repeat dose post-HD

(continued)

TABLE 6–24 Intravenous Dosages for Commonly Used Antimicrobials (continued)

Drug	Normal Adult Dose	Renal Failure Parameter	Renal Failure Dose
Ceftazidime	1–2 g q8–12h[a]	Cr Cl: 10–50	500 mg q24–48h
	2 g q8h[b]	< 10	500 mg q48–96h
		HD	1 g/week
Fluoroquinolones			
Ciprofloxacin	400 mg q12h	Cr Cl: 30–50	200–400 mg q12h
		5–29	200–400 mg q18h
		HD	200 mg q12h
Levofloxacin	500 mg q24h	Cr Cl: 10–50	250 mg q24h
		< 10	125–250 mg q24h
		HD	125 mg q24h
Trovafloxacin	200–300 mg q24h		No change
Miscellaneous			
Vancomycin	1 g q12h	Cr Cl: 40–90	q24h
		20–40	q48–72h
		< 20	Re-dose
		HD	q5–7d
Gentamicin[g]	2 mg/kg[e]	Cr Cl: 51–90	60–90% q8–12h
	1.7–2 mg/kg q8h[f]	10–50	30–70% q12h
		< 10	20–30% q24–48h
		HD	Give ½ loading dose post-HD
Imipenem	500 mg q6–8h[c]	Cr Cl: 21–40	250 mg q6h
	500 mg q6h[b]	6–20	250 mg q12h
Aztreonam	1–2 g q8h[c]		1–2 g[e]
	2 g q6h[b]	Cr Cl: 10–30	1 g q8h[f]
		HD	500 mg post-HD
Antifungals			
Fluconazole	400 mg q24h		400 mg[e]
		Cr Cl: 21–50	200 mg q24h[f]
		11–20	100 mg q24h[f]
		HD	400 mg post-HD
Amphotericin B	0.3–1 mg/kg/day	Cr Cl: < 10	0.5–1 mg/kg q24–36h
ABLC	5 mg/kg/day		No change
ABCD	3–5 mg/kg/day		No change
Liposomal	3–5 mg/kg/day		No change

[a]Moderate-to-severe disease.
[b]Severe disease.
[c]Moderate disease.
[d]Pseudomonas sp. infection.
[e]Loading dose.
[f]Maintenance dose.
[g]Follow blood levels of drug continuously.
ABBREVIATIONS: Cr Cl, Creatinine clearance, given in mL/min/1.73m^2; HD, patient on hemodialysis.

to management of these infectious diseases. With future advances in antibiotic therapy and diagnostic testing we can look forward to reducing the harm to our patients.

REFERENCES

1. Centers for Disease Control and Prevention (CDC) National Nosocomial Infections Surveillance System (NNIS). NNIS report: Data summary from October 1986 to April 1998, issued June 1998. www.cdc.gov/ncidod/hip
2. Centers for Disease Control and Prevention. Nosocomial infection surveillance, 1984. CDC surveillance summaries. *MMWR* 1986;35(1SS):17SS–29SS.
3. Vincent JL, Bihari DJ, Suter PM, et al. The prevalence of nosocomial infection in ICUs in Europe. *JAMA* 1995;274:639–644.
4. O'Grady NP, Barie PS, Bartlett JG, et al. Practice parameters for evaluating new fever in critically ill adult patients. *Crit Care Med* 1988 26:392–408.
5. Craven DE, Kunches LM, Lichtenberg DA, et al. Nosocomial infection and fatality in medical and surgical ICU patients. *Arch Intern Med* 1988;148:1161–1168.
6. Kollef MH, Silver P. Ventilator-associated pneumonia: An update for clinicians. *Respir Care* 1995;40:1130–1140.
7. Centers for Disease Control and Prevention. Guidelines for prevention of nosocomial pneumonia. *MMWR* 1997;46(No. RR-1).
8. Huxley EJ, Viroslav J, Gray WR, et al. Pharyngeal aspiration in normal adults and patients with depressed consciousness. *Am J Med* 1973;64:564–568.
9. Cook DJ, Reeve BK, Guyatt GH, et al. Stress ulcer prophylaxis in critically ill patients: resolving discordant meta-analyses. *JAMA* 1996;275:308–314.
10. Cook DJ, Guyatt GH, Leasa D, et al. A comparison of sucralfate and ranitidine for the prevention of upper gastrointestinal bleeding in patients requiring mechanical ventilation. *N Engl J Med* 1998;338:791–797.
11. Meduri GU, Mauldin GL, Wunderlink RG, et al. Causes of fever and pulmonary densities in patients with clinical manifestations of ventilator-associated pneumonia. *Chest* 1994;106:221–235.
12. Fagon JY, Chastre J, Hance AJ, et al. Evaluation of clinical judgment in the identification and treatment of nosocomial pneumonia in ventilated patients. *Chest* 1993;103: 547–553.
13. Bartlett JG, Breiman RF, Mandell LA, et al. Community-acquired pneumonia in adults: Guidelines for management. *Clin Infect Dis* 1998;26:811–838.
14. Pingleton SK, Fagon JY, Leeper KV. Patient selection for clinical investigation of ventilator-associated pneumonia. *Chest* 1992;102(5)Suppl:553S–556S.
15. Fishman A, Elias JA, Kaiser LR, et al. *Pulmonary diseases and disorders*, 3rd ed. New York: McGraw-Hill, 1998.
16. Marquette CH, Copin MC, Wallet F, et al. Diagnostic tests for pneumonia in ventilated patients: Prospective evaluation of diagnostic accuracy using histology as a diagnostic gold standard. *Am J Respir Crit Care Med* 1995;151:1878–1888.
17. Rello J, Gallego M, Mariscal D, et al. The value of routine microbial investigation in ventilator-associated pneumonia. *Am J Respir Crit Care Med* 1997;156:196–200.

18. Jourdain B, Joly-Guillou ML, Dombret MC, et al. Usefulness of quantitative cultures of BAL fluid for diagnosing nosocomial pneumonia in ventilated patients. *Chest* 1997;111:411–418.
19. Chastre J, Fagon JY, Bornet-Lesco M, et al. Evaluation of bronchoscopic techniques for the diagnosis of nosocomial pneumonia. *Am J Respir Crit Care Med* 1995; 152:231–240.
20. Papazian L, Autillo-Touati A, Thomas P, et al. Diagnosis of ventilator-associated pneumonia. *Anesthesiology* 1997;87(2):268–276.
21. Marquette CH, Georges H, Wallet F, et al. Diagnostic efficiency of endotracheal aspirates with quantitative bacterial cultures in intubated patients with suspected pneumonia. *Am J Respir Dis* 1993;148:138–144.
22. Papazian L, Martin C, Meric B, et al. A reappraisal of blind bronchial sampling in the microbiologic diagnosis of nosocomial bronchopneumonia. *Chest* 1993;103:236–242.
23. Meduri GU, Wunderink RG, Leeper KV, et al. Management of bacterial pneumonia in ventilated patients. *Chest* 1992;101:500–508.
24. Rouby JJ, Martin De Lassale E, Poete P, et al. Nosocomial bronchopneumonia in the critically ill. *Am Rev Respir Dis* 1992;146:1059–1066.
25. Luna CM, Vujacich P, Niederman MS, et al. Impact of BAL data on the therapy and outcome of ventilator-associated pneumonia. *Chest* 1997;111:676–685.
26. Kollef MH, Ward S. The influence of mini-BAL cultures on patient outcomes. *Chest* 1998;113:412–420.
27. Alvarez-Lerma F and the ICU-Acquired Pneumonia Study Group. Modification of empiric antibiotic treatment in patients with pneumonia acquired in the ICU. *Intens Care Med* 1996;22:387–394.
28. The choice of antibacterial drugs. The medical letter on drugs and therapeutics. 1998;40(1023):33–42.
29. American Thoracic Society. Hospital-acquired pneumonia in adults: Diagnosis, assessment of severity, initial antimicrobial therapy, and preventative strategies. A consensus statement. *Am J Resp Crit Care Med* 1996;153:1711–1725.
30. Raad I. Intravascular catheter-related infections. *Lancet* 1998;351:893–898.
31. Pearson ML, Hierholzer WJ, and The Hospital Infection Control Practices Advisory Committee. Guideline for prevention of intravascular device-related infections. *Am J Infect Control* 1996;24:262–293.
32. Veenstra DL, Saint S, Saha S, et al. Efficacy of antiseptic–impregnated central venous catheters in preventing catheter-related bloodstream infection. *JAMA* 1999;281: 261–267.
33. Darouiche RO, Raad II, Heard SO, et al, for the Catheter Study Group. A comparison of two antimicrobial-impregnated central venous catheters. *N Engl J Med* 1999; 340:1–8.
34. Platt R, Polk BF, Murdock B, et al. Risk factors for nosocomial urinary tract infection. *Am J Epidemiology* 1986;124(6):977–985.
35. Saint S, Elmore JG, Sullivan SD, et al. The efficacy of silver alloy-coated urinary catheters in preventing urinary tract infection: A meta-analysis. *Am J Med* 1998; 105:236–241.
36. Garner JS, Jarvis WR, Emori TG, et al. CDC definitions for nosocomial infections, 1988. *Am J Infect Control* 1988;16:128–140.
37. Warren JW. Catheter-associated urinary tract infections. *Infect Dis Clin North Am* 1997;11(3):609–621.

38. Jarvis WR. Epidemiology of nosocomial fungal infections, with emphasis on *Candida* species. *Clin Infect Dis* 1995;20:1526–1530.
39. Wenzel RP. Nosocomial candidemia: risk factors and attributable mortality. *Clin Infect Dis* 1995;20:1531–1534.
40. Walsh TJ, Chanock SJ. Diagnosis of invasive fungal infections: Advances in nonculture systems. *Curr Clin Topics Infect Dis* 1998;18:101–142.
41. Pfaller MA, Messer A, Houston A. National epidemiology of mycoses survey: A multicenter study of strain variation and antifungal susceptibility among isolates of *Candida* species. *Diagn Microbiol Infect Dis* 1998;31:289–296.
42. Nolla-Salas J, Sitges-Serra A, Leon-Gil C, et al. Candidemia in non-neutropenic critically ill patients: Analysis of prognostic factors and assessment of systemic antifungal therapy. *Intensive Care Med* 1997;23:23–30.
43. Rex JH, Bennet JE, Sugar AM. A randomized trial comparing fluconazole with amphotericin B for the treatment of candidemia in patients without neutropenia. *N Engl J Med* 1994;331:1325–1330.
44. Phillips P, Shafran S, Garber G. Multicenter randomized trial of fluconazole versus amphotericin B for treatment of candidemia in non-neutropenic patients. *Eur J Clin Microbiol Infect Dis* 1997;16:337–345.
45. Anaissie EJ, Darouiche RO, Abi-Said D. Management of invasive candidal infections: results of a prospective, randomized, multicenter study of fluconazole versus amphotericin B and review of the literature. *Clin Infect Dis* 1996;23:964–972.
46. Talmor M, Li P, Barie PS. Acute paranasal sinusitis in critically ill patients: guideline for prevention, diagnosis, and treatment. *Clin Infect Dis* 1997;25:1441–1446.
47. Shapiro G, Rachelefsky F. Introduction and definition of sinusitis. *J Allergy Clin Immunol* 1992;90:417–418.
48. Manabe YC, Vinetz JM, Moore RD, et al. *Clostridium difficile* colitis: An efficient clinical approach to diagnosis. *Ann Intern Med* 1995;123:835–840.
49. Gilbert DN, Moellering RC, Sande MA. The Sanford guide to antimicrobial therapy. Antimicrobial Therapy, Inc., Vienna, VA, 1998.
50. Hughes WT, Armstrong D, Bodey GP, et al. 1997 guidelines for the use of antimicrobial agents in neutropenic patients with unexplained fever. *Clin Infect Dis* 1997; 25:551–573.
51. Mulinde J, Joshi M. The diagnostic and therapeutic approach to lower respiratory tract infections in the neutropenic patient. *J Antimicrob Chemother* 1998;41(suppl D):51–55.
52. De Palo VA, Millstein BH, Mayo PH, et al. Outcome of intensive care for patients with HIV infection. *Chest* 1995;107:506–510.
53. Lazard T, Retel O, Guidet B, et al. AIDS in a medical ICU: Immediate prognosis and long-term survival. *JAMA* 1996;276(15):1240–1245.
54. Casalino E, Mendoza-Sassi G, Wolff M, et al. Predictors of short- and long-term survival in HIV-infected patients admitted to the ICU. *Chest* 1998;113:421–429.
55. Bartlett JG. 1998 medical management of HIV infection. Johns Hopkins University, Department of Infectious Diseases, Baltimore, MD, 1998.
56. Henson DL, Chu SY, Farizo KM, et al. Distribution of CD4+ T lymphocytes at diagnosis of AIDS: Defining and other HIV-Related Illness. *Arch Intern Med* 1995;155:1537–1542.
57. Stroud L, Srivastava P, Culver D, et al. Nosocomial infections in HIV-infected patients: Preliminary results from a multicenter surveillance system (1989–1995). *Infect Control Hosp Epidemiol* 1997;18:479–485.

58. Fishman JA, Rubin RH. Infection in organ-transplant recipients. *N Engl J Med* 1998;338(24):1741–1751.

59. Hospital Infections Program. Intensive Care Antimicrobial Resistance Epidemiology (ICARE), 1998. www.sph.emory.edu/ICARE/

60. Shlaes DM, Gerding DN, John JF. Society for Healthcare Epidemiology of America and Infectious Diseases Society of American Joint Committee on the Prevention of Antimicrobial Resistance. Guidelines for the prevention of antimicrobial resistance in hospitals. *Clin Infect Dis* 1997;25:584–599.

61. Pfaller MA, Jones RN, Doern GV, et al. Bacterial pathogens isolated from patients with bloodstream infection: Frequencies of occurrence and antimicrobial susceptibility patterns from the SENTRY Antimicrobial Surveillance Program (United States and Canada, 1997). *Antimicrob Agents Chemother* 1998;42(7):1762–1770.

62. Hospital Infections Program, National Center for Infectious Diseases, Centers for Disease Control and Prevention. NNIS Antimicrobial Resistance Surveillance Report, 1998. www.cdc.gov/ncidod/hip/SURVEILL/NNIS.HTM

63. Fagon JY, Maillet JM, Novara A. Hospital-acquired pneumonia: Methicillin resistance and ICU admission. *Am J Med* 1998;104(5A):17S–23S.

64. Moellering RC. Vancomycin-resistant enterococci. *Clin Infect Dis* 1998;26:1196–1199.

65. Campbell GD, Silberman R. Drug-resistant *Streptococcus pneumoniae*. *Clin Infect Dis* 1998;26:1188–1195.

66. Doern GV. Trends in antimicrobial susceptibility of bacterial pathogens of the respiratory tract. *Am J Med* 1995;99(6B):3S–7S.

67. Doern GV, Pfaller MA, Kugler K, et al. Prevalence of antimicrobial resistance among respiratory tract isolates of *Streptococcus pneumoniae* in North America: 1997 results from the SENTRY Antimicrobial Surveillance Program. *Clin Infect Dis* 1998;27:764–770.

68. Wright AJ. The penicillins. *Mayo Clin Proc* 1999;74:290–307.

69. Marshall WF, Blair JE. The cephalosporins. *Mayo Clin Proc* 1999;74:187–195.

70. Wilhelm MP. Vancomycin. *Mayo Clin Proc* 1991;66:1165–1170.

71. McGowan JP. Aminoglycosides, vancomycin, and quinolones. *Cancer Invest* 1998;16(7):528–537.

72. Edson RS, Terrell CL. The aminoglycosides. *Mayo Clin Proc* 1991;61:1158–1164.

73. Lacy MK, Nicolau DP, Nightingale CH, et al. The pharmacodynamics of aminoglycosides. *Clin Infect Dis* 1998;27:23–27.

74. Gilbert DN. Aminoglycosides. In Root RK, Waldvogel F, Corey L, et al, eds. *Clinical infectious diseases, A practical approach.* New York: Oxford University Press, 1999: 237.

75. Lode H, Borner K, Koeppe P. Pharmacodynamics of fluoroquinolones. *Clin Infect Dis* 1998;27:33–39.

76. Hellinger WC, Brewer NS. Imipenem. *Mayo Clin Proc* 1991;66:1074–1081.

77. Brewer NS, Hellinger WC. The monobactams. *Mayo Clin Proc* 1991;66:1152–1157.

78. Terrell CL. Antifungal agents: Part II. The azoles. *Mayo Clin Proc* 1999;74:78–100.

79. Patel R. Antifungal agents: Part I. Amphotericin B Preparations and Flucytosine. *Mayo Clin Proc* 1998;73:1205–1225.

80. Reese RE, Betts RF. *A practical approach to infectious diseases.* Boston: Little, Brown, 1996.

CHAPTER 7

Approach to Nutritional Support

PAMELA R. ROBERTS

INTRODUCTION

In the past 40 years, numerous advances in nutritional support have made it possible to provide nutrition to virtually all patients. The goals of nutritional support for critically ill patients include preserving tissue mass, decreasing usage of endogenous nutrient stores and catabolism, and maintaining or improving organ function (i.e., immune, renal, and hepatic systems; muscle). Specific goals include improving wound healing, decreasing infection, maintaining the gut barrier (decreasing translocation), and decreasing morbidity and mortality—all of which may contribute to decreasing the ICU or hospital stay and hospitalization costs.

NUTRITIONAL ASSESSMENT

Nutritional assessment begins with the patient's history (e.g., information may be available from hospital records, family members, or the patient). Recent weight loss, anorexia, nausea, vomiting, and diarrhea are key symptoms to elicit. Physical examination findings suggestive of nutritional deficiencies (e.g., dermatitis, scaling of the skin, glossitis, poor wound healing) may be present. The body weight of critically ill patients is generally of limited value, because patients may retain excess water and these weights may not correlate with nutritional status. Ideal body weights (IBWs) are frequently more useful; IBWs for adults can be obtained from published normograms or can be estimated as follows.

- IBW for men: Use 106 pounds for the first 5 feet in height and add about 6 pounds for each additional inch of height
- IBW for women: Use 100 pounds for the first 5 feet in height and add about 5 pounds for each additional inch of height
- IBW for men and women over age 50: Add an additional 10% of the calculated ideal body weight.

Anthropometric measurements, such as skin-fold thickness and midarm muscle circumference, are of limited use in critically ill patients. Skin-fold thickness measurements (from the triceps or subscapular area) are a means of estimating body fat, but they are unreliable in the presence of fluid retention. Midarm muscle circumference is used to estimate body protein stores, but this is also unreliable in patients with fluid retention.

Functional tests are traditional measures of nutritional status. Skin tests of immune function (i.e., delayed cutaneous hypersensitivity) are frequently affected by critical illness, which limits their usefulness. Muscle strength assessment of grip or respiratory muscle function correlates with nutritional status, but these assessments have limited utility in the ICU patient.

A number of laboratory tests are used in nutritional assessment. These include measurement of visceral proteins that are produced by the liver, such as albumin, transferrin, prealbumin, and retinol-binding protein (Table 7–1).

Nitrogen excretion is determined from 12- to 24-hour urine collections and measurements of total urinary nitrogen (more accurate than total urea nitrogen level). Therefore, these test results may be unreliable in patients with renal failure or if urine is incorrectly collected. The nitrogen balance is the nitrogen intake minus the nitrogen lost in urine, through the skin and stool, or from fistulas, wounds, or dialysates. The estimate for non-urinary nitrogen excretion is 2 g/day each for skin and stool losses. A negative nitrogen balance is not necessarily detrimental over the short term (i.e., 1 to 2 weeks). Improvement in nitrogen balance suggests that nutritional support is adequate. However, the nitrogen balance may improve as catabolism decreases, despite inadequate nutritional support.

Indirect calorimetry is based on the laws of thermodynamics: the use of energy involves the consumption of oxygen (i.e., $\dot{V}o_2$) and the production of carbon dioxide (i.e., $\dot{V}co_2$), nitrogenous wastes, and water. When matter is converted to heat by the body, measurement of $\dot{V}o_2$ and $\dot{V}co_2$ indirectly reflects the metabolic energy expenditure. Typical studies measure $\dot{V}o_2$ and $\dot{V}co_2$ for 15 to 30 minutes, estimate energy expenditure and respiratory quotient (RQ), and then extrapolate to 24 hours. Following measurements over time allows recognition of changes in the metabolic rate and customization of nutritional support to meet an individual's needs. RQ reflects whole body substrate utilization.

TABLE 7–1 Visceral Proteins Used in Nutritional Assessment

Visceral Protein	Half-Life	Clinical Situations that Alter Protein Needs
Retinol-binding protein	10–12 hr	Increased with renal failure (due to reduced clearance) Decreased in vitamin A deficiency, liver failure, or protein-energy malnutrition
Pre-albumin	2–3 days	Increased in renal failure (reduced clearance) Decreased during the acute response to injury and liver failure
Transferrin	7–8 days	Depends on the iron status of the patient and is affected by blood loss or replacement Decreased by the acute response to injury or liver failure
Albumin	20 days	Decreased when vascular permeability is altered, protein synthesis is decreased, metabolism is increased, resuscitation with fluid or blood products is required, or liver failure is present

Various Body Fuels and their RQ

Fat = 0.70

Protein = 0.80

Carbohydrate = 1.0

The RQ can vary between 0.70 and 1.2. Excess carbohydrate calories result in net fat synthesis and lead to high carbon dioxide production (e.g., RQ of more than 1.0), which should be avoided. Numerous problems are associated with indirect calorimetry. Inaccurate results may occur in indirect calorimetry determinations when the fraction of inspired oxygen (FIO_2) is more than 0.40. In addition, any leak in the system can introduce error (e.g., endotracheal tube cuff leak). Indirect calorimetry determinations are labor-intensive, because a steady state is needed for accurate measurements and this can take an extended period of time to obtain in a critically ill patient. In fact, some authors recommend that three to five measurements per day be averaged to obtain a daily average energy expenditure. Therefore, indirect calorimetry can be associated with high cost, especially if measured frequently.

TIMING OF NUTRITIONAL SUPPORT

Optimal timing for instituting nutritional support must be a clinical decision: it cannot be determined by nutritional assessment indexes because many of the results are altered by critical illness. Optimal timing remains controversial. Some patients tolerate short periods of starvation by using endogenous stores to support body functions. Well-nourished patients (who are not stressed) have actually survived without food for 6 weeks (ingesting only water). Critically ill patients who are hypermetabolic and hypercatabolic can probably survive only a few weeks of starvation before death. Total starvation has no benefit.

Data suggest that outcome can be improved with early and optimal nutritional support. Early nutritional support offers many advantages, such as blunting the hypercatabolic-hypermetabolic response to injury. In numerous studies, patients randomized to receive early versus delayed feeding had decreased infection rates, fewer complications, and a shorter length of stay in the hospital. Animal studies show improved wound healing, improved renal and hepatic function, and decreased bacterial translocation in injury models with early feeding. For improved outcomes, current recommendations include initiation of nutritional support within the first 24 to 48 hours after admission to the ICU.

ENTERAL VERSUS PARENTERAL ROUTE

Enteral nutrition is required for optimal gut function: maintenance of gut barrier and the gut-associated immune system and immunoglobin A (IgA) secretion. Total parenteral nutrition (TPN) contributes to immunosuppression; this is thought to be related to intravenous lipids, which are high in omega-6 long-chain fatty acids. Studies report increased infection rates compared with enteral feeding in patients who have had trauma, burns, surgery, or chemotherapy or radiation therapy for cancer. A higher mortality rate (than with enteral feeding) was reported in patients receiving TPN who have also had chemotherapy or radiotherapy or a burn injury. TPN is not superior to enteral nutrition in patients with inflammatory bowel disease or pancreatitis.

TPN may be beneficial in patients with short-gut syndromes, some types of GI fistulas, or chylothorax. Enteral nutrition is the preferred method of feeding in patients who are receiving chemotherapy and radiation therapy or who have undergone surgery, burns, trauma, sepsis, renal failure, liver failure, and respiratory failure. Parenteral nutrition is indicated when enteral nutrition is not possible (e.g., inadequate small-bowel function). Enteral nutrition is less expensive than parenteral nutrition. Table 7–2 is a comparison of the nutrient sources available in enteral and parenteral nutrition.

Enteral nutrition is the preferred route of nutritional support in both pediatric and adult patients. Delivery of enteral nutrition can be achieved by several routes: oral, gastric tube (i.e., nasogastric or gastric), or by small-bowel feeding tube (i.e., nasoduodenal, gastroduodenal, jejunal). The major complications encountered with administration of enteral nutrition are listed below:

- Aspiration (pneumonia, chemical pneumonitis, ARDS)
- Metabolic derangements (e.g., electrolyte disturbances, hyperglycemia); these are less common than with parenteral nutrition
- Diarrhea
- Misplaced feeding tubes (e.g., pneumothorax, empyema, bowel perforation)
- Overfeeding

TABLE 7–2 Differences in Composition of Parenteral and Enteral Formulations

Nutrient	Parenteral Nutrition	Enteral Nutrition
Carbohydrate sources	Dextrose	Simple sugars, complex starches, and fibers
Nitrogen sources	Amino acids[a]	Amino acids, peptides, intact proteins (whey, casein, soy)
Fats	Long-chain fatty acids (soy-based intra-lipids are primarily omega-6)	Medium-chain triglycerides, long-chain fatty acids (omega-3 or omega-6)
Vitamins	Should be added before administration	Present in formulations
Trace elements	Should be added before administration	Present in formulations

[a]Glutamine is absent; cysteine is present only in a few preparations.

TPN should be used only when enteral nutrition is not possible (e.g., short gut syndrome, chylothorax). Failure of the stomach to empty is not an indication for TPN but rather for a small-bowel feeding tube. Most patients with diarrhea can be managed with enteral nutrition. Overall TPN management is best performed by specially trained nutritional support teams. Initial TPN orders may be based on recommendations in Tables 7–3 and 7–4. TPN is delivered via peripheral or central vein. Major complications associated with TPN administration are listed below:

- Unsuccessful central line placement (pneumothorax, hemothorax, carotid artery perforation)
- Metabolic derangements (hyperglycemia, electrolyte disturbances)
- Immunosuppression
- Increased infection rates (catheter-related sepsis, pneumonia, abscesses)
- Liver dysfunction (fatty infiltration, cholestasis, liver failure)
- Gut atrophy (diarrhea, bacterial translocation)
- Venous thrombosis
- Overfeeding

In addition, TPN lacks some conditionally essential amino acids that are not stable in solution (i.e., glutamine, cysteine). The glucose-to-fat ratio is usually 3:2 to 2:3 (ratio of calories from each source). Larger amounts of glucose (more than 60% of calories) can result in several problems: increased energy expenditure, increased carbon dioxide production, increased pulmonary workload (may delay ventilator weaning), and liver steatosis and can lead to compromise of the immune system.

QUANTITY OF NUTRIENTS

Calories

Energy needs are met by the caloric content of the major nutrients. Lipids provide 9 kcal/g, carbohydrates provide 4 kcal/g, and proteins provide 4 kcal/g. Studies show that most critically ill patients expend 25 to 35 kcal/kg per day.

TABLE 7–3 **Macronutrient Requirements of Adults**

Nutrient[a]	Quantity	% of Total Calories	Initial Formula for 75-kg Patient
Total calories	25 kcal/kg/day	100	≈ 1875 kcal/day
Protein, peptides, and amino acids	1.2–2.0 g/kg/day	15–25	93.75 g/day (375 kcal/day)[b]
Carbohydrates	50% of calories	30–65	235 g/day (940 kcal/day)
Fats	30% of calories	15–30	62 g/day (558 kcal/day)

[a]Micronutrients (vitamins, minerals, and trace elements) should be provided to meet needs and are available in a variety of combination preparations.
[b]Based on 1.25 g/kg/day.

TABLE 7–4 Recommendations for Specific Clinical Situations

Patient Population	Initial Caloric Goal	Protein Goal	Considerations
Major vascular or cardiothoracic surgery	25 kcal/kg/day	1.5 g/kg/day	Immune-enhancing formulas may improve outcomes
Multiple trauma	25 kcal/kg/day	1.5–2.0 g/kg/day	Immune-enhancing formulas may improve outcomes
Severe burns	25–30 kcal/kg/day	1.5–2.5 g/kg/day	Aggressive high-protein regimens with immune-modulating nutrients such as arginine may improve outcomes
Acute renal failure (not on dialysis)	25 kcal/kg/day	1.0–1.2 g/kg/day	Concentrated formulas low in electrolytes are generally preferable
Acute renal failure (on dialysis)	25 kcal/kg/day	1.5 g/kg/day	Protein needs are higher than previously expected because of losses from dialysis
Liver failure	25 kcal/kg/day	1.0–1.2 g/kg/day	Branched-chain amino acids may improve neurologic function; try if patient fails to improve with standard therapy
Inflammatory bowel disease	25 kcal/kg/day	1.0–1.5 g/kg/day	Small-bowel feedings with a peptide-based formula are usually well tolerated
Pancreatitis	25 kcal/kg/day	1.0–1.5 g/kg/day	Jejunal feedings with a peptide-based formula should be attempted before a trial of TPN

ABBREVIATIONS: TPN, total parenteral nutrition.

Resting metabolic expenditure (RME) can be estimated by using the Harris-Benedict equation (Table 7–5).

RME can also be measured by indirect calorimetry. Some authors recommend adjusting RME by multiplying by a correction factor for stress states; however, correction factors frequently overestimate energy needs.

We prefer to initially administer 25 kcal/kg per day of a mixture in which total daily kilocalories are split into 20% protein, 30% lipids, and 50% carbohydrates (Table 7–3). Patients with organ failure or disease may have increased or decreased needs and should be considered individually. Overfeeding (with either

TABLE 7–5 **Harris-Benedict Equation**

Gender	RME (kcal/day)
Men	$66 + (13.7 \times W) + (5 \times H) - (6.8 \times A)$
Women	$665 + (9.6 \times W) + (1.7 \times H) - (4.7 \times A)$

ABBREVIATIONS: RME, resting metabolic expenditure; W, weight in kilograms; H, height in centimeters; A, age in years.

enteral or parenteral nutrients) is accompanied by more adverse side effects than slightly underfeeding during most critical illnesses.

Protein

Most critically ill patients need 1.2 to 2.5 g/kg per day of protein. Protein requirements increase in patients with severe trauma, burns, or protein-losing enteropathies (Table 7–4).

Water

Needs for water vary greatly among patients as a result of differences in insensible losses and GI and urine losses. A reasonable initial estimate of a patient's water requirement is 1 ml/kcal of energy expenditure in adults.

Vitamins

The water-soluble vitamins are ascorbic acid (vitamin C), thiamine (vitamin B_1), riboflavin (vitamin B_2), niacin, folate, pyridoxine (vitamin B_6), vitamin B_{12}, pantothenic acid, and biotin. Vitamins A, D, E, K are fat-soluble. Published recommended daily takes (RDIs) are based on oral intake in healthy individuals. Vitamin needs for critically ill patients have not been determined. Commercial enteral formulas generally supply the RDI (or more) of vitamins (if patients receive the amount of food that reflects their caloric needs). An adult parenteral vitamin formulation was approved by the FDA in 1979 and is available for addition to TPN solutions; this should be added just before administration, since degradation can occur.

Minerals

Minerals—sodium, potassium, calcium, magnesium, and phosphate—are present in sufficient quantities in enteral products; however, they must be provided as supplements with TPN. Special enteral formulas limit electrolytes for patients with renal failure.

Trace Elements

Iron, copper, iodine, zinc, selenium, chromium, cobalt, and manganese are trace elements for which the requirements in critically ill patients have not been determined. Sufficient quantities are thought to be present in enteral products, but they must be provided as supplements in TPN (all except iron can be added to the solution). Deficiencies (e.g., copper, chromium) have been reported in patients receiving long-term TPN. Specific problems are best managed by specially trained nutritional support teams.

SPECIFIC NUTRIENTS

Nitrogen Sources

Nitrogen is best delivered as intact protein (in patients whose digestion and absorption functions are intact) or hydrolyzed protein (in patients with impaired digestion). Protein is absorbed primarily as peptides (66%) and amino acids (33%). Evidence suggests that peptides generated from the diet possess specific physiologic actions. Essential amino acid formulas should be avoided, because they have been linked to a poor outcome compared with both intact protein and peptides.

Some amino acids become essential during critical illness; these are called "conditionally essential amino acids" and include glutamine, cysteine, arginine, and taurine. In addition, some amino acids appear to have specific roles. For example, glutamine is used as a primary fuel by enterocytes and immune cells, and arginine is required for optimum wound healing and immune function. Cysteine and glutamine are needed for synthesis of glutathione. Note that glutamine (and typically cysteine) are not present in TPN solutions because of stability issues. Branched-chain amino acids (BCAA) may improve mental status in patients with hepatic encephalopathy, because they are primarily metabolized by peripheral muscle instead of the liver.

Lipids

Linoleic acid is an essential fatty acid; humans need 7% to 12% of total calories supplied as linoleic acid. It is an omega-6 polyunsaturated, long-chain fatty acid (which has been shown to be immunosuppressive) and is a precursor to membrane arachidonic acid. The soy-based lipids used in TPN formulations are omega-6 fatty acids. The omega-3 polyunsaturated fatty acids (PUFA) are found in fish oils and linolenic acid; they decrease production of dienoic prostaglandins (i.e., PGE_2), TNF, IL-1, and other pro-inflammatory cytokines. The medium-chain triglycerides (MCTs) are a good energy source and are water-soluble. MCTs enter the circulation via the GI tract. Short-chain fatty acids (SCFA) (e.g., butyric and propionic acid) are a major fuel for the gut (especially the colon) and are derived from metabolizable fibers, such as pectin and guar.

Some enteral formulas have been designed as high-fat formulas and are being marketed as a product for decreasing the respiratory quotient (RQ). However, unless a patient is overfed, these have little effect on carbon dioxide production. A problem with these formulas is that they are tolerated poorly by the GI tract and may lead to bloating and diarrhea.

Carbohydrates

Starches and sugars are a good energy source. Fiber has several benefits. Metabolizable fiber is converted to SCFA by bacteria in the colon. Other fiber sources add bulk, which increases stool mass, softens stool, adds body to stool, and provides some stimulation of gut mass.

Nucleic Acids

Dietary nucleic acids (e.g., RNA) may be necessary for immune function and are added to some immunity-enhancing formulations.

NUTRITION FOR SPECIFIC CONDITIONS

This section discusses patients with specific conditions that change their nutritional needs (Table 7–4).

Acute Renal Failure

For enteral nutrition in patients with acute renal failure, use of an intact protein or peptide formula with a moderate level of fat is recommended. Protein intake should not be restricted, because adequate nitrogen is required for healing and for other organ functions. The current protein intake recommendation for a critically ill patient with acute renal failure and on hemodialysis is 1.5 g/kg per day. Patients on continuous renal replacement therapies may need more than 1.5 g/kg per day. Fluid intake may be limited with a double-strength formula (2 kcal/mL). Electrolyte levels (potassium, magnesium, phosphate) should be monitored carefully; enteral formulas with limited electrolytes are available.

Hepatic Failure

The current recommendations are to use an intact protein or peptide formula in patients with hepatic failure. Usually protein levels of 1.0 to 1.2 g/kg daily are needed to support repair and immune function. BCAA may be of value if encephalopathy persists after use of intact protein or peptide diets: these are more expensive and have not been proven efficacious.

Inflammatory Bowel Disease

Post-pyloric enteral feeding of a peptide-based diet is usually well-tolerated in patients with inflammatory bowel disease. Enteral nutrition should be attempted before initiating TPN.

Pancreatitis

Recent trials report that jejunal enteral feeding of a peptide-based diet is well-tolerated in patients with severe pancreatitis. Patients with less severe pancreatitis can frequently be managed with oral nutritional support after 1 to 3 days of bowel rest. Current evidence indicates that enteral nutrition should be attempted before initiating TPN in the overwhelming majority of these patients.

Wound Healing

Sufficient quantities of specific nutrients are needed for healing. Nutrients believed to be important in wound repair include vitamin A, vitamin C, zinc, arginine, and copper. Requirements for some of these nutrients increase in critical illness. Pharmacologic quantities of arginine improved wound healing in numerous animal studies and increased collagen deposition in humans.

Thermal Injury

Many studies have examined nutritional support in patients with thermal injury. These patients generally have higher energy expenditures and protein losses and needs than other groups of critically ill patients and are expected to need 30 to 35 kcal/kg daily and 2.0 to 2.5 grams of protein per kilogram per day. A study of standard nutritional support with and without additional protein found less morbidity and improved survival in the group fed with the high-protein formula. Others reported that patients who were fed enterally throughout all of their surgeries had decreased wound infections in comparison to patients randomized to have their food held perioperatively. Patients with severe burn injuries benefit from aggressive early enteral nutrition.

Infection and Inflammation

Combinations of nutrients with immune function activity, such as arginine, glutamine, omega-3 fatty acids, peptides, and RNA, have been available for the past 10 years. Numerous studies comparing these immunity-enhancing formulas with standard formulas have reported lower rates of infection and decreased length of time on mechanical ventilation and length of ICU stay in the immune formula groups. Several meta-analyses concur that these formulas are beneficial.

Multiple Organ Failure

Nutritional support is usually of marginal value in patients with multiple organ failure; it should be started before organ failure develops.

DETERMINING ADEQUACY OF NUTRITIONAL SUPPORT

Visceral protein levels may be useful monitors of responses to nutritional support (Table 7–1). Pre-albumin levels are responsive to short-term nutritional repletion (e.g., 7 days). Transferrin and albumin levels are slower to improve because they have longer half-lives. Visceral protein levels are affected by nutritional intake and the disease state (e.g., inflammation and renal or hepatic dysfunction). Increasing levels of visceral proteins suggest that nutritional support is adequate. Such levels usually normalize in 1 to 2 weeks if the disease process is controlled and nutritional support is adequate. If visceral protein levels fail to increase, underlying infection, inflammation, or other disease processes should be considered, in addition to re-evaluating the adequacy of nutritional support and considering the possibility of ordering nitrogen balance and energy balance (i.e., indirect calorimetry) studies.

Nitrogen balance studies can determine the level of catabolism and can provide a better estimate of protein needs. Improvement in nitrogen balance test results suggests that nutritional support is adequate. Nitrogen balance may improve as catabolism decreases, despite inadequate nutritional support. Indirect calorimetry goals are to keep the RQ at less than 1. Values over 1 suggest lipogenesis from excessive caloric intake; values of 0.7 are found in starvation and reflect fat oxidation.

GENERAL CONCERNS REGARDING OVERFEEDING

Potential complications from overfeeding have led to recent recommendations for lower total daily caloric intakes (i.e., a goal of 25 to 30 kcal/kg per day) in critically ill adult patients. Complications from overfeeding include liver compromise and increased carbon dioxide production (from lipogenesis), which results in increased ventilatory requirements. A worsened outcome in conjunction with overfeeding has been noted in a number of animal models and some human studies. Indirect calorimetry is potentially useful in prevention of these complications.

GASTROINTESTINAL DYSFUNCTION IN CRITICAL ILLNESS

Oral nutrition is the best form of nutritional support; but in many critically ill patients, this is not feasible. Decreased motility of stomach and colon are common and typically last 5 to 7 days in critically ill patients but may persist longer if patients remain critically ill. Gastric paresis is best assessed and monitored by measuring gastric residual volume. A gastric residual volume of more than 150 mL is usually considered abnormal. Patients with gastric residual volume of more than 150 mL should be fed in the small bowel (post–pyloric valve) to decrease risk of aspiration. Bowel sounds are a poor index of small-bowel motility. Motility and nutrient absorptive capability of the small bowel is usually preserved even after severe trauma, burns, or major surgery.

General Approach to Enteral Feeding in the ICU

1. Enteral nutritional support should be initiated within 12 to 48 hours of admission to ICU (Figure 7–1).
2. If oral feeding cannot be used, the gastric route is the second choice and should be tried in most patients before placing a small-bowel tube (Figure 7–2).
3. Patients at high risk for aspiration or known gastric paresis should be fed using a small-bowel tube.
4. The head of the bed should be elevated at least 30 degrees to decrease the risk of aspiration.
5. Feeding formulas should not be diluted.
6. In adults, feeding should be started at 25 to 30 mL/hr and increased by 10 mL/hr every 1 to 4 hours, as tolerated on the basis of gastric residual volumes remaining at less than 150 mL, until caloric goal is achieved.
7. Gastric residual volume should be monitored every 4 hours.
8. If gastric residual volume in adults is more than 150 mL, hold feeding for 2 hours and then resume.
9. If the protein goal level is not achieved, use a formula with a higher protein-to-calorie ratio or add protein to the formula.
10. Feeding may be increased at slower rate (i.e., 10 mL/hr every 6 to 12 hours) but often this is not necessary.
11. The goal rate of infusion should be met by the third day of therapy (and frequently earlier).
12. The adequacy of nutritional support should be confirmed after 5 to 7 days.
13. If visceral proteins or other nutritional indexes suggest that present support is inadequate, consider a nutritional support consultation.
14. Note that current formula osmolalities (300 to 600 mOsm per kilogram of water) rarely cause intolerance or diarrhea.

IMPROVING OUTCOME WITH NUTRITIONAL SUPPORT

Early nutrient administration is vital to achieving optimal results. Enteral nutrition maintains better immune function and produces better outcomes compared with TPN. Specific nutrients can modulate immune function. Recent trials of

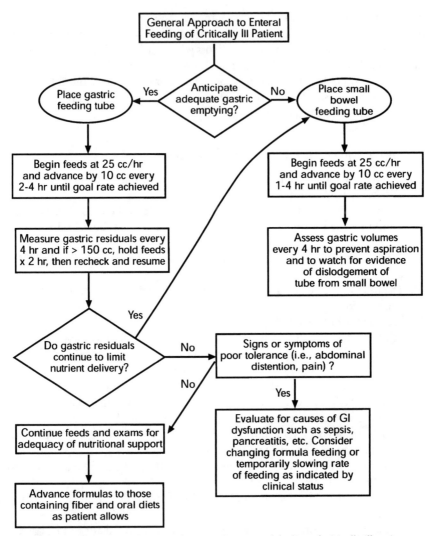

FIGURE 7–1 Flow diagram for general approach to enteral feeding of critically ill patients.

immune-enhancing formulations have reported benefits such as decreases in infections, length of stay, and time on mechanical ventilation for critically ill patients. Several analyses of these trials found improved outcomes in patients randomized to immune formulas and concluded by recommending use of immune formulas in critically ill patients. Currently, little data exists to determine if any of the current formulas are superior to others. These are the first generation of immunity-enhancing enteral formulations, and improvements are anticipated. Mortality rates do not appear to be affected by use of the current formulations. In summary, extensive review of prospective, randomized, clinical trials comparing

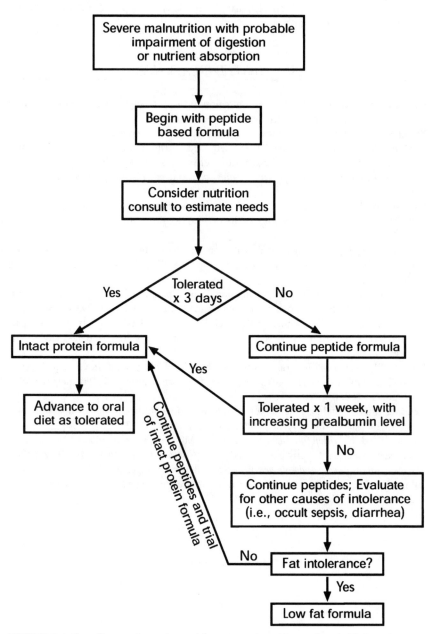

FIGURE 7–2 Flow diagram for patients with severe malnutrition and probable impairment of digestion or nutrient absorption.

early enteral feeding with immunity-enhancing compared with standard enteral diets indicates that these formulas are highly likely to improve outcome and reduce hospitalization costs.

SUGGESTED READINGS

Beale RJ, Bryg DJ, Bihari DJ. Immunonutrition in the critically ill: a systematic review of clinical outcome. *Crit Care Med* 1999;27:2799

Bower RH. Nutrition during critical illness and sepsis. *New Horizons* 1993;1:348.

Cerra FB, Benitez MR, Blackburn GL, et al. Applied nutrition in ICU patients: a consensus statement of the American College of Chest Physicians. *Chest* 1997;111:769.

Grant JP. *Handbook of total parenteral nutrition,* 2nd ed. Philadelphia: W.B. Saunders, 1992.

Kalfarentzos F, Kehagias J, Mead N, et al. Enteral nutrition is superior to parenteral nutrition in severe acute pancreatitis: results of a randomized prospective trial. *Brit J Surg* 1997;84:1665.

Klein S, Kinney J, Jeejeebhoy K, et al. Nutrition support in clinical practice: review of published data and recommendations for future research directions. *J Parent Enter Nutr* 1997;21:133.

Kudsk KA, Croce MA, Fabian TC, et al. Enteral versus parenteral feeding: Effects on septic morbidity after blunt and penetrating abdominal trauma. *Ann Surg* 1992;215:503.

Moore FA, Feliciano DV, Andrassy RJ, et al. Early enteral feeding, compared with parenteral, reduces postoperative septic complications: The results of a meta-analysis. *Ann Surg* 1992;216:172.

Roberts PR, Zaloga GP. Enteral nutrition in the critically ill patient. In Grenvik A, Ayres SM, Holbrook PR, et al., (eds). *Textbook of critical care,* 4th ed. Philadelphia: W.B. Saunders, 2000:875.

Veterans Affairs Total Parenteral Nutrition Cooperative Study Group. Perioperative total parenteral nutrition in surgical patients. *N Engl J Med* 1991;325:525.

Zaloga GP, ed. *Nutrition in critical care.* St. Louis: Mosby Year Book, 1994.

Zaloga GP, Roberts PR. Early enteral feeding improves outcome. In Vincent JL, ed. *Yearbook of intensive care and emergency medicine.* Berlin: Springer, 1997:701.

Zaloga GP. Immune-enhancing enteral diets: where's the beef? *Crit Care Med* 1998;26:1143–1146.

CHAPTER 8

Approach to Cardiac Arrhythmias

ANDREW CORSELLO

JOSEPH M. DELEHANTY

DAVID HUANG

INTRODUCTION

Cardiac arrhythmias are one of the most commonly seen manifestations of cardiac disease in critically ill patients. In patients without established cardiac dysfunction, the milieu of critical illness—with alterations in autonomic tone, electrolyte imbalance, and multiorgan system dysfunction—predisposes the patient to the development of many rhythm disturbances. If the patient has concomitant cardiac disease—such as myocardial ischemia, valvular disease, or ventricular dysfunction—the likelihood of rhythm disturbances is much higher.

BRADYCARDIA

Bradycardia is frequently encountered in the ICU. Maintenance of the heart rate in the normal range is a complex physiologic process involving many neural feedback systems that act at various levels of the cardiac conduction system.

The sinus node is located in the right atrium near the junction of the right atrium and the superior vena cava; it receives its blood supply from the sinus node artery that usually arises from the right coronary artery. The sinus node is heavily innervated by both sympathetic and parasympathetic fibers. Parasympathetic stimulation reduces the rate of depolarization of the pacemaker cells in the sinus node and thereby slows the sinus rate. Conversely, sympathetic stimulation increases the rate of depolarization of the pacemaker cells and causes an increase in the sinus rate. The sinus rate in an individual is determined by the balance of sympathetic and parasympathetic tone and by the intrinsic properties of the node itself.

Excessive vagal tone is a relatively common cause of paroxysmal sinus bradycardia in the ICU. Endotracheal suctioning, abdominal distention, and pain often cause excessive vagal tone and bradycardia. Such events may lead to hemodynamically significant bradycardia, which can be treated effectively with a vagolytic agent, such as atropine. In extreme cases, temporary pacing, either transcutaneously or transvenously, may be required.

Excessive sympathetic tone, leading to sinus tachycardia, is a common tachyarrhythmia seen in the ICU. Inadequate sympathetic tone is much less frequently encountered, but it is still a clinically significant cause of bradycardia. Certain clinical situations in which this can occur deserve mention. Patients who have high thoracic or cervical spine injuries have sustained a loss of cardiac sympathetic innervation, especially in the initial weeks after injury. This may result in profound bradycardia at rest and also in response to any vagal stimulation. This type of bradycardia can almost always be managed with either atropine or low-dose infusions of a sympathomimetic agent, such as isoproterenol, but in extreme cases, pacing, either temporary or permanent, may be necessary.

Intrinsic abnormalities of the sinus node are relatively infrequent but should be recognized. There may be idiopathic degeneration and fibrosis of the sinus node, but sinus node dysfunction may also be a result of a variety of other disease states, such as CAD, long-standing hypertension, collagen vascular disease, myocarditis, or infiltrative diseases (such as a sarcoidosis, amyloidosis, or hemochromatosis). These conditions usually result in an excessive bradycardia or failure to increase the sinus rate in response to a stimulus, such as fever, hypoxia, or release of catecholamines.

A subset of patients with sick sinus syndrome, also referred to as tachybradycardia syndrome, may have periods of supraventricular tachycardia (SVT), usually atrial fibrillation or atrial flutter, followed by a prolonged sinus pause after conversion. These patients usually require pacemaker placement to prevent severe bradycardia, which in turn allows the use of agents to control the heart rate during tachycardia.

In addition to the above-mentioned abnormalities, a variety of drugs influence sinus node function. Digoxin produces bradycardia as a result of its enhancement of vagal tone. Beta blockers, calcium channel blockers, and most of the commonly used antiarrhythmic agents directly reduce the sinus rate. Systemic processes, such as hyperkalemia and hypercapnia, hypothyroidism, increased ICP, hypothermia, and sepsis, may also interfere with normal sinus node function.

HEART BLOCK

The atrioventricular (AV) node is a distinct anatomic structure and is located in the right atrium, immediately above the septal leaflet of the tricuspid valve and anterior to the ostium of the coronary sinus. It receives its blood supply from the AV nodal artery, which in the majority (more than 90%) of cases arises from the right coronary artery. Similarly to the sinus node, both sympathetic and parasympathetic nerves heavily innervate the AV node.

Conduction of the impulse from the sinus node through the AV node is represented on the surface ECG as the PR interval. Most of the PR interval is a result of conduction through the AV node, because the conduction velocity from the sinus node to the AV node is rapid. The conduction velocity through the AV node is determined by a number of factors, including autonomic tone, electrolyte levels, the presence of ischemia, drugs that have been prescribed, and intrinsic changes within the node, such as fibrosis. Given the complexity of control of conduction through the AV node, it is not surprising that abnormalities of AV node function can occur in the critically ill patient.

First-degree AV block is usually the most benign of AV node abnormalities seen and is detected by prolongation of the PR interval on the surface ECG. It may be seen in otherwise normal individuals, but it is often a manifestation of increased vagal tone and, as such, may be seen at the same time as sinus bradycardia in the ICU. First-degree AV block is usually a response to vagotonic stimuli. It is also seen in patients who are treated with drugs that slow conduction through the AV node, particularly digoxin, beta blockers, calcium channel blockers, and most of the commonly used antiarrhythmic agents. First-degree AV block may be seen in acute inferior-wall myocardial infarction (MI) as a result of the reflex increase in vagal tone and ischemia to the AV node. Inflammatory conditions of the heart muscle, such as myocarditis, may also cause first-degree AV block, and it may be seen in endocarditis, specifically aortic-valve endocarditis, where it may be a sign of myocardial abscess formation.

Type I second-degree AV block, also referred to as Wenckebach AV block or Mobitz type I block, is characterized by a progressive lengthening of the PR interval on the surface ECG, followed by a nonconducted P wave. In addition to the progressive lengthening of the PR interval, a progressive shortening of the RR interval is usually seen in patients with type I second-degree AV block. Type I second-degree AV block can be thought of as an exaggeration of first-degree AV block and is almost always a manifestation of increased vagal tone. The block in conduction, when it occurs, is usually at the level of the AV node, and therefore, there is still a functional escape through the bundle of His. Type I second-degree AV block is commonly seen in patients with acute inferior infarction and, unless there are accompanyinig adverse hemodynamics, does not require specific treatment. If treatment is needed, atropine usually produces an adequate response. In rare cases, temporary pacing may be necessary.

Type II second-degree AV block is characterized by the abrupt onset of a nonconducted P wave that is not preceded by a lengthening of the PR interval. Unlike type I second-degree AV block, type II is an ominous event that requires treatment in almost all cases. Type II block is usually a manifestation of a block in the conduction system at or below the bundle of His, and therefore, there may not be a reliable escape mechanism. It is usually not a manifestation of just excessive vagal tone but also of a diseased conduction system.

Type II block occurs much less frequently than type I block in acute MI situations and it has a much worse prognosis. In cases in which there is 2:1 AV block, it is not possible to determine if there is progressive prolongation of the PR interval. In these cases, types I and II AV block can usually be distinguished by the duration of the QRS complex. Because the delay in conduction in type I block is within the AV node, the QRS complex duration is usually normal, whereas it is usually prolonged in Type II block (Figure 8–1).

Atropine may also be used to distinguish the level of block in this setting. If atropine is given and AV conduction improves along with an increase in the sinus rate, the level of block is at the AV node. If, however, AV conduction worsens after atropine is administered, the block is below the level of the AV node.

Complete heart block is defined as the absence of conduction of supraventricular impulses to the ventricle and is manifested on the ECG as a dissociation of atrial and ventricular activity (Figure 8–2). In patients with intact sinus node function, there are P waves at regular intervals but none of these P waves are conducted and the site of the escape mechanism determines the ECG characteristics of the escape rhythm. If the escape mechanism is at the level of the AV node or

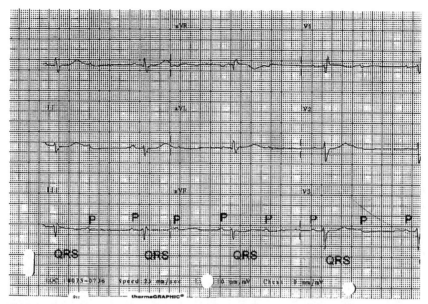

FIGURE 8–1 *Twelve-lead ECG demonstrating 2:1 AV block with wide complex QRS. Although it cannot be definitively determined whether this is type I or type II second-degree AV block, the wide complex QRS strongly suggests type II. The tracing is from an 84-year-old woman who presented with syncope. She subsequently had episodes of complete heart block (see also Figure 8–2).*

bundle of His, the QRS complex may be narrow, unless an underlying bundle branch block (BBB) is present. If the escape mechanism is below the level of the bundle of His, the QRS complex is usually wide.

As with other forms of AV block, complete heart block may be a complication of MI. Complete heart block is an ominous occurrence in the setting of an anterior infarction and is a manifestation of extensive ischemia and necrosis of the conduc-

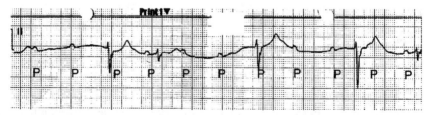

FIGURE 8–2 *Subsequent rhythm strip from patient described in Figure 8–1. The fourth and the last P waves are probably conducted, but the other P waves are nonconducted and have no constant relationship to the ventricular escape rhythm.*

tion system. When complete heart block is complicating inferior infarction, it may be responsive to atropine, but there are cases that are unresponsive to atropine and require temporary pacing (Figure 8–3). In some cases, temporary pacing may be preferable to use of atropine, because atropine may result in tachycardia that may exacerbate ischemia. Some investigators have reported cases of refractory heart block in cases of inferior infarction that responded to administration of aminophylline,[1] and it is thought that, in these cases, the heart block may have been a result of local accumulation of adenosine, which can be antagonized by aminophylline. The so-called Bezold-Jarisch reflex is usually seen in patients with inferior infarctions who are undergoing reperfusion therapy with either thrombolysis or angioplasty. This is a syndrome of profound bradycardia, AV block, and hypotension that is likely to be a result of stimulation of vagal afferent fibers in the inferoposterior wall of the left ventricle, resulting in intense vagal outflow. The hypotension is a result of not only the bradycardia but of the vasodilatory effects of vagal stimulation. This condition is managed by fluid administration, administration of atropine, and appropriate use of temporary pacing.

Complete heart block is also seen in cases of drug toxicity, electrolyte disturbances, and infiltrative diseases of the myocardium. In all such cases, temporary ventricular pacing may be necessary until either the reversible causes have been addressed or until permanent pacing can be accomplished. Some patients with complete heart block or high-grade AV block can be managed with low-dose in-

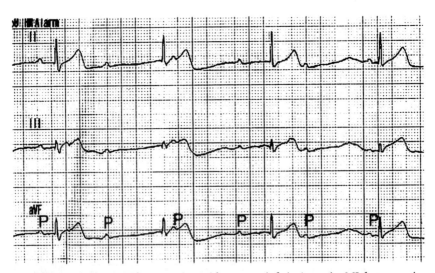

FIGURE 8–3 *Rhythm strip from a patient with an acute inferior/posterior MI demonstrating complete heart block. The heart block was refractory to therapy with atropine and aminophylline and required temporary pacing. After successful angioplasty and stenting of a dominant left circumflex artery, the patient regained normal AV conduction.*

fusions (2 mg/min) of isoproterenol, but care must be used with this agent because it may cause hypotension from peripheral vasodilation and may also precipitate ischemia in patients with underlying CAD. Patients with complete heart block may present with syncope or near syncope, but it is not uncommon to see patients who are minimally symptomatic present with complete heart block and relatively slow escape rhythms. In such patients, careful observation until permanent pacemaker placement is appropriate.

The diagnosis of heart block is definitively made electrocardiographically, but there are clues to the diagnosis on both physical examination and analysis of intravascular pressure tracings. In patients with either high-grade type II second-degree AV block or complete heart block, there are prominent pulsations of the jugular venous pulse waveform that occur when the atrium contracts against a closed tricuspid valve. This "cannon A wave" can be seen on careful analysis of the neck veins, the central venous pressure (CVP) tracing, or even a PAWP tracing in patients who have indwelling catheters.

PACING

Temporary pacing is often the preferred method of treatment for critically ill patients with symptomatic bradycardia. With the advent of transcutaneous pacemakers, pacemakers are being used more frequently. The transcutaneous pacemaker delivers electrical energy across the chest wall through large electrodes. It is effective in capturing the ventricle in most cases, but as would be expected given the fairly large impedance across the chest wall, the currents that must be used are appreciable (an average of 50 to 80 mA).[2] The current required is greater in patients with hemodynamically significant bradycardia than it is in normal patients. While the external pacemaker is a very useful device, it should be tested in all patients in whom it is being used to ensure that it can capture the ventricle. Once it has been tested, it can be set at a low back-up rate to minimize patient discomfort.

Successful capture must be documented during testing. This may be difficult in some cases, because the electrical artifact of pacing is large and may obscure the QRS complex. In these cases, it may be helpful to also document the presence of an arterial pulse accompanying each paced beat.

Transvenous temporary pacing is in general more reliable than transcutaneous pacing but is also more invasive and time-consuming. In addition, the transvenous pacemaker is associated with a higher rate of complications during insertion, including bleeding or infection, pneumothorax, cardiac perforation and tamponade, and transient arrhythmias, particularly ventricular tachycardia. Access for transvenous pacemakers is preferably from the right internal jugular vein or the left subclavian vein. If necessary, the femoral vein can be used as an access site, but it will almost always be necessary to use fluoroscopy to correctly position the pacing wire from the femoral approach. When placing a temporary pacemaker, it is prudent to recognize the patient that will likely need subsequent permanent pacemaker implantation, because that may determine the access site. We currently use a balloon-tipped pacing wire that may be inserted either blindly or by ECG guidance, but if there is time and access to fluoroscopy, we recommend that the wire be placed fluoroscopically. The ideal location is in the apex of the right ventricle, but it may be necessary to have the wire in other locations to achieve good pacing and sensing thresholds. The pacing threshold is defined as the minimal current that is necessary to capture the ventricle. It can be determined by progressively lowering the amplitude of the pacemaker, and determining the amplitude at which capture no longer occurs. This is the pacing threshold, which ideally should be less than 2 mA. The pacing threshold should be tested at least daily while the temporary pacemaker is in place, because it is not uncommon for the wire to migrate and the threshold to change. In most circumstances in the ICU, a temporary pacemaker is used in the ventricular demand mode (VVI mode). This means that the pacemaker detects the intrinsic heart rate and does not pace unless the intrinsic rate is less than the lower rate of the pacemaker. To determine the sensing threshold, set the rate of the pacemaker lower than the intrinsic rate of the patient. The sensitivity of the pacemaker is set in millivolts and is the voltage that must be sensed to inhibit the firing of the pacemaker. The lower the voltage, the more sensitive the pacemaker is. As an illustration, if the pacemaker is set to a sensitivity of 1 mV, it senses any electrical activity of more than 1 mV at the electrode and inhibits pacemaker output. If, on the other hand, the sensitivity is set at 10 mV, the pacemaker is not inhibited unless electrical activity of more than 10 mV is detected. If the sensitivity is too high (i.e., the number of millivolts is too low), it is possible that electrical activity of the heart that does not represent a QRS complex, such as a P wave or a T wave, may be sensed as a QRS complex and the pacemaker will be inappropriately inhibited. The phenomenon of "oversensing" is manifested by failure of the pacemaker to pace when it should and can be corrected by decreasing the sensitivity (i.e., increasing the number of millivolts). "Undersensing" refers to the situation in which the pacemaker does not recognize a QRS complex as such and can lead to inappropriate firing of the pacemaker when it should be inhibited. This is potentially a dangerous situation if the pacemaker fires on a T wave, because it may lead to ventricular tachycardia or fibrillation. Undersensing can be corrected by increasing the sensitivity of the pacemaker (i.e., decreasing the number of millivolts). The sensing threshold can be determined by progressively decreasing the sensitivity to the point where the pacemaker is no longer appropriately inhibited. The level of millivolts at which this occurs is the sensing threshold. The sensing threshold should be set quickly to avoid prolonged inappropriate pacing. Sudden loss of pacemaker function usually means that it's position in the ventricle has changed and requires repositioning under fluoroscopic guidance. The pacemaker should not be blindly repositioned, because this may result in damage to intracardiac structures. There are occasions where either atrial pacing or dual-chamber pacing is appropriate, but this topic is beyond the scope of this discussion.

As mentioned earlier, AV block occurs not infrequently in acute MI. When symptomatic, it requires prompt therapy with either pharmacologic agents or pacing. There are patients who present with acute MI who can be identified as being at high risk for the sudden development of high-grade AV block on the basis of varying degrees of intraventricular conduction delay. One group of investigators[3] found that most patients who develop complete heart block have preceding conduction disturbances. They were able to identify seven risk factors for development of complete heart block, which include: first-degree AV block, type I second-degree AV block, type II second-degree AV block, left anterior fascicular block, left posterior fascicular block, complete right BBB, and complete left BBB. In patients with only one risk factor, the chance of complete heart block was only 1.2%; in those with two risk factors, it was 7.8%; with three risk factors, the rate of progression to complete heart block was 25%; and, in the small number of patients with four or more risk factors, the chance was 36.4%. There is some controversy regarding the use of temporary prophylactic pacing in these patients, since the ultimate prognosis may be determined more by the site and extent of infarction rather than by the development of heart block. Heart block in anterior infarction, for example, is a marker of very extensive myocardial necrosis and the prognosis for the patient is likely to be related to this fact rather than the specific electrical disturbances. Over the past several years, guidelines have been developed for the use of temporary pacing in acute MI; these are shown in Tables 8–1 and 8–2.[4]

SUPRAVENTRICULAR TACHYCARDIA

Tachycardia of various origins occurs often in critically ill patients. Arrhythmias arising from origins above the ventricle have been grouped as SVTs. They typically manifest on ECG tracings as narrow QRS complexes, but sometimes a widened QRS, as discussed elsewhere in this chapter, also occurs. The rate of

TABLE 8–1 Indications for Temporary Transcutaneous Pacing

Class I Indications	Sinus bradycardia with symptoms of hypotension that is unresponsive to drug therapy
	Type II second-degree AV block
	Third-degree heart block
	Bilateral BBB
	Newly acquired or age-indeterminate LBBB, RBBB, and left anterior fascicle block
	RBBB and left posterior fascicle block
	RBBB or LBBB with first-degree AV block
Class IIa Indications	Stable bradycardia without hypotension of hemodynamic compromise
	New or age-indeterminate RBBB
Class IIb Indications	New or age-indeterminate first-degree AV block
Class III Indications	Uncomplicated acute MI with no evidence of conduction system dysfunction

ABBREVIATIONS: AV, atrioventricular; BBB, bundle branch block; LBBB, left bundle branch block; RBBB, right bundle branch block; MI, myocardial infarction.

TABLE 8–2 **Indications for Temporary Transvenous Pacing**

Class I Indications	Asystole
	Symptomatic bradycardia, including sinus bradycardia and type I second-degree AV block that is not responsive to atropine
	Bilateral BBB
	New or age-indeterminate bifascicular block (RBBB with LAFB or LPFB, or LBBB) with first-degree AV block
	Type II second-degree AV block
Class IIa Indications	RBBB with either LAFB or LPFB (new or age-indeterminate)
	RBBB with first-degree AV block
	LBBB, either new or age-indeterminate
	Incessant VT for overdrive pacing
	Recurrent sinus pauses > 3 sec, not responsive to atropine therapy
Class IIb Indications	Bifascicular block of indeterminate age
	New or age-indeterminate RBBB
Class III Indications	First-degree AV block
	Type I second-degree AV block with no hypotension and normal hemodynamics
	Accelerated idioventricular rhythm
	BBB or fascicular block known to exist before acute MI

ABBREVIATIONS: AV, atrioventricular; BBB, bundle branch block; RBBB, right bundle branch block; LBBB, left bundle branch block; LAFB, left anterior fascicular block; LPFB, left posterior fascicular block; VT, ventricular tachycardia; MI, myocardial infarction.

tachycardia can be quite variable, anywhere between 100 beats/min to more than 200 beats/min. Atrial activities may be present on the ECG tracing, although with some types of SVT, distinct atrial activities may not be distinguishable.

The most common forms of SVT encountered are atrial fibrillation and atrial flutter. Other types of SVT include AV nodal reentrant tachycardia, AV reentrant tachycardia that is using a bypass tract, atrial tachycardia, and sinus tachycardia. Each of these tachycardias exhibits characteristics that allow distinguishing among them; however, occasionally it may be difficult to identify the exact mechanism of a SVT on the basis of surface ECG analysis alone. Atrial tachycardia and sinus tachycardia typically have visible P waves preceding each QRS complex, if 1:1 AV conduction is preserved during the tachycardia episode. Atrioventricular nodal reentrant tachycardia and AV reentrant tachycardia often may not have visible P waves.

Atrial fibrillation has been recognized since the early twentieth century. Instead of well-organized impulse propagation through the atria during normal sinus rhythm, the mechanism of atrial fibrillation is thought to result from multiple chaotic circulating loops of electrical impulses within the atria. These reentrant circuits typically function at rapid rates, and are disorganized rapid fibrillatory activities that lead to the characteristic ECG appearance of a fine, undulating baseline without any discrete atrial electrical signals. Furthermore, because of the irregularity of the atrial rate in fibrillation, the conducted ventricular rhythm has a characteristic "irregularly irregular" response (Figure 8–4).

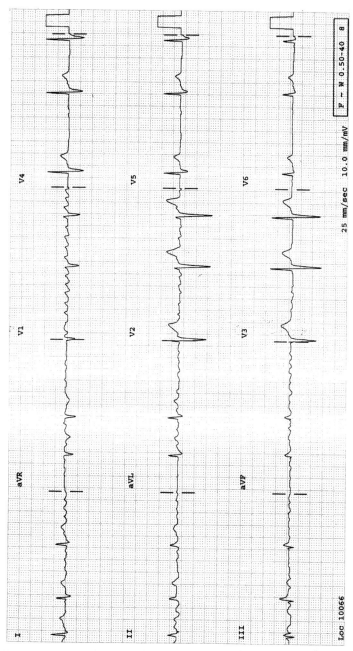

FIGURE 8–4 Twelve-lead ECG from a patient with atrial fibrillation and a controlled ventricular response. Note the chaotic baseline without defined atrial activity. There is a suggestion of a more organized pattern in the V_1 lead, but this is not seen in other leads. The ventricular response is characteristically "irregularly irregular."

Atrial flutter has also been extensively studied electrophysiologically. Unlike the disorderly atrial activities in fibrillation, it is now well-accepted that for most instances of clinically encountered atrial flutter, the electrical impulse circulates around in the right atrium in one large loop. Because atrial flutter is more organized than atrial fibrillation, it displays more organized atrial activities of larger amplitude on ECG. Atrial flutter usually has an associated "sawtooth" pattern, which represents revolving atrial activities and is best appreciated in the inferior limb leads 2, 3, and aVF (Figure 8–5). In typical atrial flutter, the reentrant circuit usually has a well-defined cycle length at about 300 beats/min. Often, there is a 2:1 AV conduction pattern during atrial flutter, leading to a consistently regular ventricular response of 150 beats/min.

Many of the impulses of a SVT can be transmitted down to the ventricle via the AV junction, especially when AV conduction is enhanced by release of catecholamines. The rapid ventricular rate is usually the main problem associated with atrial arrhythmias in the ICU. The fast rates are especially troublesome for patients who have underlying CAD or ventricular hypertrophy, because ischemia and significant hemodynamic compromise can occur rapidly. The goal of therapy in the care of patients with atrial arrhythmia is stabilization of hemodynamics and ventricular rate control. During sustained atrial arrhythmias in a patient with stable blood pressure, AV nodal blocking agents, such as beta blockers, calcium channel blockers, and digoxin, are all effective agents in slowing the ventricular response. Diltiazem can be given intravenously as a bolus at a dose of 5 to 20 mg, which may be followed by an infusion of the same drug at rates of 5 to 20 mg/hr. This allows for rapid control of heart rate and subsequent conversion to oral long-term therapy. Digoxin is also effective, but the onset of action is somewhat longer than that of diltiazem. Digoxin is typically given as a loading dose of 1 mg over the course of 24 hours. We typically give 0.5 mg initially, followed by another 0.25 mg in 4 to 6 hours and a second 0.25 mg in yet another 4 to 6 hours. If there is hemodynamic compromise, then urgent restoration of sinus rhythm with direct-current (DC) energy-synchronized cardioversion is imperative. In addition, if the rapid ventricular response rate during atrial arrhythmia is making conditions such as myocardial ischemia, infarction or congestive heart failure worse, early cardioversion is also indicated.

Pharmacologic antiarrhythmic agents are usually used for chemical cardioversion and maintenance of sinus rhythm, if the patient's blood pressure permits their use. Oral antiarrhythmic agents for atrial fibrillation include class 1a drugs, such as quinidine and procainamide; class 1c drugs, such as propafenone and flecainide; and class 3 drugs, such as sotalol and amiodarone. Procainamide has been the first-line intravenous antiarrhythmic that is traditionally used. More recently, intravenous amiodarone has also been used with success. Intravenous procainamide is typically given as a bolus of 10 to 15 mg/kg of body weight over 20 to 30 minutes, followed by a maintenance infusion at a rate of 1 to 6 mg/min. Care must be taken when administering procainamide intravenously because it may cause significant prolongation of the QT interval and the QRS duration; if given rapidly, it may also

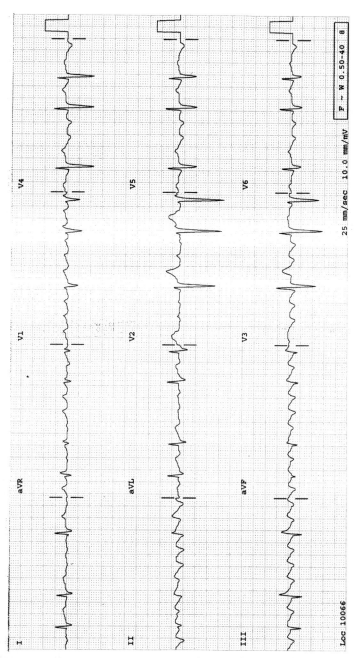

FIGURE 8–5 *Twelve-lead ECG from the same patient in Figure 8–4, now showing a characteristic "sawtooth" pattern that is especially apparent in inferior leads. This patient alternates between atrial fibrillation and "typical" atrial flutter. The rate of the flutter waves is somewhat slower than is usually seen (230/min) as a result of antiarrhythmic therapy.*

cause hypotension. Procainamide should not be given at a rate faster than 50 mg/min. Intravenous amiodarone is usually given in a 150-mg bolus over 10 minutes and may be repeated if ineffective. Then a maintenance infusion of 1 g of amiodarone every 24 hours may be given. A central venous line is recommended with the use of intravenous amiodarone to avoid phlebitis. Intravenous amiodarone has not yet been officially approved as a therapy for supraventricular arrhythmias. Both of these agents can further lower a patient's blood pressure; therefore, close monitoring of patients is mandatory when these agents are used. Intravenous ibutilide has also been reported to be an effective agent for cardioversion, although its conversion rate for atrial flutter is much higher than for atrial fibrillation. Ibutilide may lead to significant QT prolongation and should be avoided in patients with electrolyte imbalance or who are already on agents that can prolong QT intervals, such as phenothiazines. Caution and continuous ECG monitoring must be exercised with the use of ibutilide, because dramatic QT prolongation can lead to torsades de pointes, and potentially convert a nonemergent arrhythmia to one that causes immediate hemodynamic collapse. Intracardiac thrombi and systemic emboli may form in patients with atrial fibrillation or atrial flutter sustained for more than 48 hours. Therefore, if anticoagulant therapy is not contraindicated by concurrent medical problems, it should be initiated for these patients.

Precipitating factors that may lead to atrial fibrillation and atrial flutter should be sought if clinical conditions warrant such concerns. For example, it is well-documented that pulmonary embolism can lead to atrial arrhythmias, especially atrial fibrillation. This may be important in postoperative patients or patients with hypercoagulable states. Other factors that can lead to atrial fibrillation or atrial flutter include hypertensive heart disease, valvular disease, pericarditis, myocarditis, hyperthyroidism, and even fever.

Another supraventricular rhythm disturbance that is seen frequently in the critically ill patient is multifocal atrial tachycardia (MAT), which is a rapid irregular rhythm that is characterized by a rate that exceeds 100 beats/min and has at least three distinct P-wave morphologies. This is most frequently seen in patients with severe underlying lung disease, particularly those receiving inhaled bronchodilators or theophylline preparations. Treatment is difficult and should be aimed primarily toward improving the pulmonary condition. There are several reports on the use of both intravenous metoprolol and intravenous verapamil to control the rate. Caution must be used when giving beta blockers, such as metoprolol, to patients with reactive lung disease; our experience with this agent in this situation has not been successful.

Reentrant SVTs, including AV nodal reentrant tachycardia and AV reentrant tachycardia using a bypass tract, are characterized by regular, narrow complex tachycardia on the surface ECG. It may be possible to identify a retrograde P wave after the QRS complex, particularly in the case where a bypass tract is involved, but if the retrograde conduction is sufficiently rapid, it may not be visible. It may also be difficult to detect a P wave in cases of rapid sinus tachycardia. In these cases, we advise the use of adenosine injections or carotid sinus massage as therapeutic intervention and for diagnostic purposes. The initial dose of adenosine is 6 mg, given as a rapid intravenous injection. If there is no response, a dose of 12 mg may be given. In cases of reentrant SVTs or some atrial tachycardias, the response to adenosine is usually prompt termination of the tachycardia. In the case of sinus tachycardia, however, a brief slowing of the sinus rate is seen, which usually allows identification of distinct P waves.

WIDE COMPLEX TACHYCARDIA

A wide complex tachycardia may lead to serious consequences or it may be a relatively benign occurrence. The correct diagnosis of such a tachycardia is imperative, especially in the critical care setting. A wide complex tachycardia usually arises from a ventricular origin; however, an SVT with aberrant conduction can also manifest as a wide complex tachycardia. Other than ventricular fibrillation, ventricular tachycardia is the most ominous tachyarrhythmia involved in the care of patients in the ICU. Because it may lead to rapid hemodynamic collapse, prompt intervention is necessary. SVT often is better tolerated, although significant hemodynamic compromise can occur quickly as well. Hemodynamic stability in conjunction with a wide complex tachycardia does not rule out ventricular tachycardia. Equally important is an understanding of the consequences of both pharmacologic and nonpharmacologic therapy for wide complex tachycardia to avoid potentially harmful interventions. Some of the drugs used for the management of SVT, such as calcium channel blockers, may lead to adverse consequences in a patient with ventricular tachycardia. Therefore, in the ICU, all wide complex tachycardia should be assumed to be ventricular in origin until it can be ruled out with a high degree of certainty, especially in patients with known cardiac disease.

Distinguishing ventricular tachycardia from SVT with aberrant conduction on the basis of surface ECGs can be difficult, especially because recordings from only one or two leads are often all that is available. There are some findings that may be helpful in diagnosis of the origin of a wide complex tachycardia.

"Atrioventricular dissociation," or evidence of separate atrial and ventricular activities, should always be sought in the patient with a wide complex tachycardia tracing. This is manifested as P waves and QRS complexes that are temporally unrelated. The P waves, or atrial ECGs, are often difficult to discern and may be present in any part of the cardiac cycle, including parts of the QRS complex or T waves. Techniques to amplify the amplitude of the atrial activities, such as esophageal leads or even placement of a transvenous electrode, may be helpful. Although the presence of AV dissociation is not completely diagnostic for ventricular tachycardia, it does make a ventricular tachycardia highly likely. The presence of a 1:1 AV relationship is consistent with either SVT or ventricular tachycardia and cannot be used to distinguish one from the other.

Another phenomenon to look for is the presence of a "fusion" beat, i.e., a combined QRS complex resulting from impulses originating from two different areas of the heart. A combination, or fused, QRS complex between a beat originating in the ventricle and one from a supraventricular site is more reliable for the diagnosis of ventricular tachycardia (Figure 8–6). Typically, this is seen in ventricular tachycardia with relatively slower rates, allowing time for the supraventricular impulses to conduct down to the ventricle.

When possible, a 12-lead ECG should be obtained for further information in differentiating the origin of the tachycardia. There are well-tested morphologic criteria for wide complex tachycardias of both right and left BBB–type patterns in patients in whom the origins of tachycardia were confirmed by invasive electrophysiology studies.

If the QRS morphology in a wide complex tachycardia displays a right BBB–type pattern and, in lead V_1, the initial R wave (the initial positive deflection) is dominant, the tachycardia is likely to be of ventricular origin. This can be seen either as a monophasic R wave in V_1 or as the first initial positive deflection (R) being taller than the second positive deflection (r′). In a wide complex tachycardia with a right BBB–type pattern, an R wave amplitude of less than the S wave in lead V_6 suggests ventricular tachycardia. In tachycardias displaying a left BBB–type pattern delay in the initial forces with a broadened r wave (r > 0.04 sec), notches in the initial QRS downstroke in lead V_1 suggest ventricular tachycardia. Furthermore, during tachycardia with a left BBB–type pattern, a q wave present in lead V_6 makes it likely that the tachycardia is of ventricular origin.[5]

Basic premises for these criteria are that the more fragmented the initial QRS forces are and the wider the QRS duration is, the more likely there is a ventricular origin of the tachycardia. This results from muscle-to-muscle conduction during ventricular tachycardia rather than conduction down to the ventricles through specialized His and Purkinje tissues during SVT. These criteria were tested in patients who did not have existing BBBs or Wolff-Parkinson-White syndrome. Furthermore, these criteria probably cannot be relied on for patients on antiarrhythmic therapy, because many of these drugs can alter cardiac conductivity and thereby affect the initial forces of the QRS complex patterns and duration.

Another criterion on 12-lead ECGs that suggests a ventricular origin of a wide complex tachycardia is concordance of the QRS pattern in the precordial leads (V_1 through V_6).[6] Both positive concordance (i.e., all QRS complexes in V_1 though V_6 display monophasic R waves) and negative concordance (i.e., all precordial QRS complexes display monophasic QS patterns) are suggestive of ventricular tachycardia. Negative concordance is diagnostic for ventricular tachycardia, but positive concordance may, rarely, result from tachycardia involving an accessory AV bypass tract. Table 8–3 summarizes the criteria that are useful for distinguishing the cause of a wide complex tachycardia.

Cycle length variability is not a useful diagnostic criterion for wide complex tachycardias. While it is true that atrial fibrillation conducted with aberration displays an irregularly irregular pattern, the rate of a ventricular tachycardia can often

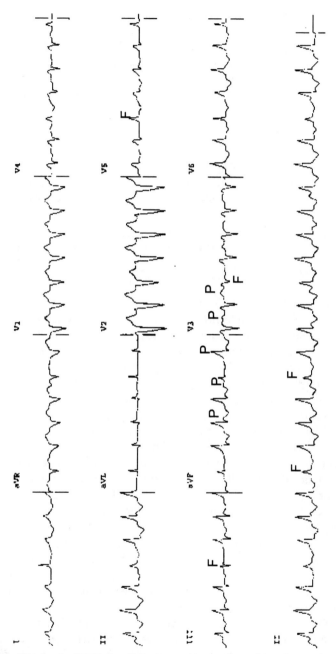

FIGURE 8-6 *Twelve-lead ECG demonstrating a wide complex tachycardia. P waves (P) can be seen dissociated from the QRS in what is termed AV dissociation. In addition, fusion beats can also be detected (F). The combination of AV dissociation and fusion beats is, in almost all cases, diagnostic of ventricular tachycardia.*

TABLE 8–3 Criteria for diagnosis of etiology of wide complex tachycardia based on Qrs morphology.[8]

	Aberration	VT
RBBB	QRS $\leq$ 0.12 sec	QRS $\geq$ 0.14 sec
	Axis: Normal	Axis: Superior
	V_1: rsR' or rR'	V_1: R, Rr', RS
	V_6: R/S > 1	V_6: R/S < 1
LBBB	QRS $\leq$ 0.14 sec	QRS $\geq$ 0.16 sec
	Axis: normal or leftward	Axis: rightward
	Lead V_1 or V_2: R < 0.04 sec	Lead V_1 or V_2: r $\geq$ 0.04 sec
	Onset to nadir: < 0.07 sec	Onset to nadir: $\geq$ 0.07 sec
	Smooth downstroke	Notch on downstroke
	V_6: No Q wave	V_6: Q wave

ABBREVIATIONS: VT, ventricular tachycardia; RBBB, right bundle branch block; LBBB, left bundle branch block.

be irregular as well. Similarly, it has been suggested that alternating cycle length may be a marker for certain forms of SVT, but alternating cycle length variations have been well described in patients proven to have ventricular tachycardia.

Always compare a patient's baseline ECG to the one obtained during wide complex tachycardia. If a BBB pattern is present during sinus rhythm and the tachycardia displays a BBB pattern of the alternate bundle, then the tachycardia is very likely to be ventricular. As mentioned, the wider the QRS duration, the more likely that the tachycardia is of ventricular origin. Interestingly, a wide complex tachycardia with QRS duration shorter than the conducted QRS is almost always caused by ventricular tachycardia. These tachycardias often are originating from a septal region, and the left and right ventricles are activated in a more simultaneous fashion than a supraventricular impulse conducted down to the ventricle with a bundle branch conduction block.

Other than ECGs, clinical physical examination may also help in distinguishing ventricular tachycardia from SVT with aberrant conduction. The presence of "cannon A waves," resulting from atrial contraction against closed AV valves, during inspection of the jugular pulse suggests the presence of AV dissociation and, therefore, ventricular origin of the tachycardia. Variations in the intensity of the first heart sound (S_1) and splitting of S_1 during auscultation as a result of ventricular dyssynchrony also suggest ventricular tachycardia.

Characteristics of a wide complex tachycardia may provide important clues about the underlying cardiac pathology. Patients with transmural scars from infarctions or cardiomyopathy from various causes have a substrate for reentrant monomorphic ventricular tachycardia, or a wide complex tachycardia displaying a consistent QRS morphology from beat to beat. On the other hand, insufficient myocardial arterial supply or increased myocardial demand may lead to electrophysiologic instability within the myocardium, resulting in ventricular fibrillation or polymorphic ventricular tachycardia, a wide complex tachycardia with varying QRS morphologies. Therefore, recognition of the different ventricular arrhythmias as manifestations of the underlying cardiac pathophysiology can help in choosing the proper therapeutic and management interventions.

Urgent intervention for a wide complex tachycardia is often needed as a result of the hemodynamic effects. If hemodynamic collapse is evident or if blood pressure is unstable, countershock with DC energy is required. There are other clinical indications for relatively urgent DC cardioversion as well. These include ischemia or infarction, angina, and severe heart failure. If a patient's blood pressure is stable, then the various criteria may be applied to distinguish ventricular and supraventricular origin of the tachycardia and a decision for appropriate therapy may be applied.

Traditionally, intravenous lidocaine is the first antiarrhythmic used for ventricular tachycardia. Under ischemic conditions, such as during the infarction period, ventricular arrhythmias often are manifested as polymorphic ventricular tachycardia (Figure 8–7) or ventricular fibrillation. Under these circumstances, intravenous lidocaine is reasonably effective and it should be considered as a first-line agent. For nonacute infarction or non–ischemia-related ventricular arrhythmias, typically manifested as a monomorphic ventricular tachycardia (with consistent beat-to-beat QRS morphology), several clinical reports have suggested that intravenous procainamide may be more effective for termination than lidocaine.[9] Intravenous amiodarone has become widely available over the past few years. Data are becoming available suggesting its effectiveness in terminating and suppressing ventricular arrhythmias.[10] Amiodarone probably is superior in comparison to lidocaine or procainamide for ventricular arrhythmia management. However, it may have a profound blood pressure–lowering effect and its use should be accompanied by cautious hemodynamic monitoring.

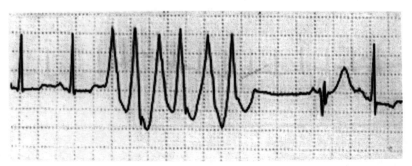

FIGURE 8–7 *Rhythm strip showing 6-beat run of polymorphic ventricular tachycardia. There is a variable morphology to the QRS complexes of the tachycardia. This is often seen in the patients with ischemia.*

The use of adenosine has been advocated as a diagnostic tool for distinguishing ventricular origins from supraventricular origins in a wide complex tachycardia. Adenosine has vasodilator effects and a possible "steal" phenomenon in the coronary circulation; this may induce myocardial ischemia and lead to further hemodynamic compromise. Even though the half-life of adenosine is brief, its effects in patients with severe CAD may trigger a cascade of hemodynamic effects that may become irreversible. Therefore, we recommend that the use of adenosine as a diagnostic measure for wide complex tachycardia must be taken with caution, especially in patients with known severe coronary disease. Unless it is absolutely certain that the diagnosis is SVT, calcium channel blockers, such as diltiazem or verapamil, should not be used to treat wide complex tachycardias because there are a multitude of reports detailing hemodynamic collapse in patients with ventricular tachycardia who were treated with these agents.[7]

TORSADES DE POINTES

Torsades de pointes is a subtype of polymorphic ventricular tachycardia that should be recognized because it has distinct diagnostic and therapeutic implications that differ from other types of wide complex tachycardia. A French term meaning "twisting of the points," torsades de pointes has an appearance similar to rapid QRS axis shifting. It is usually characterized by prolonged QT intervals, and it is often initiated with a premature ventricular extrasystole occurring on or around the T wave of the preceding beat. Known causes of torsade de pointes typically include conditions that prolong the QT interval, such as congenital long QT interval syndrome; electrolyte imbalances, such as hypokalemia, hypomagnesemia, or hypocalcemia. Drugs that prolong the QT interval are also known to lead to torsades de pointes; these include class Ia and III antiarrhythmic drugs and some antihistamines and psychotropic medications. Table 8–4 lists a number of causes of prolongation of the QT interval and torsades de pointes. Care should be paid to patients with decreased clearance of any of these suspect medications as well as any combinations that may compound the prolongation of the QT interval. Remember that bradycardia may prolong the repolarization process, and thus the QT interval. The effects of these precipitants are more pronounced and the risk of torsades de pointes is higher in patients with bradycardia.

If sustained, the acute intervention for torsades de pointes, as with all wide complex tachycardia with hemodynamic instability, is countershock with DC energy. Once a stable rhythm has been restored, the major goal of the therapy is to shorten the QT interval as much as possible. This obviously includes removal of the offending agent or correcting the underlying conditions. Sometimes cardiac pacing or the use of an isoproterenol infusion may be necessary to further decrease the ventricular repolarization time, especially if bradycardia is present. If the episodes of torsades de pointes are not sustained, then, in addition to the above interventions, empiric intravenous magnesium therapy has been suggested.

TABLE 8–4 Causes of prolongation of QT interval and torsades de pointes

Drugs	Electrolyte Abnormalities	Congenital
Quinidine, procainamide, sotalol, amiodarone	Hypokalemia	Jervell and Lange-Nielsen syndrome
Tricyclic and tetracyclic antidepressant agents	Hypocalcemia	Romano-Ward syndrome
Phenothiazines Haloperidol (Haldol)	Hypomagnesemia	
Antihistamines		
Macrolide antibiotics		
Pentamidine		
Serotonin antagonists		
Adenosine		
Cocaine		
Cisapride		
Arsenic poisoning		

TOXIC AND METABOLIC CAUSES OF ARRYTHMIAS

The medical ICU often serves as the stabilization site for patients after life-threatening overdoses and severe metabolic disturbances. These conditions can result in cardiac rhythm disturbances that require prompt recognition and treatment. Adequate suspicion, proper interpretation of the ECG, and complete knowledge of the specific emergency treatments are part of the armamentarium of the ICU physician. Some of the most commonly encountered problems, discussed here, include hyperkalemia and hypokalemia, hypercalcemia and hypocalcemia, and hypothermia; overdoses of a tricyclic agent or digitalis; and acquired torsades de pointes.

Hyperkalemia

Hyperkalemia may be caused by a number of processes, including acidosis from any cause, acute renal failure, iatrogenesis, and hemolysis. Life-threatening elevations in potassium levels can be a complication of the patient's original problem or of treatment they received during their admission. Because hyperkalemia often causes no symptoms in itself, the ECG tracing must be relied on to define the clinical implications of hyperkalemia and the urgency of treatment.

The ECG changes of hyperkalemia are variable and depend not only on the severity but also on the chronicity of the elevation in serum potassium level. Although a close correlation exists between the potassium level and ECG changes in animal models, the relation is less clear in clinical cases. Abnormal potassium levels affect P waves, the QRS complex, and T waves. P-wave voltage decreases as a result of slow intra-atrial conduction with low-amplitude atrial depolarization and the PR interval lengthens. With severe widening and attenuation of the P wave, there may be no atrial depolarization seen on the surface ECG, so the erroneous diagnosis of a junctional rhythm may be made. Type I or II second-degree AV block may also occur. As the QRS complex widens, the normally sharp contour of the QRS becomes wider and eventually merges with the T wave, until no ST segment exists. The T wave becomes symmetrically peaked, the entire QRST complex can resemble a sine wave, and the QT interval usually remains normal or short (Figure 8–8).

When any of these abnormalities are present on the ECG tracing, treatment becomes emergent. Measurement of the serum potassium level should not delay immediate treatment, which should follow within seconds of the recognition of the characteristic ECG pattern. The initial treatment of hyperkalemia should include administration of 1 to 2 amps (10 ml, 10% calcium gluconate) of calcium gluconate to promote membrane stabilization. Calcium should only be withheld in cases of digitalis intoxication or critical hyperphosphatemia. After this, intravenous insulin and glucose (10 U of regular insulin and at least 50cc of 50% dextrose, depending on the serum glucose) plus sodium bicarbonate (8.4%) should be given to drive potassium into intracellular space. Since these measures do not reduce whole body potassium level, they should be followed by treatment, such as dialysis and potassium-binding resins (e.g., sodium polystyrene sulfonate, 30 to 60 g), to drive down whole body potassium levels in situations of whole body overload.

Hypokalemia

The cardiac and ECG manifestations of hypokalemia can be subtle but the arrhythmias are life-threatening nonetheless. Mild potassium deficiency causes a prolongation of the QTU interval and increases cardiac electrical instability, predisposing the patient to atrial and ventricular arrhythmias. In patients with severe deficiency of potassium, U waves become prominent, T waves decrease in amplitude, and torsades de pointes may occur. Concurrent magnesium deficiency worsens the arrhythmic effects of potassium deficiency and creates a refractoriness to potassium replenishment. Replenishment of potassium is the only therapy for potassium depletion, and details of restoring potassium levels are discussed elsewhere.

Hypothermia

Severe hypothermia requiring ICU admission can cause characteristic ECG changes. After the body temperature falls below approximately 30°C to 32°C, patients often become bradycardic and Osborne waves (also called J waves) occur.

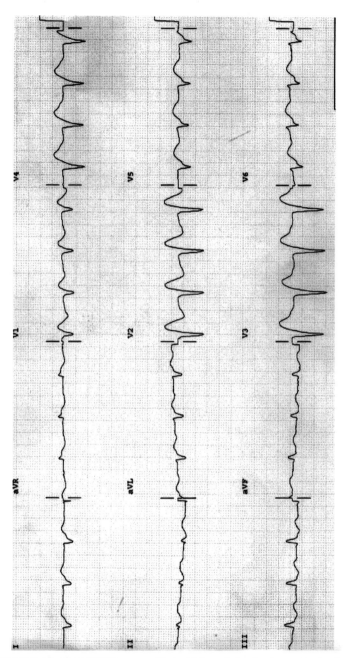

FIGURE 8–8 *Twelve-lead ECG from a patient with hyperkalemia, demonstrating loss of atrial activity, prolongation of the QRS duration, and merging of the ST segment with a prominent, peaked T wave.*

These are best seen as an upward deflection at the onset of the ST segment in leads II, III, aVF, V_5 and V_6. The QT interval is often prolonged. These ECG findings require no specific treatment beyond the treatments for severe low body temperatures.

Hypomagnesemia

Hypomagnesemia cannot be recognized on the ECG but it plays a role in the genesis of arrhythmias. Administration of magnesium may shorten the QT interval, the PR interval, and the QRS complex and speed intra-atrial conduction. Magnesium is administered as $MgSo_4$ (magnesium sulphate) and the usual dose is 2 to 4 g intravenously over 20 minutes.

Hypocalcemia

Low serum calcium levels prolong the second phase of the action potential and prolong the ST segment and QT interval. Treatment is repletion of calcium and this may be done by intravenous infusion of 100 to 200 mg of elemental calcium over 10 minutes, followed by an infusion of 1 to 2 mg/kg per hour.

Hypercalcemia

Hypercalcemia, on the other hand, shortens the QT interval, sometimes causes T-wave changes, and rarely causes J waves. Hypercalcemia can be managed acutely by forced saline diuresis to enhance urinary excretion of calcium.

ELECTRICAL CARDIOVERSION

The technique of electrical cardioversion refers to the controlled administration of electrical energy to the heart in an attempt to convert abnormal rhythms. Defibrillation refers to the administration of electrical energy to terminate ventricular fibrillation.

Cardioversion and defibrillation are performed using external devices that deliver a set quantity of energy. The cardiac effects are a direct result of the passage of electrical current through the heart. The resistance of the chest wall determines the amount of current that reaches the heart. It is imperative that material be used between the electrodes of the device and the chest wall to not only reduce the electrical resistance, but also to minimize the risk of chest wall burns. The electrical shock can be delivered in either a synchronized or unsynchronized fashion. In unsynchronized mode, the energy will be delivered independent of the electrical activity of the heart. This is appropriate in situations in which there is no organized cardiac activity, such as ventricular fibrillation, and when the patient is unstable, but it should be avoided in all other circumstances. If the electrical current is delivered to the heart during repolarization (on the T wave), it may precipitate ventricular fibrillation. In the synchronized mode the electrical current is delivered simultaneously with the QRS complex. This mode should be used in all cases except for ventricular fibrillation (in which there is no QRS complex to be identified) and hemodynamically unstable ventricular tachycardia. In the synchronized mode, there may be a delay between when the device is activated and when the shock is delivered, because the shock is delivered only on the QRS configuration. Under most circumstances, the best positioning for the electrodes is to have one placed anteriorly under the right clavicle to the right of the sternum and the other at the level of the left nipple in the midaxillary line. The recommended initial energy for various arrhythmias is summarized in Table 8–5.

SUMMARY

We have attempted to review some of the most common abnormalities of cardiac rhythm that are likely to be encountered in the critical care setting. The significance of cardiac rhythm disturbances in this setting must be understood because they may be life-threatening. Careful analysis of the rhythm is essential in making the correct diagnosis and instituting the correct therapy. While there are excellent pharmacologic agents that are available for the management of rhythm disturbances, all of these agents are potentially toxic and should be used only with caution and with an understanding of their effects and possible complications. Table 8–6 lists a number of the commonly used drugs to control cardiac rhythm in the critical care setting and the usual doses.

TABLE 8–5 **Recommended energies for cardioversion/defibrillation of various arrhythmias**

Rhythm Disturbance	Electrical Therapy
Ventricular fibrillation	Asynchronous shock with initial energy of 200 J, followed by 300 J, then 360 J
Rapid or hemodynamically unstable ventricular tachycardia	Asynchronous shock at 200 J, followed by 300 J, then 360 J
Stable ventricular tachycardia	Synchronous shock at initial energy of 50 J
Atrial fibrillation	Synchronous shock at initial energy of 200 J, followed by 360 J if unsuccessful
Atrial flutter	Synchronous shock at 50 J
Reentrant supraventricular tachycardia	Synchronous shock at 100 J

TABLE 8–6 Recommended doses for anti-arrhythmic agents commonly used in the critical care setting

Drug	Indication	Dosage
Lidocaine	Ventricular tachycardia or fibrillation	1.0–1.5 mg/kg as initial dose, followed by 1–4 mg/min infusion; may give second bolus of 50–100 mg, 5 min after initial bolus
Procainamide	Ventricular tachycardia, atrial fibrillation, or supraventricular tachycardia	15 mg/kg, no more than 20 mg/min bolus, followed by 1–4 mg/min infusion
Ibutilide	Conversion of atrial fibrillation or flutter	1.0 mg over 10 min, may be repeated once, if there is no effect
Amiodarone	Refractory ventricular tachycardia or fibrillation	Bolus of 150 mg over 10 min, followed by 1 mg/min for 6 hr, followed by 0.5 mg/min, may repeat bolus as needed
Adenosine	Termination of supraventricular tachycardia	6 mg as rapid bolus, followed by 12 mg as rapid bolus, if no response
Diltiazem	Atrial fibrillation or flutter to control ventricular response and supraventricular tachycardia	5–20 mg bolus, followed by 5–20 mg/hr continuous infusion
Verapamil	Termination of supraventricular tachycardia	5–10 mg over 5 min
Esmolol	Atrial fibrillation or flutter, to control ventricular response	500 μg/kg over 1 min followed by infusion of 50 μg/kg/min (initial infusion rate)
Magnesium	Torsades de pointes	2 grams of magnesium sulfate over 20 min
Digoxin	Atrial fibrillation or flutter, to control ventricular response	0.5 mg initially, followed by 0.25 every 4–8 hrs to maximum of 1-mg loading dose.

REFERENCES

1. Altun A, Kirdar C, Ozbay G. Effect of aminophylline in patients with atropine-resistant late advanced atrioventricular block during acute inferior myocardial infarction. *Clin Cardiol* 1998;21:759–762.
2. Falk RH, Zoll PM, Zoll RH. Safety and efficacy of noninvasive cardiac pacing: A preliminary report. *N Engl J Med* 1983;309:1166–1168.
3. Lamas GA, Muller JE, Turi ZG, et al. A simplified method to predict occurrence of complete heart block during acute myocardial infarction. *Am J Cardiol* 1986;57:1213–1219.
4. 1999 update: ACC/AHA guidelines for the management of patients with acute myocardial infarction: Executive summary and recommendations. *Circulation* 1999;100:1016–1030.

5. Kindwall E, Brown J, Josephson ME. Electrocardiographic criteria for ventricular tachycardia in wide QRS complex left bundle branch morphology tachycardia. *Am J Cardiol* 1988;61:1279–1283.

6. Wellens HJJ, Bar FWHM, Lie K. The value of the electrocardiogram in the differential diagnosis of a tachycardia with a widened QRS complex. *Am J Med* 1978; 64:27–33.

7. Buxton AE, Marchlinski FE, Doherty JU. Hazards of intravenous verapamil for sustained ventricular tachycardia. *Am J Cardiol* 1987;59:1107–1110.

8. Miller JM, Hsia HH, Rothman SA, et al. Ventricular tachycardia versus supraventricular tachycardia with aberration: electrocardiographic distinctions. In Zipes DP, Jalife J, eds. *Cardiac electrophysiology: From cell to bedside*, 3rd ed. Philadelphia: WB Saunders, 2000:696–705.

9. Gorgels AP, van den Dool A, Hofs A et al. Comparison of procainamide and lidocaine in terminating sustained monomorphic ventricular tachycardia. *Am J Cardiol* 1996; 43–46.

10. Helmy R, Herree JM, Gee G et al. Use of intravenous amiodarone for emergency treatment of life-threatening ventricular arrythmias. *J Am Coll Cardiol.* 1988;12: 1015–1022.

Approach to Acute Myocardial Infarction: Diagnosis and Management

SETH M. JACOBSON

JOSEPH M. DELEHANTY

INTRODUCTION

Each year approximately 1.5 million people in the United States experience acute MI. The mortality rate approaches 30%, with more than half of those deaths occurring before reaching the hospital.[1] The diagnosis and treatment of acute MI has evolved considerably in recent years with the advent of new diagnostic markers and new therapeutic options for early reperfusion. In addition, evidence-based adjuvant medical therapy has reduced both short-term and long-term mortality rates and the risk of future coronary events. In the past 25 years, a 47% reduction in age-adjusted coronary mortality rates has been seen. Patient education, early reporting of symptoms, prompt recognition and medical therapy, and rapid reperfusion therapies will further reduce cardiac mortality in the coming years. This chapter is a current summary of the diagnosis and treatment of acute MI.

Acute MI is generally a consequence of coronary atherosclerosis. It occurs when there is a sudden decrease in coronary blood flow to an area of viable myocardium. In a coronary artery, an atherosclerotic plaque fissures, ruptures, or ulcerates and a thrombus forms at the site. This may lead to complete coronary artery occlusion. Fewer than 5% of MIs occur in the absence of CAD. Instead, these MIs may be invoked by coronary vasospasm, coronary embolization, or other unknown causes. Ultimately, myocyte death results within 2 to 4 hours, unless perfusion is restored. Time and the territory of myocardium supplied by the occluded vessel determines the degree of myocyte death and the resulting ventricular dysfunction. Therefore, rapid diagnosis is essential in the management of acute MI.

DIAGNOSIS

The triad of diagnosis depends on clinical presentation, ECG analysis, and serum levels of cardiac markers. In many cases of acute MI, no precipitating factors can be blamed and many of these events occur at rest. In roughly 40% to 50% of cases, a precipitating factor may be found, such as vigorous physical activity, emotional stress, or a medical or surgical illness. The incidence of MI is highest within a few hours of awakening (6 AM to 12 noon). There also seems to be a seasonal component: more MIs occur in the winter months (even in temperate climates). Major risk factors for CAD include cigarette smoking, diabetes, hypercholesterolemia, hypertension, obesity, sedentary lifestyle, age over 50, male sex, and a family history for premature CAD in a first degree relative.

Chest pain is the most common and most important symptom of acute MI. It is typically described as a retrosternal heaviness, crushing, or squeezing sensation, which may radiate to the left shoulder and arm or to the neck and jaw. It is often accompanied by diaphoresis, nausea, dyspnea, weakness, syncope, or a sense of "impending doom" and typically lasts more than 20 minutes. Approximately 50% of patients have unstable anginal symptoms hours to days before their MI. Other less common presentations may be silent (especially in diabetic patients), or patients may present with pulmonary edema or new arrhythmias such as ventricular fibrillation, ventricular tachycardia, or atrial fibrillation. Women often have a more atypical presentation for acute MI which often delays diagnosis and worsens prognosis.

Physical examination is rarely diagnostic by itself but may help indicate the severity of the MI. Most patients lie still in bed and appear pale and diaphoretic. Tachycardia is common in anterior-wall MIs, and bradycardia may be indicative of an inferior-wall MI with heart block. Hypotension can indicate shock or right ventricular infarction. A new murmur consistent with a ventricular septal defect or papillary muscle rupture can be an ominous sign and may require immediate imaging studies (such as an echocardiogram).

The 12-lead ECG is the initial diagnostic test of choice, since it can be completed and read within minutes of presentation. The nomenclature of transmural versus nontransmural MI has a pathologic basis and is rarely used in clinical cardiology. Even the more common Q-wave versus non–Q-wave MI classification is beginning to fall out of favor in the rapid reperfusion era. This is because the ECG's of many patients with MI do not go on to show Q-waves, and even if they do, these waves are usually not present at the moment when therapeutic decisions need to be made. A more current differentiation is ST elevation MI versus non–ST elevation MI, because the former may indicate a need for urgent revascularization with thrombolytics or angioplasty. All patients presenting with ST elevation MI should be considered for immediate reperfusion therapy.

Classic ECG patterns of acute ST elevation MI include more than than 1-mm ST elevations in 2 or more contiguous leads or a new onset of BBB. This almost always indicates a total occlusion of the affected artery. ECG findings present in MI without ST elevation include ST segment depression, T-wave inversions or flattening, or even a normal ECG. Unfortunately, the ECG analysis is diagnostic in less than half of patients with acute MI. Reviewing a previous ECG, especially if abnormal, is important when attempting to evaluate for acute MI. Many times this step is overlooked or not completed because there is not enough time. This oversight can cause considerable confusion, misinterpretation, and delay, putting a patient at higher risk. The ECG abnormalities may evolve over days after an acute MI. Therefore, daily ECG tracings are indicated for the first 3 days. This is especially helpful after reperfusion when recurrent chest pain requires reassessment.

Serum cardiac markers (sometimes called "enzymes") have become the gold standard for the diagnosis and quantification of acute MI. However, these markers are less helpful in the triage and management of acute MI in the emergency department, since they take time for analysis. Levels of these markers do not begin to rise for 2 to 6 hours after the onset of symptoms.

Troponins I and T levels have virtually replaced creatine kinase–MB (CK-MB) levels as markers of cardiac injury, because of their higher sensitivity and specificity for myocardial damage. The initial rise of troponin levels occurs approximately 3 hours after myocardial injury, but it may occur several hours later in many patients. Therefore, it is essential that the use of troponin levels for the diagnosis of acute MI includes at least two measurements with one being 6 to 10 hours after the onset of symptoms. Troponins peak at 12 to 24 hours and are detectable for up to 7 to 10 days. If troponins are not present 10 hours after symptoms have resolved, it is extremely unlikely that myocardial damage has occurred. The role of CK-MB measurement in the acute setting is now limited to assisting in the timing of a recent MI, to evaluate recurrent chest pain occurring after MI or cardiac surgery, and to correlate with the extent of myocardial damage. Another rarely used serum cardiac marker is myoglobin levels, which begin to rise within 2 hours of acute MI and peak at approximately 6 hours after onset, but the utility of this marker is limited by its low specificity for cardiac injury.

Occasionally, when the diagnosis of acute MI remains in doubt, other diagnostic tests may be used. Echocardiography can be performed to evaluate for a new wall-motion abnormality. Nuclear testing, including pyrophosphate infarct scintigraphy, Tc-99m sestamibi perfusion imaging, and radiolabeled antimyosin antibody scans, can also be used to make the diagnosis of acute MI.

TREATMENT

When a patient comes to the emergency department complaining of typical chest pain, a complete assessment needs to be performed quickly. According to the 1999 American College of Cardiology (ACC) and American Hospital Association (AHA) guidelines for the management of patients with acute MI, a targeted clinical examination and interpretation of a 12-lead ECG tracing should be completed in the first 10 minutes.[2] One or more intravenous lines should be established. Supplemental oxygen and continuous ECG monitoring should be provided to all patients with acute ischemic chest discomfort. Aspirin, 160 to 325 mg, should be administered and chewed by the patient. Blood samples for electrolyte levels, CBC count, coagulation times, and serum cardiac markers should be sent for analysis. On the basis of clinical presentation and the 12-lead ECG results, a decision on whether or not to perform urgent reperfusion therapy can be made. A flowchart depicting the management of patients presenting with ischemic chest pain is shown in Figure 9–1.

Thrombolytic Agents versus Percutaneous Transluminal Coronary Angioplasty

Reperfusion therapy is the cornerstone of treatment for acute MI with ST elevation and ischemic chest pain of less than 12 hours' duration. Rapid re-establishment of flow is the goal. The key to success depends more on the efficiency of delivery than the choice of reperfusion modality (Tables 9–1 and 9–2). If an institution can provide both percutaneous transluminal coronary angioplasty (PTCA) and pharmaceutical thrombolysis, the PTCA is the preferred approach. Multiple trials have

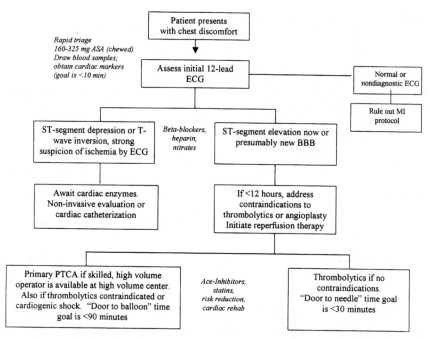

FIGURE 9–1 *Flowchart depicting managment of patients presenting with ischemic chest pain.* ABBREVIATIONS: *ASA, aspirin; ECG, electrocardiogram; MI, myocardial infarction; BBB, bundle-branch block; PTCA, percutaneous transluminal coronary angioplasty; ACE, angiotensin-converting enzyme.*

TABLE 9–1 **Direct Percutaneous Transluminal Coronary Angioplasty**

Advantages	Disadvantages
• Excellent reperfusion rates; 80%–90% TIMI-3 flow for > 90% of patients	• Requires 24-hour access to catheterization lab
• Facilitates access for placing hemodynamic support devices (e.g., intra-aortic balloon pump)	• Requires skilled personnel in a center with a high volume of these procedures
• Treats underlying stenosis and occlusion	• Requires large arterial sheaths
• Reperfusion promptly discerned	• Requires access to emergent CABG surgery
• Facilitates diagnosis; enables assessment of extent and severity of CAD	• Costly (initially)
• Effective in the setting of hemodynamic instability	• May delay treatment unacceptably
• Low mortality	• Restenosis rates fairly high
• Few contraindications	• Traumatic (as perceived by patient)

ABBREVIATIONS: CAD, coronary artery disease; CABG, coronary artery bypass graft.

TABLE 9–2 Thrombolytic Therapy

Advantages	Disadvantages
• Widely available, no catheterization lab or CABG capabilities needed	• Given in only 30% to 35% of acute MIs, use limited by age or contraindications
• Treats the underlying acute problem; dissolves the occluding thrombus	• Effectiveness in the setting of hemodynamic instability is unproven
• Significantly decreases 30-day mortality rates (large, well-controlled trials)	• Slightly increases overall risk of stroke and hemorrhagic stroke
• Significantly decreases 5-year mortality rates (large, well-controlled trials)	• Early (90-min) patency in 55% to 80% of cases; later (3–24 hr) patency in 80%–90% of cases; some patients fail to reperfuse
• Fast setup; short time to initiate	• With standard regimens, early TIMI-3 flow achieved in only about 50% of patients
• Can be given by nursing or emergency medical staff	• Reliable assessment of reperfusion involves extra steps
	• Does not alter residual stenosis or plaque

ABBREVIATION: CABG, coronary artery bypass graft.

compared the two methods. Primary PTCA is recommended if it can be performed quickly (from admission to balloon inflation time in less than 90 minutes) by skilled interventionists (who perform more than 75 procedures per year) and is supported by experienced personnel in a center where there is a high volume of such cases (200 to 300 procedures per year). A major advantage of PTCA over thrombolysis is apparent in the setting of cardiogenic shock.

Thrombolytic therapy is the primary mode of reperfusion therapy in approximately 80% to 90% of hospitals in the United States. Contraindications to thrombolytics are shown in the following lists.

Absolute Contraindications to Thrombolytic Therapy

• Active internal bleeding
• History of hemorrhagic stroke (any time), other stroke (less than 1 year before MI), intracranial neoplasm, or recent head trauma
• Suspected aortic dissection
• Major surgery or trauma less than 2 weeks before MI

Relative Contraindications to Thrombolytic Therapy

• Blood pressure higher than 180/110 mm Hg on two readings
• Active peptic ulcer disease
• History of stroke
• Known bleeding diathesis (e.g., hemophilia) or current use of anticoagulants
• Prolonged or traumatic cardiopulmonary resuscitation

- Diabetic hemorrhagic retinopathy
- Pregnancy
- History of chronic severe hypertension

Approved thrombolytic regimens and patency rates, are shown in Table 9–3. Multiple strategies of reperfusion therapy are being compared in research studies, including new thrombolytic agents, half-dose thrombolytic agents with platelet glycoprotein IIb/IIIa inhibitors, and facilitated percutaneous coronary intervention (FPCI). FPCI is a combination of drugs, angioplasty, and stenting and may become the intervention of choice in the future.

Platelet Glycoprotein IIb/IIIa Inhibitors

The benefit of platelet glycoprotein IIb/IIIa inhibiting agents in non-ST elevation MI, acute coronary syndrome, and angioplasty is well described. Briefly, IIb/IIIa inhibitors block the final common pathway involved in platelet adhesion, activation, and aggregation. Contraindications for IIb/IIIa inhibitors are similar to thrombolytics but also include thrombocytopenia as a relative contraindication. These agents are now commonly used in the setting of MI without ST segment elevation and as an adjunct to primary angioplasty. Recommended doses of IIb/IIIa inhibitors are:

- Abciximab (ReoPro), confirmed dose 0.25 mg/kg bolus, then 0.125 µg/kg/minute (to a maximum of 10 micrograms/min)
- Eptifibatide (Integrilin), 180 µg/kg bolus, followed by an infusion of 2 µg/kg per minute
- Tirofiban (Agrastat), 0.4 µg/kg bolus, followed by an infusion of 0.1 µg/kg per minute

TABLE 9–3 Approved Thrombolytic Regimens, Patency Rates, and Estimated Costs

Thrombolytic Agent	Regimen	Patency rate* (at 90 min)
Streptokinase	1.5 million U, infused over 30–60 min	~51%
Alteplase (t-PA)	15 mg bolus; 0.75 mg/kg over 30 min (max, 50 mg); 0.5 mg/kg over 1 hr (max, 35 mg)	~84%
Anistreplase (APSAC)	30 U injected slowly over 2–5 min	~70%
Reteplase (r-PA)	10 U injected over 2 min, then 10 U injected over 2 min, 30 min later	~83%

Aspirin

Aspirin inhibits cyclooxygenase, an enzyme involved in the formation of thromboxane A_2. Thromboxane plays a powerful role in stimulating platelet aggregation. By inhibiting this enzyme, aspirin promptly inhibits platelet aggregation. Many patients have taken aspirin at home or have received it in the ambulance on the way to the emergency department, but this needs to be confirmed. The role of aspirin cannot be overstated; it has been found to reduce mortality rates by 23%. A dose of 160 to 325 mg should be given, unless absolutely contraindicated (by well-documented anaphylaxis or active bleeding). Clopidogrel or ticlopidine may be substituted for or added to aspirin for increased antiplatelet effects.

Heparin

All patients presenting with acute MI should receive intravenous unfractionated heparin or low-molecular-weight heparin (LMWH) in the emergency department unless contraindicated (by anaphylaxis or active bleeding). However, heparin is not recommended for use with streptokinase if a patient is not at high risk for systemic embolism. A typical dose of intravenous unfractionated heparin is a 5000-U bolus (80 U/kg for patients with low body weight) followed by a continuous intravenous drip at 18 U/kg per hour.

The role of LMWH in acute MI is expanding because of its possible advantages over unfractionated heparin in non-ST-elevation MI and unstable angina. However, LMWH has not been extensively studied for ST-elevation MI or in combination with thrombolytics, IIb/IIIa inhibitors, or primary angioplasty. Intravenous administration of unfractionated heparin is preferred for ST-elevation MI, but LMWH is currently preferred for non-ST-elevation MI. The most commonly used and best studied of the LMWHs is enoxaparin. It is used at a dose of 1 mg/kg given by subcutaneous injection twice daily. It should be used cautiously or not at all in patients with renal insufficiency because standard doses may lead to excessive hemorrhagic complications.

Beta Blockers

Beta blockers are used in the early hours of acute MI in an attempt to limit the size of the infarct and to reduce the likelihood of ventricular arrhythmias. Beta blockers also relieve pain, reduce myocardial oxygen demand by decreasing heart rate and blood pressure, and most importantly, reduce mortality. All patients should be considered for early therapy with beta blockers unless contraindicated (by heart failure, systolic blood pressure of less than 90 mm Hg, heart rate of less than 60 beats/min, or heart block with a PR interval of more than 0.24 seconds). However, caution should be used in acute inferior-wall MI to avoid possible bradycardia. A common dosage is three 5-mg boluses of intravenous metoprolol given 5 minutes apart. If hemodynamic stability continues, oral therapy is started and continued indefinitely. The heart rate goal is less than 70 beats/min and a systolic blood pressure of from 100 to 140 mm Hg.

Beta blocker therapy has been shown to decrease mortality rates after MI in nearly every risk-factor subgroup, including patients with advanced age, chronic heart failure, and COPD. Beta blockers can be used in patients with COPD and asthma, unless active bronchospasm is present.

Angiotension-Converting Enzyme Inhibitors

There is a great deal of evidence that angiotension-converting enzyme (ACE) inhibitors should be started in all patients after MI, unless contraindicated (by hypotension or renal insufficiency). Therapy should commence in the first 24 hours, especially in patients with anterior-wall MI, left ventricular dysfunction with an ejection fraction (EF) of less than 40%, and clinical evidence of heart failure. Initially, short-acting ACE-inhibitors, such as captopril, are used. Before discharge, captopril can be changed to a long-acting ACE inhibitor that is taken once daily to improve compliance. In patients who have an impaired EF of less than 40%, ACE inhibitors should be continued indefinitely. ACE inhibitors seem to prevent future ischemic coronary events in patients at high risk in addition to their hemodynamic effects in patients with heart failure after infarction.[3]

Additional Medical Therapy

Sublingual nitroglycerin followed by intravenous nitroglycerin infusion is useful for patients with acute MI, especially if pulmonary edema, hypertension, or persistent ischemia exists. Although no data indicate a reduction in mortality with nitrate agents, they do relieve chest pain and postinfarct ischemia. Nitroglycerin should be used cautiously if there is hypotension or evidence of right ventricular infarction. Current randomized trial data does not support the long-term use of oral or topical nitrates after MI in asymptomatic patients. However, all patients discharged should be given a prescription for sublingual nitrates on an as-needed basis.

Morphine is the drug of choice for relief of the pain of acute MI. Pain relief reduces cardiac workload and myocardial oxygen demand. Morphine also reduces pulmonary edema and relieves the anxiety experienced during acute MI. There are no documented decreases in mortality rates with morphine therapy, but it is used empirically and for humane reasons.

Individual trials and meta-analysis reveal no clear benefit in terms of mortality rates with calcium channel blocker therapy. They are not recommended as standard therapy in patients with acute MI.

Intravenous magnesium is not recommended as standard therapy for acute MI, except to replenish subtherapeutic levels or in the presence of polymorphic ventricular tachycardia.

The role of interventions to reduce plasma lipid levels in acute MI is currently being investigated. There is clear evidence of the benefit of aggressive treatment of hypercholesterolemia in the months after MI. It is current practice to obtain fasting lipid profile results in all patients within 24 hours of admission and to strongly consider the initiation of therapy with an HMG-CoA reductase inhibitor in patients with a total cholesterol level of more than 200 mg/dL and a low-density lipoprotein (LDL) cholesterol level of more than 100 mg/dL.

COMPLICATIONS OF ACUTE MYOCARDIAL INFARCTION

Multiple complications can occur immediately following acute MI. Mechanical complications include cardiogenic shock, acute and chronic heart failure, ventricular aneurysm, intra-cardiac thrombus, stroke, right ventricular infarction, pericarditis, mitral regurgitation caused by papillary muscle dysfunction or rupture, recurrent chest pain or reinfarction, and rupture of the interventricular septum or left ventricular free wall. Electrical complications include ventricular fibrillation, ventricular tachycardia, atrial fibrillation, sinus arrest, and heart block. Careful monitoring and frequent examinations may be helpful in detecting these complications before they become life-threatening. Often forgotten, complications of MI are the psychological and socioeconomic effects on the patient. Depression after MI is a powerful independent risk for mortality in the months after discharge.

CARDIOGENIC SHOCK

Like other forms of shock described in this text, cardiogenic shock is characterized by inadequate oxygen delivery to tissue. In most cases, this is accompanied by systemic hypotension with a systolic blood pressure of less than 90 mm Hg in spite of pressor support, low cardiac output with adequate or high intracardiac filling pressures, and signs of tissue hypoperfusion, such as mental confusion, impaired renal function, and peripheral vasoconstriction. Patients who are in cardiogenic shock after acute MI usually have had very extensive infarction, particularly in the anterior distribution. Exceptions to this are patients who go into cardiogenic shock after a mechanical complication, such as ventricular septal rupture as a result of acute mitral regurgitation that is secondary to papillary muscle rupture. These two complications may occur several days after presentation and are characterized by the abrupt onset of hypotension and pulmonary edema. A loud systolic murmur is usually heard in both situations and the two can be best distinguished by echocardiography. In both cases, treatment is emergency surgery to repair the septal defect or mitral valve.

The more typical patient with cardiogenic shock presents with evidence of an acute anterior infarction with ST segment elevation in the anterior precordial leads. Such patients may initially present with relatively preserved hemodynamics because the initial phases of acute infarction are characterized by a very high catecholamine drive that may serve to support the failing heart. Over the course of the next hours to days, however, it is common for the patient to develop progressive hemodynamic impairment and overt shock. The extensive loss of contracting myocardium leads to elevations in cardiac filling pressures. The high sympathetic tone is an attempt to compensate for the loss of myocardium but often leads to more ischemia as the myocardial oxygen consumption rises during a period of impaired myocardial blood flow. This leads to more ventricular dysfunction and a vicious cycle of progressive cardiac dysfunction and circulatory insufficiency.

In addition to evidence of extensive infarction on presentation, the patient at risk for cardiogenic shock is often older, female, and diabetic. A very ominous finding at presentation is a relatively low systolic blood pressure of about 100 mm Hg in combination with tachycardia. These patients should be considered to have an impending shock state.

Management of the patient with cardiogenic shock presents a major challenge. In the initial phase, circulatory support with intravenous inotropic agents and possibly intra-aortic balloon counterpulsation are commonly used. Therapy is best guided by measurement of hemodynamics, and therefore arterial catheters and pulmonary artery catheters are frequently placed. The question of whether revascularization should be undertaken in patients with cardiogenic shock remains somewhat controversial. A recent randomized trial of revascularization (both surgical and percutaneous) showed a nonsignificant improvement in short-term survival in patients who were treated with revascularization, but at 6 months after MI this improvement did achieve statistical significance.[4] In this trial, the mortality rate at 30 days was 47% in the group treated with revascularization compared with 56% in the group treated with medical therapy. This illustrates the grave prognosis linked to cardiogenic shock, no matter how it is treated. My center's current approach is to be very aggressive with consideration of revascularization in this high-risk population. We proceed with early cardiac catheterization in all such patients and usually place intra-aortic counterpulsation devices and pulmonary artery catheters in most patients. In institutions where cardiac catheterization facilities are not available, emergent transfer to such an institution as soon as possible is recommended. As mentioned earlier, cardiogenic shock is one clinical situation in which primary PTCA has been shown to be superior to thrombolysis.

Primary right ventricular infarction is a clinical scenario that results in cardiogenic shock. This is almost always a result of acute occlusion of the proximal right coronary artery and is manifested by signs of shock with relatively clear lung fields but elevation in venous pressure. In addition to evidence of inferior infarction on the ECG, there is often ST segment elevation in the right-sided precordial leads, and a finding of ST elevation of more than 1 mV in lead V_{4R} has a high diagnostic yield. Management of cardiogenic shock from right ventricular infarction consists of judicious volume balancing and infusion of dobutamine. Early revascularization has also been shown to be critical in this patient population, and this is another clinical scenario in which primary PTCA should be considered as superior to thrombolysis.

PROGNOSIS, RISK STRATIFICATION, AND SECONDARY PREVENTION

Patients who have an uncomplicated MI after reperfusion therapy can generally be discharged in 3 to 6 days. The long-term prognosis is affected by age, extent of coronary disease, ability to revascularize, left ventricular function, arrhythmias during hospital stay, and comorbid conditions. Before discharge, a patient's risk should be stratified noninvasively. This is typically done by exercise ECG stress test, stress thallium(exercise or pharmacologic), or stress echocardiogram (exercise or dobutamine). If ischemia still exists, then revascularization by angioplasty or coronary artery bypass graft is indicated. In addition, evaluation of left ventricular systolic function is helpful for medical management in the period after MI and for determining if long-term anticoagulation is necessary.[5]

During hospitalization, secondary preventative measures and risk factors should be addressed. These include smoking cessation, dietary modification and weight loss, controlling stress or changing lifestyle, education about symptoms and disease, exercise regimens, and control of blood glucose levels (in patients with diabetes), blood pressure, and blood lipid levels. Upon discharge, all patients who do not have contraindications should be taking aspirin, beta blockers, ACE inhibitors, lipid-lowering agents and should be enrolled in a comprehensive cardiac rehabilitation program.

SUMMARY

Diagnosis and treatment of acute MI is considerably different today then it was just 5 years ago. Troponin levels, IIb/IIIa inhibitors, new thrombolytic agents, stents, and lipid-lowering agents have dramatically changed the way acute MI is managed. This area continues to rapidly evolve as new studies become available. Now more than ever the statement that "time is tissue" is relevant. The Rs of acute MI to remember are:

- Recognize
- Relieve symptoms
- Reperfuse
- Reduce complications
- Reduce recurrent events
- Rehabilitate

REFERENCES

1. American Heart Association. 1998 heart and stroke statistical update. Dallas: AHA; 1999.
2. Ryan TJ, Anthman EM, Brooks NH, et al. ACC/AHA guidelines for the management of patients with acute MI: executive study and recommendations. A report of the American College of Cardiology/American Heart Association task force on practice guidelines (committee on management of acute myocardial infarction). *Circulation* 1999;100:1016–1030.
3. Yusef S, et al. Effects of angiotensin-converting-enzyme inhibitor, ramipril, on cardiovascular events in high-risk patients (The HOPE Study). *NEJM*, 2000;342(3):145–153.
4. Hochman JE, Sleeper LA, Webb JG, et al. Early revascularization in acute myocardial infarction complicated by cardiogenic shock. *N Engl J Med* 1999;341(9):625–634.
5. Moss AJ, Benhorin J. Prognosis and management after a first myocardial infarction. *N Engl J Med* 1990;322:743–753.

Approach to Endocrine Disease

David Kaufman

INTRODUCTION

Many endocrine abnormalities that are found in critically ill patients are actually appropriate responses to illness and not diseases that require treatment. A real endocrinopathy, as opposed to a response or marker of illness, can present as a lone disorder or complicate another disease. The astute clinician is aware of both the primary presentations of endocrinopathies and the subtle development of a disorder that may elude diagnosis. These disorders are also common outside of the ICU, but they may present to the intensivist in their extreme form or may be masked by a critical illness.

The most sensible approach to endocrinology during critical illness is to divide the diseases and adaptive responses into categories by their most relevant organ. Since endocrine regulation tends to span more than a single organ, these divisions may seem fragmented. However, this approach will help organize an intricate topic. The topic of endocrinology is broad and the less common disorders found in the ICU are beyond the scope of this chapter. Thyroid function is altered by critical illness, and hypothyroidism and thyrotoxicosis are often-considered diagnoses in the ICU. Cortisol level is also altered by critical illness, and relative or absolute adrenal failure is also commonly entertained in the evaluation of the ICU patient. The body is unable to significantly store adenosine triphosphate (ATP) and utilizes glucose as substrate for its immediate production. The blood concentration of glucose that should be maintained in the critically ill patient remains controversial. Patients with acute disorders of diabetes, such as diabetic ketoacidosis and hyperglycemic hyperosmolar nonketotic coma, also frequently require admission to an ICU.

THYROID GLAND

General Considerations

There are three thyroid conditions that are important in the ICU. The first is referred to as the euthyroid sick syndrome, or nonthyroidal illness, and is the most common endocrinologic finding in the ICU. Originally, the euthyroid sick syndrome was presumed to be a disorder, but it is now believed to be an adaptive response. The euthyroid sick syndrome is not a single adaptive response to critical illness but actually a programmed interaction that must be evaluated in relation to the phase and severity of the patient's illness. The other two conditions, namely hypothyroidism and thyrotoxicosis, are familiar in the outpatient arena as well and, in their extremes, present to the ICU as myxedema coma and thyroid storm, respectively. More commonly, however, other illnesses supersede hypothyroidism and thyrotoxicosis, making it difficult for all but the astute clinician to make the diagnosis. Remember that the body has a limited repertoire of phenotypic responses, despite the plethora of diseases that inflict humankind.

Since these endocrine disorders are often seen in the ICU in conjunction with another illness or, more likely, are subclinically present before the development of the critical illness, the signs and symptoms of the primary disease may significantly overlap with the endocrinopathy.

Anatomy

The thyroid gland consists of two lateral lobes connected by a portion of thyroid tissue, called the isthmus, and a developmental remnant of thyroid tissue, called the pyramidal lobe. The isthmus sits over the second and fourth tracheal rings. The lateral lobes extend from the side of the thyroid cartilage and reach the sixth tracheal ring on each side. The pyramidal lobe is variably present but usually arises from the isthmus toward the left side. The thyroid gland weighs 15 to 20 g. Thyroid blood flow is fairly high at 4 to 6 mL/min per gram of thyroid tissue.

Physiology

The thyroid gland contains follicles, and it is the cells surrounding these follicles, or the follicular cells, that produce the thyroid hormones. Thyroxine (T_4) is a prohormone with one-half to one-quarter the activity of the active hormone, triiodothyronine (T_3). In addition to a difference in activity, T_4 produces its effects on end organs within days, while T_3 effects can be measured in hours. The thyroid hormones are stored in the colloid of the follicles bound to a glycoprotein, thyroglobulin. Ninety percent of the stored hormone and released hormone are in the form of T_4, which is monodeiodinated (a single iodide ion is removed from the outer phenol ring) to T_3 in the liver and kidneys. If T_4 is monodeiodinated on the inner phenol ring, reverse T_3 (rT_3) is produced, an inactive metabolite. The ratio of T_4 to T_3 in plasma is 100:1, and both are bound to the plasma protein thyroxine-binding globulin (TBG), transthyretin, and albumin. TBG binds 80% of the thyroid hormones and TBG's affinity for T_4 is tenfold higher than its affinity for T_3.

Thyroid hormone production and release is under the control of thyroid-stimulating hormone (TSH), which is produced in the anterior pituitary gland and governed by thyrotropin-releasing hormone (TRH) from the hypothalamus. TSH release is controlled by positive and negative feedback loops via free hormone concentrations. TSH is suppressed by endogenous and exogenous glucocorticoids, dopamine, and somatostatin. These drugs are all used in the ICU for various indications, and it is unknown whether the purported benefits of these drugs in certain marginal situations truly offsets the unknown risks of TSH suppression.

Thyroid hormone is taken up by target cells and directly acts on nuclear receptors for gene transcription, leading to an increase in mitochondrial number and cristae. Oxygen use and heat production are positively and negatively influenced by thyroid hormone directly and indirectly by facilitating or diminishing the activity of other hormones, such as insulin and epinephrine.

Laboratory Testing

As with many organic compounds, the ring structure of thyroid hormone makes it relatively insoluble in plasma and, therefore, transport proteins are required to reach target organs. Although the concentration of free thyroid hormones is tightly controlled, the total amount of hormone can vary greatly with protein concentration. Only 0.03% of T_4 and T_3 are not bound to protein. Total and free thyroid hormone and TSH levels can be measured directly. The T_3 resin-uptake test (T_3RU) measures TBG saturation, and the amount of TBG can be measured directly.

Euthyroid Sick Syndrome

During illness, thyroid hormone concentration in the plasma decreases. This response occurs in a wide range of illnesses and is not specific to an underlying disease. The body has a limited repertoire of responses to illness, and thyroid hormone alterations during critical illness are no exception to this rule. This hormonal response is not limited to thyroid hormones but, during critical illness, the concentration of gonadotropin and sex hormones decreases while the plasma concentrations of adrenocorticotropic hormone and cortisol increase. Changes in thyroid hormone regulation actually can predict the severity of illness in the critically ill patient.

In mild illness, the decrease in thyroid hormone concentration is only seen with the active hormone T_3. The mechanism behind this finding is an acute inhibition of the deiodinase that removes the iodide ion to convert T_4 to T_3. Free T_4 plasma concentrations may actually rise initially, because there is less peripheral conversion of T_4 to T_3 before other pathways for T_4 degradation prevail and free T_4 plasma concentration returns to normal. The same deiodinase that converts T_4 to T_3 also degrades rT_3, leading to an accumulation of this inactive metabolite.

In severe illness, T_4 and T_3 concentrations are low, but not free T_4 levels, only the total prohormone T_4 levels. Total T_4 includes both bound and free hormone. This observation in which both hormones are at low levels in critical illness is frequently referred to as the "low T_3 and low T_4 syndrome." The mechanisms underlying the low T_4 part of the syndrome are obviously related to changes in binding proteins and not free hormone concentration. Although TBG concentration may increase in critical illness, transthyretin and albumin concentrations actually decrease, and there is an acquired defect in T_4 binding to TBG, which is presumed to result from a factor released from injured tissues.

TSH concentrations also decrease during critical illness, and this phenomenon may be cytokine-mediated. Because it is difficult to isolate a cytokine in vivo, it has not been possible to designate one specifically. Often interleukin-6 (IL-6) is noted, because blood concentrations are elevated in a wide range of disease severity. As the patient recovers from their illness, TSH levels tend to rise out of the normal range and, finally, thyroid hormone levels recover. This recovery phase can frequently be measured in months.

The best strategy when evaluating the pituitary-thyroid axis in the critically ill patient is to maintain a high index of suspicion and correlate laboratory data with strong clinical evidence of primary thyroid disease. A TSH and free T_4 assay are most appropriate to obtain when the clinical suspicion is high. Normal results in critically ill patients virtually exclude disease. A low free T_4 level and a TSH level of more than 20 mU/L, along with a high index of suspicion, is indicative of hypothyroidism. A high free T_4 level and a very low TSH level, along with a high index of suspicion, is indicative of hyperthyroidism. Routine assays of thyroid function in the critically ill patient should be avoided.

The overwhelming question is whether euthyroid sick syndrome represents an adaptive or maladaptive response. Even if the process is adaptive, it is likely that a superimposed critical illness will exacerbate undiagnosed hypothyroidism. There is no convincing evidence in any disease state to treat the euthyroid sick syndrome. A teleologic explanation would be that the organism is conserving energy by suppressing a metabolic hormone that is causing increased energy expenditure.

The diagnosis of hypothyroidism is commonly entertained well into the patient's ICU stay, usually because of failure to thrive, including inability to be weaned from mechanical ventilation. At this time, the patient is usually recovering from their illness and TSH levels tend to be high and thyroid hormone levels tend to be low. The free T_4 level remains normal, however, and the TSH level rarely exceeds 20 mU/L. Another strategy is to repeat TSH and hormone levels at weekly intervals without intervention, because the euthyroid sick syndrome should dissipate over time if the patient is recovering.

Hypothyroidism

Autoimmune thyroiditis is the most common cause of primary hypothyroidism, and diagnosis is determined by the presence of thyroid autoantibodies (Table 10–1). Hypothyroidism may also be caused by thyroid ablation in the treatment of hyperthyroidism, either surgically or radiologically. The other common cause of primary hypothyroidism is drugs, most commonly amiodarone and lithium. Secondary hypothyroidism is commonly caused by a mass or lesion in either the hypothalamus or pituitary gland.

The signs of hypothyroidism are best categorized by organ system.

1. Skin: It is the dermal accumulation of hyaluronic acid, which binds water, that leads to the classic nonpitting edema of hypothyroidism. The coolness and pallor of the skin result from the circulatory effects of hypothyroidism.
2. Cardiovascular: Hypothyroidism leads to both a negative inotropic and chronotropic state, evidenced by lowered stroke volume and heart rate. The systemic vascular resistance (SVR) increases. ECG changes include a pro-

longed PR interval, ST segment alterations, and flattening or inversion of the T-waves. A pericardial effusion may develop and lead to low voltage on the EKG as well.

3. Respiratory: Pleural effusions are common but rarely lead to dyspnea. There is an impaired ventilatory response to both hypoxemia and hypercapnia, and alveolar hypoventilation is present.
4. Renal: An impairment in renal water excretion may lead to clinically significant hyponatremia.
5. GI: Weight gain occurs because of the accumulation of fluid, and appetite is usually lost. Pernicious anemia may accompany hypothyroidism, lending credence to the view that hypothyroidism is an autoimmune disease. Bowel atony may cause pseudo-obstruction, and a search for mechanical obstruction may delay the appropriate diagnosis.
6. Nervous: CNS effects such as lethargy or the classic "myxedema madness" may be noted. The slow relaxation phase ("hung-up reflexes") of the deep-tendon reflexes are routinely observed.
7. Hematopoietic: If pernicious anemia does not lead to a macrocytic anemia, decreased erythropoietin levels cause a normocytic normochromic anemia.

Hypothyroidism is usually insidious, and if it is severe and longstanding, can present as myxedema coma, which is a syndrome not a laboratory diagnosis. Usually, signs and symptoms of hypothyroidism precede myxedema coma and go unchecked. The physical characteristic that is most prominent is the facial and periorbital puffiness, or myxedema facies. Patients usually present during the winter months and coma, hypothermia, severe bradycardia, and hypotension are found. Temperatures as low as 23.3°C have been reported. The diagnosis is made using clinical criteria along with the finding of low free T_4 serum concentrations and high TSH serum concentrations. If hypothyroidism is confirmed without myxedema coma and differentiated from the euthyroid sick syndrome, levothyroxine (T_4) can be started at 50 μg/day and TSH levels should be monitored monthly to look for resolution of the hormonal abnormalities and to follow the clinical course.

TABLE 10–1 Thyroid Hormone Interpretation in Thyroid Illnesses

| | Euthyroid Sick Syndrome | | | | |
	Early	Late	Recovery	Hypothyroidism	Hyperthyroidism
TSH	↓	↓	↑	↑	↓
Free T_4	Normal	Normal	↓	↓	↑
Total T_4	Normal	↓	↓	↓	↑
T_3	↓	↓	↓	↓	↑

ABBREVIATIONS: TSH, thyroid stimulating hormone; T_4, thyroxine; T_3, triodothyronine; ↑, increases; ↓, decreases.

If the hallmarks of myxedema coma are present—coma, hypothermia, hypotension, and bradycardia—start levothyroxine, 500 μg intravenously, followed by daily doses of 100 μg. The mortality rate for myxedema coma is 20%.

Thyrotoxicosis

Thyrotoxicosis refers to the biochemical and pathophysiologic manifestations of increased concentrations of free thyroid hormone, whereas hyperthyroidism specifically defines the thyroid gland as the origin of the increased hormone level. The form of thyrotoxicosis of most concern to the intensivist is thyrotoxic crisis, or "thyroid storm." The underlying thyroid disease is usually Grave's disease or, less frequently, multinodular goiter (in patients with severe but compensated thyrotoxicosis). The general symptoms of thyrotoxicosis are exaggerated in thyrotoxic crisis and include the following:

1. Skin: The skin is moist and warm from excessive vasodilation and diaphoresis.
2. Eyes: Retraction of the upper eyelid may give the patient a "fish-eye" appearance and should be distinguished from infiltrative orbitopathy, which is found only in Grave's disease.
3. Cardiovascular: Thyrotoxicosis leads to both a positive inotropic and chronotropic state, evidenced by raised stroke volume and heart rate. The SVR decreases. Both tachycardias and tachyarrhythmias are common.
4. Respiratory: Dyspnea is common in severe states and is caused by muscle weakness.
5. GI: Appetite is increased but not enough to keep pace with the metabolic demand, and weight loss is common.
6. Nervous: Emotional lability and tremor are cardinal features of thyrotoxicosis.
7. Hematopoietic: If the cause of thyrotoxicosis is Grave's disease, pernicious anemia may also be present. Red cell mass is increased secondary to increased levels of erythropoietin.

Patients with thyrotoxic crisis may present postoperatively or after a medical illness that, similar to surgery, is associated with cytokine production. The actual mechanism of the decompensation may be a sudden increase in free thyroid hormone released from binding proteins. Infection is the most characteristic medical illness. Severe hypermetabolism with tachycardia, diaphoresis, fever, and delirium are prominent features of the disease. The tachycardia is usually more than expected for the degree of fever. Tachyarrhythmias such as rapid atrial fibrillation are particularly common in the elderly. These tachycardias and tachyarrhythmias are frequently resistant to standard doses of heart rate–controlling medications. The elderly may alternatively present with apathy and myopathy accompanied by significant weight loss. Coma and shock may develop, which obviously portends a poor prognosis. Since another illness usually precipitates thyroid storm, it is easy to attribute the symptoms to the primary disease and miss the diagnosis of hyperthyroidism in the ICU.

Acute management of thyrotoxic crisis consists of:

- Large oral doses of propylthiouracil, 300 to 400 mg every 4 hours, to inhibit synthesis of thyroid hormone.
- Iodine to immediately prevent the release of thyroid hormone: saturated solution of potassium iodide (SSKI), 5 drops orally every 6 hours; iopate, 0.5 g orally twice daily; or sodium iodide, 0.250 g intravenously every 6 hours.
- Dexamethasone, 2 mg orally or intravenously every 6 hours, is given to prevent glandular release and peripheral conversion of T_4 to T_3.
- A beta blocker is given to ameliorate the manifestations of the hypermetabolic state. Although many experts advocate the use of propranolol, the choice of a particular agent is less important than titrating to the effect required.
- Patients in thyroid storm usually have associated volume depletion and require titration of a crystalloid infusion to replenish their extracellular volume.

ADRENAL GLANDS

Hypoadrenal crisis in the ICU is frequently evoked and investigated but less frequently found. Relative or associated adrenal failure is a complex problem since, once again, it is unclear whether low cortisol levels are a maladaptive response or a marker of severe disease. Since cortisol levels rise with acute illness it is probably not an adaptive response to have low cortisol levels during critical illness. Primary adrenal failure is obviously an adrenal disease and secondary adrenal failure a pituitary or, less frequently, a hypothalamic disease although the manifestations are mostly adrenal. Secondary adrenal failure is most commonly due to withdrawal from chronic steroid use and is usually avoided rather than diagnosed by the attentive clinician.

Anatomy

The adrenal glands sit on top of the kidneys medially and are sometimes referred to as the suprarenal gland. Although given one name, the adrenal gland really houses two organs derived from distinct embryologic tissue. The medulla is derived from neural crest ectodermal cells and is a neurosecretory organ. The cortex derives from mesodermal cells along the urogenital ridge and manufactures the corticosteroids, including the ubiquitous glucocorticoid hormone cortisol, from the two inner zones of the cortex (the zona fasciculata and zona reticularis) and the major mineralocorticoid hormone aldosterone from the outer zone of the cortex (zona glomerulosa). Each whole gland only weighs 4 to 5 g.

Physiology

The hypothalamic-pituitary-adrenal axis plays a pivotal role in homeostasis during stresses such as infection and surgery. The hypothalamus is responsible for the production of corticotropin-releasing hormone (CRH) and vasopressin and, in addition to classic negative feedback loops, is regulated by other areas of the brain, particularly the limbic system. CRH and vasopressin stimulate the release of corticotropin hormone (ACTH) from the anterior pituitary gland, which stimulates the adrenal gland to secrete cortisol.

In addition to ill-defined effects, such as a sense of well-being and appetite, cortisol assists in the maintenance of blood pressure, is a necessary hormone for the vasopressor effects of catecholamines, promotes gluconeogenesis, stimulates protein breakdown for gluconeogenic substrate, and inhibits antidiuretic hormone (ADH) through a classic feedback loop on the hypothalamus.

The mineralocorticoid hormone aldosterone is controlled by angiotensin, which in turn is released by the hormone renin, which regulates the renal glomerular baroreceptor. The renin-angiotensin-aldosterone (RAA) system is a major component of volume regulation. Aldosterone directly stimulates sodium and hydrogen reabsorption and potassium secretion in the distal nephron.

Laboratory Testing

There are two tests of adrenal function that are commonly ordered in the ICU. The first is measurement of a random cortisol level. Given the fact that there is no exact correlation between the clinical measurement (e.g., Apache scores) of stress and cortisol levels, only an extremely high level safely rules out a component of adrenal failure.

The second test is a corticotropin stimulation test; normal values are defined for outpatients with single-organ disease but not for critically ill inpatients. If the test is used in the ICU, most commonly a baseline cortisol level is measured and the patient is given 250 μg of synthetic corticotropin, followed by the measurement of a second cortisol level 1 hour after stimulating the adrenal gland. If the result is 20 μg/dL or more, it is usually safe to exclude the possibility of adrenal failure. A result of between 15 and 20 μg/dL requires judgment in determining the possible component of adrenal failure. If the result is less than 15 μg/dL and the increment from baseline to stimulated value is less than 7 μg/dL, associated adrenal failure may be an appropriate diagnosis. If the increment from baseline to stimulated value is more than 7 μg/dL, it is necessary to reexamine the patient to assess whether he or she is as critically ill as initially suspected. If treatment with corticosteroids is necessary before completing the stimulation test, a pure glucocorticoid, dexamethasone, 4 mg intravenously, may be given before cortisol tests, since dexamethasone does not interfere with the assay. Since these patients are receiving a crystalloid infusion, it is reasonable to give a corticosteroid like dexamethasone without mineralocorticoid activity. Once the cortisol tests are completed then hydrocortisone may be given.

Adrenal Function and Critical Illness

As with thyroid function, there is precious little evidenced-based data to guide corticosteroid replacement in the critically ill patient. For the usual complicated ICU patient, it is difficult to determine what the appropriate cortisol level should be for a given situation. What is the best cortisol level during a critical illness? Often, it is relatively easy to determine what value contributes to the best survival but not be able to determine whether the abnormal level is the cause of the disorder or just a marker of the severity of disease. More specifically, does endogenous replacement of a corticosteroid improve outcome or at least a secondary effect such as hypotension?

Critical illnesses, such as sepsis, are characterized by an elevated cortisol level secondary to activation of the hypothalamic-pituitary-adrenal (HPA) axis, decreased cortisol clearance, and decreased protein binding. Since it is known that there are many competing cytokines and that cytokines can directly influence the HPA axis, it is appropriate to target them as potential mediators, but it is unlikely that a single "smoking gun" will be found.

Primary Adrenal Failure

Primary adrenal failure may present acutely or chronically or the patient may have subclinical or undiagnosed hypoadrenalism and shock may develop with a superimposed acute illness. Many of the symptoms of hypoadrenalism are non-descript and include weakness, fatigue, weight loss, anorexia, and orthostatic hypotension. Abdominal complaints can also be presenting symptoms and include nausea, vomiting, pain, and diarrhea. Pigmentation of the skin (particularly the soles of the hands and feet) occurs with the increased corticotropin levels of primary hypoadrenalism, but pallor is more common with secondary adrenal failure. Eosinophilia, normocytic anemia, lymphocytosis, hyponatremia, and hypoglycemia can be seen with both primary and secondary adrenal failure.

In the ICU, acute primary adrenal failure or hypoadrenal crisis usually presents as hypotension unresponsive to vasopressors. The major problem is that, in the ICU, the disorder frequently complicates sepsis, another disease that may present with hypotension. The hemodynamic pattern of adrenal failure mimics sepsis, and patients have a low systemic vascular resistance and a high cardiac output after fluid replacement, with a normal to high pulmonary artery wedge pressure (PAWP). The manifestation is usually hemorrhage into the adrenal glands, although thrombosis of the adrenal arteries along with adrenal infarction may occur in conjunction with the antiphospholipid antibody syndrome or some other thrombotic disorder.

Since fever and abdominal pain are accompanying features, patients have been taken to the operating room for an exploratory laparotomy for which the results are negative. The surgical stress along with adrenal failure can easily lead to their demise. The diagnosis is also problematic because it is unclear whether a relatively low cortisol level in a critically ill patient is a factor contributing to morbidity and mortality or just a sign of disease severity. Chronic adrenal failure is most often the result of autoimmune adrenalitis, but other causes include opportunistic infections such as AIDS, fungal infection, tuberculosis, lymphoma, or metastatic carcinoma of the lung, breast, or kidney.

Secondary Adrenal Failure

Obtaining a thorough history is essential to avoiding secondary adrenal failure. Patients may self-prescribe corticosteroids that they have at home from an old illness, making it hard to easily determine who needs corticosteroid replacement. As in primary adrenal failure, a high index of suspicion is necessary for any patient with unexplained hypotension. It may be difficult to differentiate primary from secondary adrenal failure. Patients can actually have primary adrenal failure without hyperpigmentation. Hyponatremia can be manifested with both primary and secondary adrenal failure, since it is not only a mineralocorticoid effect but also cortisol deficiency that leads to hyponatremia. Co-secretion of ADH with CRH from the paraventricular nucleus in the hypothalamus occurs with cortisol deficiency because both hormones are under negative feedback control. In addition, the effective circulating volume depletion characteristic of adrenal failure potentiates ADH release through baroreceptor-mediated pathways. Other signs of cortisol deficiency are the same as in primary adrenal failure.

Corticosteroid Replacement

During critical illness and surgery, corticosteroids are given to prevent and to treat adrenal failure. After surgery, the cortisol levels rise rapidly but usually return to baseline within 48 hours. If the patient is not presently taking corticosteroids but has taken them recently, time to recovery of the HPA axis is unpredictable. If the patient is currently taking corticosteroids for an inflammatory disease, they may need just their usual dose or may need supplementation, with higher doses for several days. Patients taking corticosteroids for primary adrenal failure need the higher doses for several days postoperatively or during a critical illness. Hydrocortisone, 100 to 150 mg/day in divided doses or as a continuous infusion is an appropriate high dose of a corticosteroid for stress.

LIVER AND PANCREAS

Glucose derangements in the ICU are the most difficult to place within a single organ, but because the pancreas produces insulin and the liver is the major gluconeogenic organ, this categorization seems the most appropriate. The kidney is also a gluconeogenic organ and, especially under stress, may contribute significantly to total body glucose levels. The specific disorders of diabetic ketoacidosis and hyperglycemic hyperosmolar nonketotic coma are addressed here.

Anatomy

The liver is the largest glandular organ in the body. The usual weight in the adult human is 1500 grams, or approximately 2.5% of the total body weight. The liver has a dual blood supply, receiving blood from both the hepatic artery and portal vein. The basic structure of the liver consists of a portal triad (i.e., portal vein, hepatic artery, and bile duct) and central vein, with hepatocytes lining the road in between. Both the portal vein and hepatic artery drain into the central vein, and the fenestrated sinusoidal endothelial cells allow for rapid exchange of metabolic products between the interstitial fluid and the liver's blood supply.

The pancreas, like the adrenal gland, is functionally made up of two organs, the endocrine pancreas and exocrine pancreas. The pancreas is 13 to 15 cm long, with the head nestled into the loop of the duodenum and the tail bordering the spleen. The cells in the islets of Langerhans produce insulin and glucagon.

Physiology

Five hormones must be considered in any discussion of carbohydrate metabolism. Insulin is the primary regulatory hormone for glucose homeostasis. Increased insulin levels promote glucose use. The other hormones—glucagon, cortisol, epinephrine, and growth hormone—prevent hypoglycemia. They are counter-regulatory because they prevent the actions of insulin.

Laboratory Testing

In addition to glucose level measurements, the presence of ketosis is frequently investigated when there is hyperglycemia and an anion-gap metabolic acidosis. The most accurate determination is to measure serum ketone bodies with a nitroprusside test. The same test is part of the qualitative measurement performed with the urine dipstick. Only acetoacetate and one of its metabolites, acetone, are measured with the nitroprusside test, but the ketone body beta-hydroxybutyrate is not measured with this test. A patient may have a significant level of ketoacidosis, but the nitroprusside reaction does not reflect this disorder if the ketone body is largely beta-hydroxybutyrate.

Glucose and Critical Illness

Humans are unable to store significant amounts of ATP but are exquisitely designed to produce large amounts on demand through the tricarboxylic acid cycle and the oxidative phosphorylation chain. Oxygen and glucose are required for these biochemical reactions. Humans are prone to hypoxemia but not to hypoglycemia, thus oxygen is always considered as first-line therapy in the critically ill patient but not glucose. Insulin is the only hormone that causes hypoglycemia, however, because all the other glucose-related hormones are counter-regulatory and an increase in blood glucose level.

Since critically ill patients are prone to hyperglycemia, insulin is used to keep them euglycemic. Although severe hyperglycemia causes increased carbon dioxide production and steatosis and increases the incidence of infections, there are not compelling in vivo data to suggest how tightly to control the glucose in the ICU patient. The usual range that is chosen is between 150 and 250 mg/dL. There are many continuous-infusion protocols for insulin, but the central themes are the same:

1. The goal is to control the glucose concentration over hours, not minutes, so intravenous boluses are usually not necessary.
2. If the glucose concentration is dropping rapidly the infusion rate should decrease accordingly.
3. If the glucose concentration is dropping slowly and remains high, the infusion rate may be increased more aggressively.
4. Glucose levels should be monitored frequently when the patient is unstable and until a steady glucose concentration is obtained.
5. Hypoglycemia is more worrisome than hyperglycemia and should not occur from the use of exogenous insulin in the ICU.

Diabetic Ketoacidosis

Patients with diabetic ketoacidosis (DKA) present with lethargy or coma, Kussmaul respirations (rapid and deep), and signs of hypovolemia. The patients usually have type 1 diabetes and present with hyperglycemia (glucose 400 to 800 mg/dL) and an anion-gap metabolic acidosis with the anions acetoacetate and beta-hydroxybutyrate being the anions that create the gap. Acetoacetate can be metabolized to acetone or beta-hydroxybutyrate, and it is the volatile acetone excreted by the lungs that gives patients with DKA their characteristic fruity odor.

Both the urine and the serum can be tested for the presence of ketone bodies. Osmotic diuresis usually causes severe volume depletion in these patients with accompanying potassium losses, although the extracellular potassium may be at a normal level initially, as a result of cellular shifts from the acidemia. Although a lack of insulin alone and a resultant rise in glucagon direct the free fatty acids to the ketogenic pathway and lead to DKA, an underlying infection or some other inflammatory process must be considered.

The mainstay of therapy for DKA is crystalloid (with a 0.9% sodium chloride content) infusion and insulin. The volume depletion associated with DKA is usually in the range of 3 to 6 L, and 1 to 2 L should usually be given over 30 to 60 minutes. During this initial infusion of 0.9% sodium chloride, insulin can be withheld because it may exacerbate the extracellular volume depletion as glucose is driven inside cells and water follows. Extracellular potassium levels may appear normal, because acidemia drives potassium out of cells in exchange for hydrogen ions but serum potassium rapidly falls as the acidemia is corrected. In other words, the total body potassium stores are usually low despite the normal extracellular potassium concentration. Regular insulin can be given as a bolus 15 to 20 U, which saturates the insulin receptors, making larger doses unnecessary, and then infused to maintain the blood glucose between 150 to 200 mg/dL. Glucose (dextrose) and potassium are added, once these levels are between 200 and 300 mg/dL and 4.0 mEq/L, respectively. Phosphorus follows the same fate as potassium but should not be replaced until low levels are measured.

Hyperosmolar Hyperglycemic Nonketotic Coma

Severe hyperglycemia with dehydration and coma may occur in elderly patients with type II diabetes. Patients who develop hyperosmolar hyperglycemic nonketotic coma (HHNC) make enough insulin to prevent ketosis but not enough to prevent hyperglucagonemia. The increased glucagon levels lead to hyperglycemia through glycogenolysis and gluconeogenesis. A limited substrate for ketosis may also play a role in the lack of ketoacidosis in these patients.

Blood glucose levels in HHNC are much higher than in DKA and can range form 600 to 2000 mg/dL. Typically, patients have renal impairment, which exacerbates the hyperglycemia because less glucose is filtered and excreted. They also do not respond appropriately to the hyperosmolality by increasing water intake, often secondary to dementia.

The major electrolyte abnormality in HHNC is relative hyponatremia, secondary to the hyperglycemia. The glucose level increases the extracellular osmolality and causes cellular dehydration and secondary hyponatremia. For each 100 mg/dL of glucose above 100 mg/dL, the sodium level can be expected to decrease by approximately 1.6 mEq/L. This is a real hyponatremia and should not be confused with pseudohyponatremia, a laboratory phenomenon caused by dilution of the specimen without accounting for lipids or proteins that are not present in the re-suspension.

The initial treatment of HHNC is to focus on fluid and electrolyte replacement, beginning with 0.9% sodium chloride solution until the effective circulating volume is restored. Particular attention must be paid to potassium supplementation. Insulin is given, but the goal should be a gradual resolution of hyperglycemia. Remember that the neurons produce idiogenic osmoles to prevent cerebral cellular dehydration and if too much electrolyte free-water is given and the glucose corrected too rapidly, the patient develops cerebral edema.

SUMMARY

Appropriate diagnosis and management of endocrine dysfunction in the ICU requires the knowledge to differentiate among a primary disorder, a secondary disorder, and a response to illness. It is essential to consider these three possibilities when faced with a potential endocrinopathy in the critically ill patient.

SUGGESTED READINGS

De Groot LJ. Dangerous dogmas in medicine: The nonthyroidal illness syndrome. *J Clin Endocrin Metab* 84;1:151–164.

Irwin R, Cerra F, Rippe J. *Intensive care medicine.* Lippincott–Raven: New York, 1999.

Nesse RM, Williams GC. *Why we get sick.* Random House: New York, 1994.

Oelkers W. Adrenal insufficiency. *N Engl J Med* 1996;335;16:1206–1213.

Rose BD. *Uptodate.* Vol. 8, no. 1. www.uptodate.com

Smallridge RC. Metabolic and anatomic thyroid emergencies: A review. *Crit Care Med* 1992;20:276–291.

Wilson J, Foster D, Kronenberg H, et al. Williams textbook of endocrinology. W.B. Saunders: Philadelphia, 1998.

Wood A. Corticoidsteroid therapy in severe illness. *N Engl J Med* 1997;337;18:1285–1292.

Approach to Gastrointestinal Problems in the Intensive Care Unit

James R. Burton, Jr.

Thomas A. Shaw-Stiffel

INTRODUCTION

A wide variety of gastrointestinal (GI) problems result in admission to the ICU or arise during a patient's stay there. This chapter focuses on the GI disorders that are seen most frequently in the ICU and that require expert management to improve patient outcome. More than the usual emphasis is placed here on disorders involving the liver. There is an alarming rise in the number of patients admitted with cirrhosis and its complications related to chronic viral hepatitis, especially hepatitis C virus, which is estimated to infect over 4 million Americans, only 200,000 of whom have been identified to date. A systematic approach to evaluating abnormal liver test results is also essential when managing patients in the ICU; this topic is discussed in detail.

ACUTE GASTROINTESTINAL BLEEDING

Bleeding in the GI tract is a common reason for admission to the ICU. The approach to acute GI bleeding should be systematic, with special attention given to intravascular resuscitation, recognition of the factors that caused bleeding, and aggressive investigation and treatment of any identified causes.

General Approach

Regardless of the apparent source of bleeding, the initial management of patients with acute GI bleeding is generally the same. The first step is thorough patient assessment. The urgency of the situation relates to the degree of blood loss, which may be determined by the presence of tachycardia, hypotension, orthostasis, confusion, diaphoresis, and pallor.

INITIAL INTRAVASCULAR RESUSCITATION Large-bore intravenous access is of the utmost importance. To permit rapid infusion of crystalloid or blood products, it is best to insert two large-bore (14- to 16-gauge) peripheral intravenous lines or a central catheter introducer (e.g., Swan-Ganz catheter). A central venous catheter offers no advantages in comparison to large-bore peripheral access.

If more rapid intravascular volume resuscitation is needed, it should begin with normal saline or lactated Ringer's solution while the patient's blood is being cross-matched. Restoration of hemodynamic stability should take precedence over other considerations. Thus, normal saline solution should be used even in patients who have excessive levels of body sodium, such as those with cirrhotic ascites or CHF.

To assure adequate tissue perfusion, vital signs and urine output volume should be determined at frequent intervals. Central venous pressure monitoring may be necessary in elderly patients or those with cardiovascular disease, to assess for early evidence of intravascular fluid overload.

NASOGASTRIC INTUBATION All patients with acute GI bleeding should initially have a nasogastric tube inserted. Not only does it assist in identifying an upper GI source of bleeding, but it also helps to monitor the rate of upper GI bleeding and to remove gastric contents and blood to facilitate subsequent endoscopy. It may also contribute to hemostasis by allowing the walls of the stomach to collapse.

Inserting a nasogastric tube of routine caliber is not contraindicated in patients with known or suspected varices, since major bleeding from varices has rarely been linked to this procedure. In addition, many patients with portal hypertension bleed from sources other than varices and the nasogastric tube may help in assessment.[1]

Blood aspirated from the nasogastric tube usually confirms that the source of bleeding is in the upper GI tract. A bloodless nasogastric aspirate, however, does not rule out an upper tract source, since in 10% of patients duodenal bleeding may be present.[2] Lavage of the stomach with tap water clears it of clots before endoscopy, and it may also improve coagulation. Ice water was once thought to help reduce gastric or duodenal bleeding causing local vasoconstriction, but this is no longer believed to be the case.[3]

ENDOTRACHEAL INTUBATION In patients with massive hematemesis or decreased mental status, endotracheal intubation is required to prevent pulmonary aspiration, especially before endoscopy.

DETERMINING THE SOURCE The source of GI bleeding can usually be determined with some accuracy be means of a thorough history and physical examination. The color and consistency of the stool is often helpful. Melena generally indicates moderate bleeding (50 mL/day) from a source in the upper GI tract (above the ligament of Treitz), although bleeding in the right side of the colon can also present in this manner. Hematochezia usually indicates bleeding from the lower GI tract (below the ligament of Treitz) but can also be seen with a massive upper GI tract bleed. Hematemesis virtually ensures an upper GI tract source. Rapid or recent bleeding appears bright red in color, whereas earlier bleeding has a "coffee ground" appearance. (Nasopharyngeal bleeding should always be excluded in patients with hematemesis.)

The age of the patient makes some diagnoses more likely than others. This is especially true with regard to bleeding from the lower GI tract, which tends to occur more often in older patients than younger ones. In addition, advanced age worsens the prognosis of patients with an acute GI bleed. Recent ingestion of alcohol, aspirin, or NSAIDS all raise the possibility of erosive gastritis or peptic ulcer disease. Aspirin also inhibits platelet adhesion, which may aggravate any underlying bleeding tendency. A previous history of GI bleeding should also be sought.

Patients with medical conditions characterized by bleeding are at increased risk of mortality from GI bleeding. Patients with liver disease are at risk for esophageal varices. Previous radiation therapy to the abdomen or pelvis makes radiation enteritis or colitis a distinct possibility. A history of surgery on the abdominal aorta or an unrepaired abdominal aneurysm raises the potential of an aortoenteric fistula.

A thorough physical examination should initially focus on the degree of blood loss by examining for signs of shock. Stigmata signs of liver disease should be sought. A careful abdominal examination may provide relevant information as to the source of bleeding. Other aspects should be addressed, such as the general health of the patient, with particular attention to cardiopulmonary status.

LABORATORY TESTING Initial laboratory data should be sent immediately and include a CBC count, platelet count, PT time, partial thromboplastin time (PTT), liver enzyme levels, serum electrolyte levels, blood urea nitrogen (BUN) level, creatinine level, and a type and cross-match for blood transfusion. Care should be used in interpreting the patient's initial hematocrit, since it represents the volume of RBCs as a percentage of total blood volume and it does not drop until blood volume has been restored. Repletion of blood volume from extravascular fluid sources or exogenous intravenous resuscitation may take hours to occur. Therefore, the decision to transfuse should not be based solely on the patient's hematocrit. Unstable vital signs and evidence of active bleeding are better indicators.

TRANSFUSION OF BLOOD PRODUCTS Blood loss of less than 500 mL rarely causes systemic manifestations, except in elderly patients or in patients who were anemic to begin with. Orthostatic hypotension suggests a 20% reduction in blood volume. When blood loss approaches 40% of volume, shock is usually present and tachycardia and hypotension rapidly ensue. If a patient remains hemodynamically unstable after receiving 2 to 3 L of crystalloid, transfusion of blood products is indicated.

A target hematocrit of 30% is ideal for elderly patients and those with cardiac or pulmonary disease, but in young healthy patients, a hematocrit of 20% is acceptable. Packed RBCs are the preferred type of blood transfusion. Mortality from GI bleeding is high in patients who present with shock and require more than 5 U of blood.[3]

Fresh frozen plasma may also be necessary to replace clotting factors in patients who need massive transfusions and those with coagulopathies. Platelet transfusions may be indicated when the platelet count is less than 50,000/μL and for suspected platelet dysfunction after recent aspirin ingestion. In patients with rapid fluid shifts caused by GI bleeding and the infusion of multiple blood products and copious intravenous fluids, frequent monitoring of serum electrolyte, calcium, phosphate, and magnesium levels is necessary.

MEDICAL THERAPY Medical therapy to suppress gastric acid secretion is often initiated, because this reduces the harmful effects of acid and pepsin on any upper GI tract lesion that is bleeding and may also improve platelet aggregation. In patients suspected of having esophageal or gastric varices, the use of octreotide or somatostatin should be initiated before diagnostic endoscopy to reduce portal pressures and stem bleeding.

Bleeding in the Upper Gastrointestinal Tract

CAUSES The major causes of bleeding in the upper GI tract include acid-peptic disease (gastric or duodenal), gastritis, Mallory-Weiss tears, and esophageal or gastric varices. Other less common sources are portal hypertensive gastropathy, Dieulafoy's malformation, and gastric carcinoma. Acid-peptic disease is the most frequent cause of upper GI bleeding and accounts for 50% of cases,[4] with a mortality rate of about 10%. However, in certain inner city populations, esophageal sources and gastritis are more prevalent.[5] Overall, the mortality rate for acute GI bleeding is about 5% to 12%.[6,7] This increases significantly with a patient over age 60 and in patients with severe bleeding or cirrhosis.[7]

RISK FACTORS Upper GI tract bleeding is associated with a variety of risk factors. Aspirin and NSAIDs are responsible for many cases of benign gastric or duodenal ulcers and gastritis. The risk of major bleeding is increased in elderly patients and in those with significant co-morbidities. A history of peptic ulcer disease also increases the risk of bleeding, particularly in those with chronic renal disease.[2]

In hospitalized patients, acute bleeding in the upper GI tract often arises from stress-induced ulcers, secondary to the "stress" of critical illness and distinct from routine acid-peptic ulcers.[8] Risk factors for stress ulcers and GI bleeding include head injury, severe burns, major trauma, shock, sepsis, coagulopathy, hepatic or renal disease, and mechanical ventilation. Two specific risk factors that have been shown to be the most predictive for clinically important nosocomial GI bleeding are coagulopathy and respiratory failure that requires mechanical ventilation.[9] About 75% of patients admitted to the ICU show some evidence of bleeding on endoscopy, as early as 24 hours after admission.[10] Those with bleeding from nosocomial stress-induced ulcers have a worse prognosis than those admitted with routine bleeding ulcers.[11,12]

DIAGNOSTIC AND THERAPEUTIC ENDOSCOPY Fiberoptic and now videoendoscopy have revolutionized the management of acute upper GI tract bleeding. Routine upper GI endoscopy is usually recommended as the initial diagnostic procedure, since the site and severity of bleeding dictates the specific treatment approach taken. For example, the therapy of variceal bleeding is markedly different from the management of bleeding from acid-peptic disease.

All patients who are unstable hemodynamically should undergo urgent endoscopy, once they have been stabilized sufficiently. Patients with less significant upper GI tract bleeding should also have an upper tract endoscopy done within 48 hours to confirm the diagnosis and consider further management.

Specific aspects of the clinical presentation (e.g., hemodynamic instability and bright red blood suctioned by means of the nasogastric tube) offer both prognostic and therapeutic significance, as do the endoscopic findings. Brisk bleeding, spurting of blood, slow oozing, adherent clots, a visible vessel, or ulcers larger than 1 to 2 cm, are all associated with a high risk of uncontrollable bleeding or rebleeding.[2] These patients are more likely to require urgent intervention by therapeutic endoscopy or surgery. The NIH Consensus Panel on Therapeutic Endoscopy and Bleeding Ulcers currently recommends that patients with active bleeding or those with a visible vessel should undergo appropriate therapeutic interventions at the time of endoscopy.[13]

Endoscopic therapy for hemorrhage secondary to acid-peptic disease is usually successful in stopping active bleeding and decreasing the risk of recurrent bleeding and the need for transfusions or surgery. Endoscopic methods to treat ulcer bleeding include thermal and bipolar electrocoagulation, laser photocoagulation, and injection of ethanol, hypertonic solutions, or epinephrine. The combination of epinephrine injection and thermocoagulation for initial endoscopic control of bleeding yields significantly better results than either treatment alone.[14,15]

MEDICAL TREATMENT The routine treatment of documented gastroduodenal ulcers or gastritis includes the withdrawal of any inciting factors or drugs (e.g., NSAIDs or alcohol), acid suppression, and eradication of *Helicobacter pylori* (Table 11–1). The presence of *H. pylori* can be confirmed at the time of upper endoscopy by urease testing, histopathologically with silver or Giemsa staining of antral biopsies, or by serologic or urea breath tests. Intragastric pH should be maintained above 4.0 with either antacids via a nasogastric tube or intravenous administration of H_2-antagonists. Hemorrhagic gastritis secondary to aspirin, NSAIDs, or alcohol typically resolves with the removal of the offending agent, although healing may be enhanced with acid suppression. A Mallory-Weiss tear usually heals without any specific treatment, but H_2-antagonists are often used.

TABLE 11–1 FDA-Approved Oral Regimens in the Treatment
of *Helicobacter pylori* Infection

Bismuth subsalicylate, 525 mg qid for 14 days and Metronidazole, 250 mg qid for 14 days and Tetracycline, 500 mg qid for 14 days and Ranitidine, 150 mg bid for 14 days
Lansoprazole, 30 mg bid for 10 days and Clarithromycin, 500 mg bid for 14 days and Amoxicillin, 1 g bid for 14 days

SOURCE: Adapted from Guidelines for the management of *Helicobacter pylori* infection, by Howden CW, Hunt GH. *Am J Gastric Enterol* 1998;93:2330.

REPEATED BLEEDING Rebleeding of ulcers occurs in about 15% to 20% of nonvariceal upper GI tract bleeds, with the highest rate of rebleeding documented in the first 48 to 72 hours after initial treatment.[16] Patients who rebleed should undergo a repeat endoscopy before proposed surgery. There appears to be no significant difference in achieving hemostasis with surgery versus repeat therapeutic endoscopy, in terms of the need for transfusions, length of hospital stay, or mortality.[17,18] However, patients who proceed to surgery tend to have a higher risk of complications. Second-look endoscopy remains a controversial issue, because no studies to date have shown any clear benefit in favor of this approach, except perhaps for patients whose initial bleeding episodes are severe.

Stress-Induced Ulcers

Prophylaxis for stress-induced ulcers has generally been recommended for all critically ill patients.[19,20] However, while GI bleeding occurs in 20% of patients who do not receive prophylactic treatment, only in 2% to 6% is the GI bleeding significant enough to cause hypotension or necessitate a blood transfusion.[10] Therefore, we recommend stress ulcer prophylaxis only in a select group of critically ill patients[9] (Table 11–2). H_2-antagonists have been shown, in randomized trials, to prevent clinically important GI bleeding in patients compared with patients in whom no such prophylaxis is used.[9] Proton-pump inhibitors (soon to be available with intravenous formulations) may have the same effect.

There is controversy regarding whether or not the use of acid-suppressing agents may increase the risk of ventilator-related pneumonia by enhancing the growth of bacteria in the upper GI tract as a result of acid suppression. Since sucralfate does not alter gastric pH, it has been thought to be an effective alternative for stress-induced ulcer prophylaxis. However, the effectiveness of sucralfate in preventing clinically important GI bleeding has recently been questioned.[21] Enteral nutrition by itself may prevent GI bleeding, since the pH of most commercially available enteral nutritive formulations is between 6 and 7.[22] Although the overall incidence of GI bleeding appears to decrease no matter what form of prophylaxis is used, there has been no study to date which clearly demonstrates a reduction in mortality.[9,23]

TABLE 11–2 Indications for Stress Ulcer Prophylaxis

Coagulopathy (INR > 1.5; PTT > 2 times control or greater; platelet count < 50,000/μL)
On mechanical ventilation for more than 48 hours
Recent history of GI bleeding
Major burns (> 35% TBSA)
Major trauma (ISS > 15)

ABBREVIATIONS: INR, international normalized ratio; PTT, partial thromboplastin time; GI, gastrointestinal; TBSA, total body surface area; ISS, injury severity scale.

Upper Gastrointestinal Tract Hemorrhage in Liver Disease

Bleeding from varices in the upper GI tract accounts for about 20% of all admissions to the ICU for upper GI tract bleeding.[24] However, in patients with chronic liver disease who present with upper GI bleeding, variceal bleeding accounts for almost 50% of cases, acid-peptic disease for around 15%, and portal hypertensive gastropathy for only 5%.[25] In most studies, about 50% of patients with cirrhosis are found to have esophageal or gastric varices at routine upper endoscopy, and close to 50% of these patients develop an upper GI tract bleed at some point in time.[24]

Mortality from variceal bleeding is high. In patients with cirrhosis and esophageal varices the risk of variceal bleeding is 25% to 35%.[26] The risk of dying from variceal hemorrhage within 1 year of diagnosis of varices is 10% to 15%.[26] For patients who survive their first variceal bleed, the risk of recurrent bleeding is nearly 70% within the first 6 months and the mortality rate with each bleeding episode is about 30% to 50%.[26] Predictors of mortality include ongoing GI bleeding at the time of endoscopy; documented large varices, ascites, and encephalopathy; and a serum bilirubin level of more than 2.5 mg/dL, a serum aspartate aminotransferase (AST) level of more than 100 U/L, and a PT of more than 14 seconds.[27]

Gastric varices are a relatively infrequent source of upper GI bleeding compared to esophageal varices. Although gastric varices tend to bleed less often, when they do bleed, they usually hemorrhage massively and respond poorly to endoscopic or medical therapy.[28] Portal hypertensive gastropathy is another important source of bleeding in patients with liver disease, but this entity presents more often as chronic blood loss rather than massive hemorrhage.

SUSPECTED VARICEAL BLEEDING The approach to bleeding in the upper GI tract in patients with liver disease should be the same as for any other group of patients, although even more careful attention should be given to judicious intravascular volume resuscitation efforts before diagnostic or therapeutic endoscopy. Resuscitative measures include the establishment of proper intravenous access and blood volume replacement with packed red blood cells and fresh frozen plasma, when appropriate. In general, patients should be slightly undertransfused to a hematocrit of 30 to 34 mL/dL. In unstable patients or those who hemorrhage vigorously, endotracheal intubation should be performed to secure the airway before endoscopy. This is especially important in patients with an altered sensorium secondary to alcohol intoxication or hepatic encephalopathy.

In patients with liver disease and a recent history of GI bleeding, an upper tract endoscopy must be performed on an urgent basis to determine whether varices are present. If they are but not actively bleeding, specific endoscopic signs may suggest a recent episode of bleeding. These signs include large varices rather than small ones and the presence of certain stigmata, such as red wales, red hematocystic spots, and cherry-red spots, the "red color" signs of recent hemorrhage from large varices.[24] If there are multiple or large (e.g., grade 3 or 4) varices, even though no active bleeding is present, specific therapeutic measures are warranted at the time of endoscopy, as discussed in more detail later.

MEDICAL TREATMENT OF VARICEAL BLEEDING The treatment of bleeding esophageal varices differs substantially from the approach used for other lesions of the upper GI tract. Initial pharmacologic therapy centers around the use of vasoactive drugs, such as vasopressin, octreotide, or somatostatin, all of which decrease splanchnic blood flow, total hepatic blood flow, hepatic wedge pressure, and variceal wall pressures. Since varices develop whenever the hepatic venous pressure gradient (defined as portal pressure minus inferior vena cava pressure) rises to a value 12 mm Hg or higher, the goal is to lower the gradient to a level of less than 12 mm Hg.

Before the availability of somatostatin and its analog octreotide (Sandostatin), vasopressin or glypressin (with or without nitroglycerine) were the only agents available for patients with acute variceal bleeding. Their use should now be abandoned because of their significant adverse effects (e.g., coronary spasm, skin necrosis after extravasation) and the negligible effects that octreotide and somatostatin have on systemic hemodynamics.

Octreotide is given initially as a 50 µg IV bolus, followed by an infusion of 50 µg/hr, whereas somatostatin is given as a 250 µg IV bolus, followed by an infusion of 250 µg/hr. In cases of severe bleeding, boluses of these drugs may be repeated and the infusion rate may be doubled. Octreotide has been shown to improve survival and lead to less morbidity than balloon tamponade.[29] The medical literature does not yet support the use of octreotide or somatostatin infusion before endoscopy in patients with bleeding in the upper GI tract. However, these drugs have few if any side effects, and it is therefore advisable that all patients with a major hemorrhage of the upper GI tract and evidence of liver disease be started empirically on octreotide or somatostatin while awaiting endoscopy.

Vasoactive drugs, such as octreotide and somatostatin, are also the primary form of medical therapy for nonesophageal causes of bleeding secondary to portal hypertension, such as portal hypertensive gastropathy and gastric varices more than 2 to 3 cm below the gastroesophageal (GE) junction. Gastric varices less than 2 to 3 cm from the GE junction can often be managed via therapeutic endoscopy in a manner similar to those in the esophagus proper (as discussed later).

ENDOSCOPIC TREATMENT OF VARICES The endoscopic treatment of bleeding from esophageal (or "high-riding" gastric) varices consists of either sclerotherapy or band ligation (banding), or a combination of both. Sclerotherapy involves injecting sclerosing agents, such as sodium morrhuate or ethanolamine, directly into or, more often, adjacent to the varices under endoscopic control. Unfortunately, these agents are quite toxic and lead to local problems, such as esophageal ulcers, bleeding, and strictures, and systemic complications, including bacteremia, mediastinitis, and pulmonary edema.

However, sclerotherapy remains the treatment of choice when variceal bleeding is torrential and visualization of the esophagus is poor, because banding is technically more difficult under these circumstances. The advantage of endo-scopic sclerotherapy also lies in its low cost, widespread availability, and ease of use. Sclerotherapy is thought to be equally as effective as octreotide or soma-tostatin in controlling acute variceal bleeding.[30-32] The use of octreotide in combination with sclerotherapy has been shown to be more effective than sclerotherapy alone in controlling further bleeding and in survival without bleed-ing at 4 days.[33] However, sclerotherapy carries a higher morbidity rate compared with vasoactive drugs as a result of the complications noted earlier.

However, banding is much better tolerated; it is a technique whereby small elastic bands are sequentially placed onto the varices under endoscopic control. The blebs of variceal tissue become necrotic and slough off, leaving small residual ulcers. Compared with sclerotherapy, band ligation has been shown to lead to less rebleeding, lower mortality rates, and fewer complications.[34-39] Banding also achieves obliteration of the varices more rapidly and with fewer endoscopic ses-sions.[35] However, combining sclerotherapy with band ligation has not been shown to produce better results than banding alone.[40] Compared to band liga-tion alone, banding combined with octreotide significantly reduces the risk of re-current variceal bleeding and the need for balloon tamponade.[41]

BALLOON TAMPONADE Seventy-five percent to 90% of patients with variceal bleeding stop bleeding with pharmacologic or endoscopic treatment, or both.[26] For those who do not stop, other options must be considered. Balloon tamponade can be helpful to control acute, particularly torrential, bleeding, but this is only a tem-porary measure, because its use beyond 24 hours results in a high risk of local com-plications and rebleeding. The Sengstaken-Blakemore or Minnesota tube consists of a long flexible catheter with two inflatable balloons, an elongated esophageal bal-loon and a round gastric one toward the end. The tube is inserted either through the nose or the mouth. After determining that the gastric balloon is in the stomach by auscultating in the left upper quadrant for the insufflation of air, the gastric bal-loon is inflated with 50 mL of air and its placement is then confirmed to be in the stomach by x-ray films. Following this, the balloon is inflated with 250 to 300 mL of air and pulled back to be positioned snugly against the GE junction. If bleeding persists, the esophageal balloon can be gently inflated, but only when using a pres-sure monitor device to ensure a maximum pressure of 30 to 40 mm Hg.

To avoid pulmonary aspiration, the Minnesota tube should be placed only after endotracheal intubation. Furthermore, the esophageal and gastric balloons should be deflated after 24 hours to avoid the complications of local esophageal or gastric ischemia and rupture. The use of balloon tamponade is most helpful when en-doscopy is not readily available or pharmacologic therapy fails and especially when severe bleeding is present, which prevents endoscopic visualization.

TRANSJUGULAR INTRAHEPATIC PORTACAVAL SHUNT Another important option for stabilizing the patient and preventing recurrent bleeding is the trans-jugular intrahepatic portacaval shunt (TIPS). This is an ideal means of controlling acute variceal bleeding (especially from gastric varices) whenever medical or endo-scopic therapy fails and a surgical shunt is not feasible because of the advanced de-gree of the patient's liver disease or other contraindications. A TIPS is usually performed by an interventional radiologist, who first inserts a needle-tipped catheter via the right internal jugular vein down through the right atrium and into the liver, whereupon a connection is created between the portal vein and the hepatic vein. An expandable metal stent is then inserted over the guide wire, deployed and expanded within this intrahepatic connection, thus creating a direct portosystemic shunt. The goal is to reduce the hepatic venous pressure gradient to less than 12 mm Hg, below which the risk of further variceal bleeding is negligible. However, because of enhanced portosystemic shunting, hepatic encephalopathy often worsens and acute liver failure is not unusual, prompting the need at times for urgent liver trans-plantation. Recurrent clotting or stenosis of the TIPS is also a common problem.

SURGICAL SHUNTS For a patient whose liver disease is less advanced and deemed to be Child's class A (see section on cirrhosis), a surgical shunt (selective or total) is a reasonable alternative because of its excellent long-term patency rates compared with those of TIPS. Surgical shunts, particularly selective ones, are no longer a contraindication to liver transplantation as they were in the past, although technical concerns persist.

LIVER TRANSPLANTATION Liver transplantation continues to offer the best long-term solution for the complications of portal hypertension, such as bleeding from varices or portal hypertensive gastropathy, but transplantation is limited by donor availability.

PREVENTING RECURRENT VARICEAL BLEEDING Because of the high risk of rebleeding, patients with varices who eventually stop bleeding should be consid-ered for prophylaxis with nonselective beta-blockers (propranolol or nadolol). They are well tolerated and have been shown to prevent recurrent bleeding sec-ondary to portal hypertension, especially in patients who are Child's class A or B.[26] There may also be additional benefit with the combination of nonselective beta-blockers and long-acting nitrates or alpha-blockers.

Although combining pharmacologic and endoscopic therapy (i.e., sclerother-apy or banding) appears to be a reasonable approach, there have been no defini-tive studies to date and more data from randomized controlled trials are needed. Unfortunately, neither pharmacologic or endoscopic treatment appears to de-crease overall mortality in patients with liver disease, even though band ligation has been shown to reduce mortality rates from bleeding compared with scle-rotherapy.[37]

Many experts suggest that all patients with cirrhosis should undergo an upper GI tract endoscopy to determine the presence and severity of varices or portal hy-pertensive gastropathy. Patients confirmed to have large (i.e., grade 3 or 4) varices should be started on pharmacologic treatment with a beta-blocker and continued on this indefinitely. Although beta-blockers have been shown to prevent the first variceal bleed, they do not improve overall survival.[26] The use of endoscopic therapy to prevent a first bleed remains controversial and at present this approach is not recommended. In some studies sclerotherapy actually caused more bleeding.[24,26] In one study, however, band ligation was shown to prevent the first bleed in cirrhotic patients who were at high risk of bleeding from esophageal varices.[42] Although a recent comparison of banding and propranolol for primary prevention suggested that banding was more effective,[43] current recommendations are to give nonselective beta-adrenergic blockers and reserve banding for patients with contraindications or intolerance to these drugs.

Lower Gastrointestinal Tract Hemorrhage

Lower GI tract bleeding is defined as any bleeding which occurs distal to the ligament of Treitz. On the whole, it occurs less often than upper GI tract bleeding. Most cases of lower GI tract bleeding originate in the colon and present with hematochezia, although bleeding from the small intestine or proximal colon can sometimes lead to melena. Diverticulosis, angiodysplasia, neoplasm, ischemia, inflammatory bowel disease, and infectious colitis cause significant GI bleeding. The most common source for bleeding in the lower GI tract is from the upper GI tract.

CAUSES Diverticulosis accounts for about 40% of all cases of lower GI bleeding.[44] The bleeding is often acute and painless but can be massive. Although diverticular disease occurs primarily in the left colon, diverticulae in the right colon tend to bleed more vigorously, for unknown reasons. Patients with benign or malignant neoplasms rarely present with massive hemorrhage; they develop chronic blood loss instead. Inflammatory bowel disease is the most frequent cause of lower GI tract bleeding in young adults who have small-to-moderate amounts of bright red blood mixed with diarrheal stool. Rarely does inflammatory bowel disease present as a life-threatening hemorrhage, except occasionally in patients with Crohn's disease. Aortoenteric fistula can cause a sudden, massive GI bleed; these fistulas occur most often in patients who have had previous surgery on their abdominal aorta or who have unrepaired aortic aneurysms.

EVALUATION Eighty percent of lower GI bleeds stop spontaneously and do not require any therapy.[45] The initial evaluation of a patient with a lower GI bleed includes a rectal examination and anoscopy to evaluate the perianal tissues, the anus, and anal canal for fissures or hemorrhoids. A flexible sigmoidoscopy is also recommended to assess for bleeding in the rectum, sigmoid colon, and lower descending colon.

Colonoscopy

The role of colonoscopy in acute bleeding remains controversial, since ongoing bleeding and stool in the unprepared colon often obscures the endoscopist's view. If a colonoscopy is planned, adequate bowel preparation with an osmotically balanced electrolyte solution is required. Inadequate preparation of the bowel for examination is the most common reason for failure to identify the source of bleeding at colonoscopy. This procedure should not be performed in patients who are in shock or in those who have active bleeding, since the patient may be too unstable for the examination and the accuracy in diagnosis is compromised.

Radiographic Studies

If a colonoscopy cannot be performed or if it fails to identify the source of bleeding and moderate or intermittent bleeding occurs, a technetium-labeled RBC scan should be considered. The study involves first tagging the patient's RBCs with technetium pertechnetate, injecting them back into the patient, and then imaging the abdominal area every few minutes. Sites with bleeding rates as low as 0.05 to 0.1 mL/min can be identified. Another option is selective angiography, which can localize the site as long as the rate of bleeding is more than 0.5 mL/min. In fact, this is the test of choice in patients with massive lower GI bleeding, since vasopressin can also be infused selectively or the bleeding vessel may be embolized. However, perforation secondary to ischemic damage has been reported. CT scanning or surgery are the next steps, if all other diagnostic tests are unrevealing.

ACUTE PANCREATITIS

Acute pancreatitis is a potentially life-threatening disorder characterized by inflammation of the pancreas that may also involve peripancreatic tissues or remote organ systems, or both. There are many causes of acute pancreatitis: excess alcohol intake, gallstones, trauma, infection, drugs, toxins, hyperlipidemia, or hypercalcemia, but on occasion, no apparent cause is found, despite an extensive workup. Although the mortality rate with most cases of acute pancreatitis is 5% to 10%,[46] when complications arise, the risk of death approaches 35%.[47] Thus, it is important to grade the severity of this condition as soon as possible after presentation and to manage patients aggressively based on the apparent acuity of their illness. It is also essential to recognize and treat any complications as soon as they arise.

Clinical Presentation

In most instances, patients with acute pancreatitis complain of abdominal pain, ranging from mild, tolerable discomfort to severe incapacitating distress. The onset of pain is usually acute in onset and persists for hours without relief. The pain is most intense in the epigastrium or periumbilical region, and often radiates to the back. Nausea and vomiting are also common.

Key aspects of the physical examination are signs of shock, namely tachycardia and hypotension. Fever is another common feature. Pulmonary findings include basilar rales, atelectasis, and pleural effusions. Abdominal tenderness is almost always present. A pancreatic pseudocyst may be palpable. Ecchymoses in the periumbilical area (Cullen's sign) or flanks (Turner's sign) indicate hemorrhagic pancreatitis.

The differential diagnosis of acute pancreatitis includes a variety of other disorders, such as mesenteric ischemia, perforated duodenal or gastric ulcer, acute cholecystitis or biliary colic, inferior-wall MI, dissecting aortic aneurysm, renal colic, and diabetic ketoacidosis.

Laboratory Diagnosis

Elevated serum levels of amylase and lipase in excess of three times the upper limit of normal suggest the diagnosis of acute pancreatitis,[48] although mild elevations of these enzymes can be seen with perforated duodenal or gastric ulcers, mesenteric ischemia, and tubo-ovarian pathology. The degree of the amylase or lipase elevation does not correlate with the severity of the pancreatitis. Serum amylase level has a low sensitivity (~ 70%)for diagnosis when the upper limit of normal is used as the cutoff.[49] Lipase level is a preferable test to amylase level, since the latter enzyme may be elevated with salivary disease, in diabetic ketoacidosis, and with some carcinomas.

In acute pancreatitis, the serum amylase level typically returns to normal within 48 to 72 hours, since the kidney rapidly clears the enzyme. In contrast, serum lipase levels may remain elevated for 1 to 2 weeks, which makes the lipase level a useful "historical" marker of previous disease. Once the diagnosis of acute pancreatitis has been made, it is usually not necessary to measure amylase and lipase levels on a daily basis, since they have little, if any, value in predicting clinical outcome or prognosis.

One instance in which measuring daily levels of lipase and amylase may be useful is in gallstone-induced pancreatitis. A rapid return of elevated levels to normal suggests that the gallstone has passed into the duodenum or moved back up the common bile duct and that it is now safe for the patient to undergo a cholecystectomy.

A recently developed noninvasive method to detect acute pancreatitis is a urine dipstick test for trypsinogen-2, a precursor of trypsinogen. It has a sensitivity of about 94%, so if negative, this test is helpful in ruling out acute pancreatitis.[50] In most cases of acute pancreatitis, leukocytosis is present along with hyperglycemia, hypocalcemia, and transient elevations in liver enzymes. Measurement of liver enzymes may be helpful in differentiating gallstone-induced pancreatitis from other causes. A serum alanine aminotransferase (ALT) level of more than 80 U/dL is very specific for biliary pancreatitis, but the sensitivity is only 50%.[51] The positive predictive values of an elevated serum alkaline phosphatase level and total bilirubin level are about 80%, while the negative predictive values are 40% and 48%, respectively.[52] The presence of hypoxemia (PaO_2 of 60 mm Hg or less) may signal the onset of acute respiratory distress syndrome (ARDS).

Radiologic Diagnosis

Plain films are simple to obtain, but they have a sensitivity of less than 50% in detecting acute pancreatitis.[53] Their main utility is in ruling out other causes of acute abdominal pain (e.g., free air from a perforated ulcer). Ultrasonography is most useful in identifying biliary disease or gallstone-induced pancreatitis. In fact, all patients who have mild-to-moderate acute pancreatitis of unclear cause should have an abdominal ultrasound examination within 48 hours of admission to rule out gallstones as the cause. Ultrasonography can also provide important information on pancreatic edema and inflammation as well as identify pancreatic pseudocysts. CT scanning permits detailed visualization of the pancreas and its surrounding structures. In particular, contrast-enhanced dynamic CT scanning provides additional information on the severity of pancreatitis and helps to establish a prognosis (as discussed later).

Determining Severity

A concerted effort should be made at the time of presentation to categorize the severity of acute pancreatitis and to identify patients with severe pancreatitis, since they appear to do best when managed in an ICU. Organ failure and local complications are the most important predictors of a poor outcome in acute pancreatitis (Table 11–3).[54] Local complications include pancreatic necrosis, pseudocysts, and abscesses. Organ failure and local complications may not be apparent at the time of presentation, and physicians must remain vigilant to identify patients with complications resulting from severe disease. The one factor that appears to lead most often to organ failure, and hence plays a major role in determining the severity of acute pancreatitis, is third-space losses. Evidence of significant losses includes hypotension, oliguria, azotemia, tachycardia, and a hematocrit value of more than 50%.

RANSON CRITERIA A variety of scoring systems have been developed to help categorize the severity of acute pancreatitis and predict outcome. Ranson et al[55] developed 11 diagnostic criteria (5 at admission and 6 at 48 hours after admission) (Table 11–4). Studies have shown that there is an increased risk of mortality when three or more Ranson criteria are identified, either at admission or 48

TABLE 11–3 **Signs of Organ Failure**

Shock (BP < 90 mm Hg or HR > 130 beats/min)
Pulmonary insufficiency ($PaO_2 \leq 60$ mm Hg)
Renal failure (creatinine level > 2 mg/dL or urine output < 50 mL/hr)
GI bleeding (> 500 mL/day)

ABBREVIATIONS: BP, blood pressure; HR, heart rate; GI, gastrointestinal.

TABLE 11–4 Ranson's Criteria of Pancreatitis Severity

At Admission	During initial 48 hours
Age > 55	Hematocrit decreases > 10 mg/dL
WBC count > 16,000/mm^3	BUN level increase of > 5 mg/dL
Glucose level > 200 mg/dL	Ca^{++} < 8 mg/dL
LDH level > 350 U/L	PaO$_2$ < 60 mm Hg
AST level > 250 U/L	Base deficit > 4 mEq/L
	Fluid sequestration > 6 L

ABBREVIATIONS: WBC, white blood cell; BUN, blood urea nitrogen; LDH, lactate dehydrogenase.

hours after admission.[56,57] The mortality rate rises from approximately 10% to 20%, when three to five criteria are met, to more than 50%, when six or more are present. The main limitation with the Ranson criteria is that the assessment is not complete until 48 hours after presentation.

APACHE II SCORE The Acute Physiology and Chronic Health Evaluation II (APACHE II) score uses 12 physiologic measures, along with age and general health status to determine disease severity. It has a high sensitivity and specificity for distinguishing mild from severe cases of pancreatitis on the day of admission.[58,59] The APACHE II score identifies two-thirds of severe cases at admission, and after 48 hours, the prognostic accuracy of APACHE II scores is comparable to that of the Ranson criteria. The patient usually survives if the APACHE II score is eight or less. A major advantage of APACHE II over the Ranson criteria is that severity of disease and prognosis can be determined at the time of admission rather than waiting a full 48 hours. However, the main disadvantage with APACHE II scoring is its complexity.

GRADING SEVERITY WITH CT CRITERIA All patients with severe pancreatitis as determined by the presence of organ failure, a high APACHE II score, or three or more Ranson criteria should have a dynamic contrast-enhanced CT scan. This is the best available test to distinguish interstitial (benign) from necrotizing (severe) pancreatitis. If significant renal impairment (a serum creatinine level of more than 2 mg/dL) is present or if a history of contrast sensitivity exists, a non–contrast-enhanced CT scan should be done, but the distinction between interstitial and necrotizing pancreatitis is less readily evident. With non–contrast-enhanced scans, the Balthazar-Ranson grading system (Table 11–5) can be applied instead. The most severe forms of acute pancreatitis are seen with grades D or E; these grades are associated with organ failure and pancreatic necrosis.[60] If a contrast-enhanced CT scan is feasible, the degree of any pancreatic necrosis can be used to determine the CT severity index (Table 11–6). Patients with a total score of 7 to 10 have a higher morbidity and mortality than those with scores of less than seven.[60]

TABLE 11–5 Balthazar-Ranson Grading System

A = Normal-appearing pancreas
B = Focal or diffuse enlargement of the pancreas
C = Pancreatic gland abnormalities characterized by mild peripancreatic inflammatory changes ("stranding")
D = Fluid collection in a single location, usually within the anterior pararenal space
E = Two or more fluid collections near the pancreas (such as within the anterior pararenal space and within the lesser sac) and/or the presence of gas in or adjacent to the pancreas

Treatment

HYDRATION The medical management of acute pancreatitis is largely supportive, except when specific complications arise. The most important aspect of supportive care is aggressive intravenous fluid repletion, given the common problem of extravascular fluid sequestration in the retroperitoneum and elsewhere. However, excessive intravenous hydration to maintain renal perfusion and cardiac output may compromise pulmonary function, leading to endotracheal intubation and mechanical ventilation. Despite this, intravenous fluids should not be withheld, unless specifically contraindicated.

ANALGESIA Supportive therapy also includes narcotic analgesia for adequate pain relief. Meperidine is preferred over morphine to prevent spasm of the sphincter of Oddi. However, care should be taken with meperidine, since its toxic metabolites may accumulate, especially in patients with renal failure. There is no evidence to suggest that fentanyl cannot be used for analgesia in acute pancreatitis. Likewise, there is no evidence to suggest that propofol cannot be used as a sedative for ventilated patients with acute pancreatitis.

NUTRITION Patients should receive nothing by mouth until their symptoms of nausea, vomiting, and abdominal pain have begun to resolve. The use of nasogastric suctioning provides no additional benefit, unless there is protracted nau-

TABLE 11–6 CT Severity Index

CT Grade	Score	Necrosis	Score
A	0	None	0
B	1	< 33%	2
C	2	33–50%	4
D	4	> 50%	6

NOTE: Total score = CT grade (0–4) + Necrosis score (0–6)
ABBREVIATION: CT, computed tomography.

sea and vomiting.[61,62] If a patient is not expected to take anything orally for more than 5 days, TPN is recommended because nutritional depletion may slow recovery time. When TPN is instituted, there appears to be no specific formulation that benefits the patient most. The use of lipid formulations is contraindicated only in patients with acute pancreatitis from hypertriglyceridemia.

INFECTION AND ANTIBIOTIC THERAPY Prophylactic antibiotics play no discernible role in acute pancreatitis, except in patients with documented pancreatic necrosis or infected pseudocysts in which prophylaxis may reduce the risk of sepsis. Fever in patients with acute pancreatitis early in their course should prompt an immediate workup to exclude pancreatic necrosis, infected pseudocyst, cholangitis, or pneumonia. If the patient is severely ill, broad-spectrum antibiotics with coverage for bowel flora should be instituted as soon as possible after cultures have been obtained. The development of a fever 2 weeks into the course of acute pancreatitis should raise the suspicion of a pancreatic abscess and lead to an aggressive workup.[63]

OTHER CONSIDERATIONS The use of somatostatin in patients with acute pancreatitis has not been shown to alter outcome in terms of mortality or in the prevention of complications.[64] However, patients with acute pancreatitis are at significant risk for stress-induced ulceration and intravenous H_2-receptor antagonists are clearly indicated for this reason.

All patients with biliary obstruction or cholangitis should undergo endoscopic retrograde cholangiopancreatography (ERCP). In this setting, ERCP has been shown to improve morbidity and mortality rates if performed within 24 to 72 hours.[65,66] In patients with acute biliary pancreatitis, but no evidence of biliary obstruction on imaging tests, early ERCP has not been shown to be of any benefit and may actually lead to a higher risk of complications.[67]

Complications

Patients with severe pancreatitis, those who fail to improve after 72 hours, and those who deteriorate despite aggressive management should have a dynamic contrast-enhanced CT scan to assess for pancreatic necrosis. Necrosis may be either infected or sterile. Patients with fever, tachycardia, leukocytosis, severe pain, and bacteremia usually have infected areas of necrosis. Any patient suspected of having this should undergo an immediate CT-guided needle aspiration for cultures and sensitivities, and if confirmed, the patient requires urgent surgical debridement. As mentioned earlier, the use of antibiotics in patients with necrotizing pancreatitis that is yet infected may reduce the risk of sepsis.

Pseudocysts, defined as collections of pancreatic juice that lack an epithelial lining, often resolve spontaneously. However, drainage is indicated if the pseudocyst enlarges to a diameter of more than 6 cm or begins to cause pain. Infection or hemorrhage involving a pseudocyst warrants decompression, either surgically or percutaneously. Other complications of acute pancreatitis include acute respiratory distress syndrome (ARDS), pericardial effusion, acute renal failure, DIC, and portal vein thrombosis with variceal bleeding or encephalopathy.

EVALUATION OF ABNORMAL LIVER ENZYME LEVELS

The term "liver function tests" (LFTs) refers to a battery of blood tests that reflect evidence of liver disease; they include aspartate aminotransferase (AST), alanine aminotransferase (ALT), alkaline phosphatase (ALP), total bilirubin, and albumin with or without total protein concentrations.[68,69] The prothrombin time (PT), while not typically part of the LFT panel, is an important element in assessing hepatic function.

However, most of these tests do not represent liver "function" in a strict sense. Instead, they more often reflect hepatic injury. Even measures of "hepatic function," such as serum albumin level or prothrombin time, are influenced by extrahepatic factors, including the patient's nutritional status, antibiotic therapy, or the administration of fresh frozen plasma. The term "liver tests" is therefore recommended. More quantitative LFTs, such as galactose, caffeine, or aminopyrine clearance tests, are available but not widely performed at present.

Serum Aminotransferases

Serum aminotransferases (transaminases) are derived from the cellular enzymes involved in the transfer of the amino acids aspartate (AST) and alanine (ALT) to ketoglutaric acid. Since ALT is present almost exclusively in the liver, whereas AST is found in both cardiac and skeletal muscle and liver, brain, and kidney tissue, elevations in serum ALT levels are more specific indicators of hepatic injury.

The ratio of serum AST to ALT levels can also be useful in diagnosing specific liver disorders. The AST enzyme is found in both the cytosol and the mitochondria of hepatocytes, whereas ALT is found only in the cytosol. In alcoholic hepatitis, toxic damage occurs primarily to the mitochondria, leading to a larger increase in AST level than ALT level. Furthermore, the enzymatic reaction with ALT requires pyridoxal 5'-phosphatase as a co-factor. Since the level of this co-factor is often deficient in alcoholics, the apparent activity of ALT is reduced compared to that of AST. In alcoholic hepatitis, the AST:ALT ratio is typically more than 2.0, with an AST level of not more than 400 U/L. In contrast, a ratio of less than 1.0 is typically seen in viral hepatitis.

The degree of transaminase elevation can also be helpful in the differential diagnosis of liver disease. The highest serum levels (over 10,000 U/L) are encountered in acute viral, toxin-mediated, and ischemic or congestive hepatopathy. In patients with symptomatic choledocholithiasis, the first laboratory abnormality is often an elevation in serum AST level, usually to no more than three to five times the normal level, but sometimes to more than 10 times the normal level in cholangitis.

If liver disease is suspected, correlation of an elevated serum AST concentration with an elevated serum ALT level should always be tried. An increase in AST level in the absence of an elevated ALT level suggests cardiac or skeletal muscle injury and can be confirmed by measuring creatine kinase isoenzyme levels.

Alkaline Phosphatase

Alkaline phosphatase (ALP) is an enzyme that catalyzes the hydrolysis of phosphate esters. It is present in a wide variety of tissues, including liver, bone, placenta, intestine, and kidney. Most of the enzyme is found in liver and bone, except during pregnancy, when the majority of it is derived from the placenta. Elevated ALP levels can also be seen in malignancies of the liver and bone. Ideally, ALP measurements should be done when the patient is fasting, since serum ALP levels may rise after a fatty meal as a result of the release of the intestinal isoenzyme. Bile duct epithelial cells synthesize hepatic ALP. In response to bile duct obstruction, the cells increase their synthesis and release of ALP.

In confirming the source of an elevated serum ALP level, the ALP can either be fractionated into isoenzymes or serum levels of gamma-glutamyl transferase (GGT), 5'-nucleotidase (5'-NT), or leucine aminopeptidase (LAP) can be measured. All three of these enzymes are useful in differentiating hepatobiliary from bone disease and obstructive from hepatocellular jaundice and in detecting the presence of infiltrative diseases of the liver. However, GGT is also elevated in pancreatitis and MI. In addition, since GGT is a microsomal enzyme, its tissue levels rise in response to enzyme induction by drugs, such as ethanol, barbiturates, and phenytoin. GGT also has a long half-life of 3 weeks.

An elevated ALP level of hepatic origin usually indicates either intrahepatic or extrahepatic causes of cholestasis. The most common cause of intrahepatic cholestasis is drugs, although other causes include infiltrative processes, such as lymphoma, sarcoidosis, primary biliary cirrhosis (PBC), TPN, tuberculosis, and fungal or systemic infections. Causes of extrahepatic cholestasis include common bile duct obstruction by gallstones, tumor, or stricture; acalculous cholecystitis; or localized obstruction in the liver by carcinoma. An elevated ALP level may or may not be accompanied by an elevated bilirubin level. An elevated ALP level with a normal bilirubin level suggests an infiltrative process involving the liver or a nonhepatic cause, such as cardiac failure or hyperthyroidism.

Bilirubin

Bilirubin is the end-product of hemoglobin degradation. The total bilirubin level represents a balance between production of bilirubin and its excretion by the liver. Normally, the total bilirubin level consists mostly of indirect (unconjugated) bilirubin, which accounts for 50% to 80% of total bilirubin. If more than 80% of the total bilirubin is indirect, this suggests hemolysis. Hemolysis is also characterized by an elevated reticulocyte count, an abnormal peripheral smear, and a low serum haptoglobin level. In most cases of hemolysis, given normal liver function, serum levels of total bilirubin often do not exceed 6.0 mg/dL. An elevated indirect bilirubin level can also be seen with Gilbert's syndrome, a common benign condition of no prognostic significance, which is characterized by a relative deficiency of glucuronyl transferase.

If more than 50% of the total bilirubin is direct (conjugated) bilirubin, this indicates either hepatocellular dysfunction or cholestasis. With a hepatocellular process, the ALP level is typically two to three times normal, whereas with cholestasis, the ALP level is often more than three to five times normal. Since direct bilirubin is water-soluble, the kidney, in cases of extrahepatic cholestasis, easily excretes it. Consequently, when the total bilirubin level is found to exceed 25 mg/dL, extrahepatic cholestasis is unlikely except in cases with simultaneous renal failure and/or hemolysis.

In sepsis, an elevated total bilirubin level is often seen, especially when the degree of elevation is out of proportion to the elevations in ALP or ALT levels. The clinical presentation and appropriate culture data help to differentiate sepsis from intrinsic liver disease. An elevation in serum bilirubin level without an elevation in ALP or ALT levels suggests an underlying cardiac disorder rather than an intrinsic hepatocellular cause.

Albumin

Albumin is a plasma protein that is synthesized exclusively by the liver. It has a half-life of approximately 21 days, so a decrease in serum albumin levels suggests liver disease of more than 3 weeks' duration. However, severe illness and malnutrition can also adversely affect albumin synthesis. Albumin may be lost in the urine in patients with nephrotic syndrome or into the GI tract in patients with protein-losing enteropathy. In addition, the volume of distribution of albumin affects serum albumin levels, so hypoalbuminemia is not specific to liver disease. The PT is a far more sensitive index of liver synthetic function than is albumin level.

Prothrombin Time

The liver synthesizes clotting factors I (fibrinogen), II (prothrombin), V, VII, IX, and X. Vitamin K is a necessary cofactor for the carboxylation of glutamic acid residues for the formation of factors II, VII, IX, and X. The PT is a measure of the vitamin K-dependent clotting factors, of which factor VII has the shortest half-life, at around 24 hours. A prolonged PT is not specific for liver disease, since it can also result from congenital disorders, DIC, drugs that antagonize vitamin K, or vitamin K deficiency. The PT may be prolonged in patients with liver disease for two reasons: vitamin K malabsorption secondary to cholestasis or hepatocellular synthetic dysfunction. A means of differentiating between these is to administer parenteral vitamin K. If the prolongation in PT is from cholestasis, at least a 30% correction in the PT should be seen after 24 hours. If no correction occurs, synthetic liver failure is the most likely cause of a prolonged PT.

In the ICU, a prolonged PT is most likely related to dietary vitamin K deficiency, not liver disease. In patients with acute or chronic liver disease, the degree of PT prolongation is a good prognostic tool. In fact, the PT is part of the King's College Hospital criteria for assessing the severity of acute liver failure, and the PT remains an important aspect of the Child-Turcotte-Pugh grading system for chronic liver disease.

Patients with Abnormal Liver Test Results

HISTORY As in any evaluation, an accurate history is essential. Often symptoms of liver disease are nonspecific and offer little assistance in the differential diagnosis. Important elements of the history include questions about prescription and over-the-counter medications, alcohol and illicit drug use, family, transfusion, sexuality, travel, employment, and past medical and surgical histories. Drug-induced liver injury is important to consider in any patient, and it may present as a hepatocellular picture or a cholestatic one. A family history of hemochromatosis, Wilson's disease, or alpha$_1$-antitrypsin deficiency is most helpful. Genetic factors may also play an important role in primary sclerosing cholangitis (PSC), PBC, or autoimmune hepatitis.

CONFIRMATION OF ABNORMAL TEST RESULTS Given an abnormal liver test result, the first step is to confirm that it does indicate some form of liver disease. Correlating each abnormal test result with another (Table 11–7) does this.

TABLE 11–7 Tests To Confirm Liver Disease

Test	Confirmation Test
AST level	ALT level
Alkaline phosphate level	GGT or alkaline phosphatase isoenzymes or 5'-nucleotidase level
Bilirubin level	Rule out hemolysis with direct bilirubin level, reticulocyte count, haptoglobin level, and peripheral blood smear
Albumin level	Prothrombin time
Prothrombin time	Trial or vitamin K to rule out malabsorption

NOTE: An elevated level on these tests should prompt the confirming test listed opposite.
ABBREVIATIONS: AST, asparate aminotransferase; ALT, alanine aminotransferase.

Similarly, various nonhepatic factors that may lead to abnormal liver tests (e.g., serum AST levels may be elevated after MI) must be considered.

CLASSIFICATION The second step in making a correct diagnosis is to classify the patient's liver condition as hepatocellular, cholestatic (either intrahepatic or extrahepatic), or mixed. The hallmark of hepatocellular disorders is an elevation in aminotransferase levels (i.e., AST and ALT), whereas cholestatic disorders are associated with an elevated ALP level, with or without abnormalities in other liver test results, such as total bilirubin level. Some liver problems, such as infiltrative disease or infections, lead to a mixed pattern of abnormal liver test results.

Hepatocellular Disease

Patients with evidence of hepatocellular injury (i.e., serum ALT levels more than three to five times normal) without any obvious cause, such as a recent cardiac arrest or acetaminophen overdose, should have additional laboratory tests, including hepatitis A, B, and C viral serology, antinuclear antibody (ANA) and anti–smooth muscle antibody (ASMA) for autoimmune hepatitis, cholestatic disease, ceruloplasmin level for Wilson's disease, iron studies (serum iron level, total iron binding capacity, percent iron saturation, serum ferritin level) for hemochromatosis, and alpha$_1$-antitrypsin levels to rule out deficiency (Table 11–8). Any and all drugs should be suspected, since they are among the most common causes of hepatocellular injury. Patients with serum ALT elevations of less than three times normal and an elevated ALP or bilirubin level who are symptomatic and have had persistently elevated ALT levels for more than 6 months should undergo additional laboratory testing, along with an abdominal ultrasound examination.

Cholestatic Disease

Patients who have an elevated ALP level that is more than two to three times normal likely have a cholestatic disorder, and they should have an abdominal ultrasound or CT scan to assess the biliary tree, liver, and pancreas (Figure 11–1). Biliary tract dilation suggests the presence of choledocholithiasis, bile duct stricture, cholangiocarcinoma, pancreatitis with edema of the head, pancreatic can-

TABLE 11–8 Laboratory Tests for Evaluation of Hepatocellular Dysfunction

Anti-nuclear antibody (ANA)
Hepatitis A, B, and C serology
Anti–smooth muscle antibody (ASMA)
Serum iron level, total iron binding capacity, and ferritin level
Ceruloplasmin level
Alpha$_1$-antitrypsin level

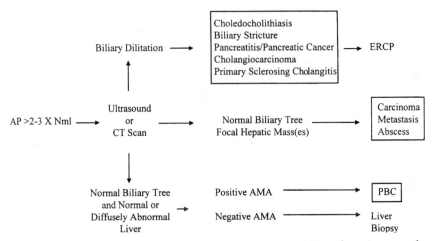

FIGURE 11–1 Approach to Cholestatic Disease. ABBREVIATIONS: ERCP, endoscopic retrograde cholangiopancreatography; AMA, antimitochondrial antibody; PBC, primary biliary cirrhosis.

cer, or PSC. Further evaluation should include ERCP to evaluate the site of obstruction and intervene with stone extraction or stent placement. In contrast, a normal biliary tract with focal hepatic mass or masses on imaging studies should raise the question of hepatocellular carcinoma, metastatic cancer, or abscess. Lastly, a normal biliary tree and either a normal liver or a diffusely abnormal liver on imaging tests should lead to suspicion of other conditions, such as fatty infiltration or the more aggressive nonalcoholic steatohepatitis (NASH), infiltrative processes, metabolic diseases (such as Wilson's disease), autoimmune hepatitis, or PBC. The anti-mitochondrial antibody (AMA) is highly sensitive for the diagnosis of PBC. A liver biopsy is indicated in other cases.

ACUTE LIVER FAILURE

Acute liver failure (ALF) is a clinical syndrome of massive liver necrosis that leads to severe impairment of liver function and progressive hepatic encephalopathy. Although uncommon, it is not rare; more than 2,000 cases occur annually in the United States with a mortality rate of almost 80% if left untreated.[70] However, with the availability of orthotopic liver transplantation, survival now approaches 50% to 75%.[71,72] Since patients with ALF can deteriorate rapidly and unexpectedly, they require close monitoring in the ICU with prompt intervention whenever necessary. A thorough understanding of the causes, clinical presentation, and natural history of ALF is paramount in managing these patients correctly and improving their outcome.

Causes of Acute Liver Failure

Viral hepatitis and drug-induced liver injury account for most cases of acute liver failure (ALF) worldwide, although the reported causes of ALF vary significantly between countries. For example, in the United Kingdom, acetaminophen is by far the most common reason for development of ALF; 50% to 60% of all cases are related to this drug.[73] In Asian countries, the foremost cause of ALF is viral hepatitis. There are many other identifiable causes of ALF, but almost half of cases remain unexplained.

Viral hepatitis is the primary cause of ALF in most parts of the world with hepatitis A virus (HAV) and hepatitis B virus (HBV) together accounting for about 70% of all cases.[74] There is an increased risk of ALF in conjunction with HAV infection in elderly patients and in those who use intravenous drugs.[74] However, overall, HAV rarely leads to ALF, and when it does, it usually has a favorable prognosis. Acute liver failure is most often seen with HBV, although ALF is an unusual manifestation of HBV, since this complication occurs in only 1% of all patients acutely infected with HBV.[75]

Acute liver failure due to viral hepatitis results from a massive immunologic assault against infected and adjacent "bystander" hepatocytes. The cause for this remains uncertain but likely relates to a unique host immunologic response directed against HBV. One-third to one-half of those with HBV infection in whom ALF develops become seronegative for hepatitis B surface antigen (HBsAg) within a few days as a result of this aggressive immunologic response.[76] Patients with rapid viral clearance have a more favorable prognosis than those who are slow to clear the virus.[77] On occasion, ALF occurs in patients with chronic HBV infection who develop reactivation of viral replication after immunosuppression or when they become superinfected with hepatitis D virus (HDV). In some countries, superinfection with HDV contributes to more than one-third of all cases of ALF.[70]

Hepatitis C virus (HCV) is a rare cause of ALF in Western countries, but it may play a more important role in Japan.[78] Dual infection with HBV and HCV results in a poor prognosis.[79] Hepatitis E virus (HEV) is an important cause of ALF in South and Central Asia and in Central America. HEV infection has a high case-fatality rate, especially in pregnant women.[80] Other viruses reported to cause ALF include cytomegalovirus (CMV), Epstein-Barr virus (EBV), and herpes viruses 1, 2, and 6.

The other main cause of ALF is drug-induced hepatotoxicity. One of the most important drugs implicated in acute hepatic necrosis is acetaminophen, the leading cause for ALF in some areas of the world, such as the United Kingdom. In most healthy individuals, 12 g of acetaminophen is the minimum amount required to produce hepatocellular necrosis. However, as little as 4 g may cause significant hepatic damage if taken concomitantly with alcohol or drugs that induce cytochrome P-450 enzymes. Other drugs that are intrinsically toxic to the liver include hydrocarbons and white phosphorus. Acute toxic hepatitis may also result from an idiosyncratic hypersensitivity reaction to certain drugs, such as halothane, isoniazid, rifampin, valproic acid, sulfonamides, propylthiouracil, alpha-methyldopa, and phenytoin.

There are other unusual causes of ALF. Rarely, Wilson's disease can present with ALF. Hepatic ischemia or congestion resulting from MI, cardiac arrest, cardiomyopathy, or pulmonary embolism may also lead to ALF. Sinusoidal obstruction from infiltrative malignancies can cause acute hepatic decompensation. Similarly, ALF may result from obstruction of venous outflow, either from the Budd-Chiari syndrome (hepatic vein thrombosis) or veno-occlusive disease after systemic chemotherapy or bone marrow transplantation. Other rare causes of ALF include the ingestion of the mushroom *Amanita phalloides*, acute fatty liver of pregnancy, or Reye's syndrome. Idiopathic ALF (in which tests for HAV, HBV, and other known causes reveal negative results) constitutes 20% to 40% of all cases.[70]

Clinical Presentation and Diagnosis

Acute liver failure is characterized by rapidly worsening hepatocellular dysfunction with abnormalities in hepatic protein synthesis, metabolism, and detoxification. Patients usually present with jaundice, coagulopathy, and altered mental status. Jaundice develops secondary to decreased bilirubin excretion and coagulopathy caused by altered synthesis of coagulation factors. Hypoglycemia results from decreased glucose synthesis and lactic acidosis from the increased synthesis of lactate, which is related to anaerobic metabolism and decreased hepatic clearance of this compound.

Encephalopathy is a characteristic feature of ALF, which may begin with mild confusion, irritability, or psychosis. The patient's mental status may fluctuate widely, but in some cases, cerebral edema may occur suddenly and lead to uncal herniation and death within minutes. However, most cases of cerebral edema occur in patients with ALF who have progressed to the more advanced stages of hepatic coma (Table 11–9). The pathogenesis of cerebral edema in ALF remains unknown.

Nonspecific complaints such as nausea, vomiting, fatigue, and malaise are common in ALF. The diagnosis is easily made in patients who have features of acute hepatitis along with confusion or agitation and a prolonged PT, or both. A

TABLE 11–9 Hepatic Encephalopathy Grading Scale

Grade	Neurologic Status
0	No abnormality detected
1	Trivial lack of awareness, shortened attention span
2	Lethargy, disoriented, personality changes, inappropriate behavior
3	Somnolent, responsive to painful stimuli
4	Coma, unresponsive to painful stimuli

careful history from the patient and family should include in-depth questions regarding possible drug or toxin exposures, intravenous drug use, foreign travel, and acetaminophen ingestion. If acetaminophen ingestion is considered, note the exact amount and time of the ingestion.

On physical examination, bruising or bleeding related to coagulopathy, an altered mental status, or a small or shrinking liver may be found. Patients usually have a markedly elevated total bilirubin level, moderately elevated AST and ALT levels, and a prolonged PT. Viral serology should include, at a minimum, hepatitis A IgM antibody, HBsAg, and IgM antibody to hepatitis B core antigen (HBcAg).

Classification and Prognosis of Acute Liver Failure

The clinical presentation and prognosis of ALF vary widely depending on the cause. One relatively accurate predictor of outcome is the time interval between the onset of jaundice and the onset of encephalopathy.[70,81] Patients with a shorter interval tend to have a better prognosis than those who develop encephalopathy more slowly. A recent classification of ALF uses the terms hyperacute, acute, and subacute to reflect different patterns of illness, cause, and most importantly, prognosis (Table 11–10).[81]

The ability to predict a patient's outcome is essential, since those with a poor prognosis should be considered as early as possible for liver transplantation. When prognostic data suggest a less than 20% chance of survival without transplantation, liver transplantation is advisable. The King's College Hospital (KCH) criteria[82] and other scoring systems have been used with some success to identify patients with severe hepatic failure who should be considered for liver transplantation. The fulfillment of KCH criteria usually predicts a poor outcome, but lack of fulfillment does not predict survival.[83]

TABLE 11–10 Classification of Acute Liver Failure

Hyperacute liver failure

Encephalopathy develops within 7 days of the patient becoming jaundiced. This subgroup has a high incidence of cerebral edema and marked prolongation of the PT. Paradoxically this group has the highest likelihood of recovery with medical management.

Acute liver failure

Encephalopathy develops 8 to 28 days after the onset of jaundice. This group has a high mortality rate with a high incidence of cerebral edema and marked prolongation of the PT.

Subacute liver failure

The interval between the onset of jaundice and encephalopathy is 4 to 12 weeks. This group has a high rate of mortality, despite a low incidence of cerebral edema and prolongation of the PT.

TABLE 11–11 Selection Criteria For Liver Transplantation

Cause of Acute Liver Failure	Criteria
Acetaminophen overdose	Arterial pH < 7.30 *or* INR > 6.5 *and* Creatinine > 3.4 mg/dL *and* Grade 3 or 4 encephalopathy
All other causes	INR > 6.5, regardless of the grade of encephalopathy *or* Any three of the following:
	1) Age < 10 or > 40 years
	2) Liver failure caused by nonviral hepatitis
	3) Halothane-induced hepatitis or idiosyncratic drug reation
	4) Duration of jaundice before encephalopathy, more than 7 days
	5) INR > 3.5
	6) Serum bilirubin level > 17.5 mg/dL

ABBREVIATION: INR, international normalization ratio.

Medical Management of Acute Liver Failure

The overall management of ALF is similar to that used for other patients with multiorgan failure: maintenance of normal vital signs and cardiovascular support, while managing any complications that arise until either hepatic regeneration occurs or liver transplantation is performed.

ACETAMINOPHEN OVERDOSE There are few toxins, apart from acetaminophen, that damage the liver in a dose-related fashion and for which an antidote is available. All patients suspected of having acetaminophen intoxication should receive N-acetylcysteine (NAC) at the earliest juncture, since there is little harm in using it and a definite risk in withholding it. N-acetylcysteine appears to work by replenishing the hepatocyte storage pool of glutathione, an important scavenger of acetaminophen's toxic metabolites.

Nomograms have been used to determine whether NAC is required, but their value has been questioned because the exact time of ingestion is not always known and the ingestion may have occurred in multiple stages. Treatment is most effective if started within 8 to 10 hours, although there may still be some benefit to using NAC up to 36 hours after the ingestion,[84] because of its vasodilatory effect on the microcirculation of other organs, accompanied by increased oxygen delivery and consumption.[85]

The loading dose of NAC is 140 mg/kg, followed by a maintenance dose of 70 mg/kg every 4 hours for a total of 17 doses, although it is often continued for longer than this, for the reasons mentioned above. The FDA has not yet approved an intravenous formulation because anaphylaxis remains a concern. The risk of this can be overcome by using a filter during the infusion of NAC. The intravenous dosing of NAC is 150 mg/kg, given in 5% dextrose over 1 hour, followed at 4-hour intervals by 70 mg/kg given over 1 to 4 hours.

GENERAL MANAGEMENT Patients with ALF require close observation in an ICU, preferably one at a tertiary care center with a liver transplant program. All patients should have large-bore intravenous access, an arterial line (unless severely coagulopathic), a urinary catheter, and a nasogastric tube to administer oral medications and to assess for upper GI bleeding. Careful attention should be paid to the patient's vital signs, cardiac rhythm, and fluid status, with maintenance of adequate intravascular volume and the use of inotropic agents as needed. Acute respiratory distress syndrome is common in patients with ALF and occurs in close to 33% of patients when acetaminophen is implicated as the cause.[86]

Patients should receive stress-induced ulcer prophylaxis because they are at higher than usual risk of upper GI tract bleeding as a result of severe coagulopathy, endotracheal intubation, and the added "stress" of their illness. Hypoglycemia is common and, if present, a 10% dextrose solution should be given intravenously. Particular attention should also be given to maintaining adequate nutrition.

Careful monitoring is required for other metabolic and hematologic abnormalities related to renal failure and DIC. Patients with ALF who go on to have grade 3 or 4 hepatic encephalopathy require endotracheal intubation to protect their airway and prevent aspiration. The remainder of intensive care management is directed at the specific complications of ALF; infection, bleeding, renal failure, and cerebral edema.

INFECTION Infection is a common problem in patients with ALF, likely related to the impairment of neutrophil function, decreased complement production, and the frequent need for invasive procedures. In one prospective study, 80% of patients with ALF were found to have a bacterial infection at some point during their hospitalization.[87] The risk of infection tends to be higher in patients who develop encephalopathy than in those who do not.[88] Uncontrolled infection occurs in about 25% of patients with ALF, which then excludes them from liver transplantation.[70]

Pneumonia accounts for 50% of infections, whereas bacteremia and UTIs account for 20% and 25%, respectively.[89] The most common causative bacteria include *Staphylococcus aureus,* streptococci, and gram-negative rods. Fungal infections are also common and occur in one-third of patients,[89] with *Candida* species the most frequent fungus detected. All patients with ALF should have surveillance cultures performed, and ascitic fluid or wounds should be cultured regularly. Catheter sites should also be checked frequently and changed regularly.

There is continued debate regarding the role of prophylactic antibiotics in patients with ALF. Their use may mask infection and possibly increase the risk of fungal infections. The use of enteral decontamination has not been shown to be of any benefit in preventing infection.[88] Although prophylactic parenteral antibiotics may decrease the number of infections and thereby lead to a higher likelihood of transplantation, their use does not appear to improve survival.[90]

(Whether this would still be true now that liver transplantation has become more acceptable in the treatment of ALF remains to be determined.) A high suspicion for infection and a low threshold to treat should always be maintained. Empiric antibiotics should include vancomycin, a third-generation cephalosporin, and fluconazole. Aminoglycosides should be avoided because these antibiotics appear to be more nephrotoxic in patients with liver disease. Furthermore, many patients with ALF already have some degree of concomitant renal impairment.

COAGULOPATHY Severe coagulopathy and intractable hemorrhage are common in ALF. However, the prophylactic use of fresh frozen plasma (FFP) was not shown to be of any benefit in a randomized controlled trial.[91] Instead, prophylactic FFP may contribute to fluid overload and increase the risk of developing pulmonary edema. It also makes the PT less reliable as a measure of disease severity and the need for liver transplantation. The main reason for using FFP should be when a patient is bleeding actively or before any invasive procedures. However, the use of parenteral vitamin K is appropriate.

RENAL FAILURE Renal failure is also common in ALF. Both acute tubular necrosis with a high urine sodium concentration and hepatorenal syndrome with a low urine sodium concentration occur. Renal failure secondary to the hepatorenal syndrome does not usually resolve unless there is improvement in hepatic function. Renal dialysis is often more difficult in patients with ALF because of hemodynamic instability and bleeding. Common indications for dialysis include volume overload, acidosis, and hyperkalemia.

HEPATIC ENCEPHALOPATHY AND CEREBRAL EDEMA In ALF, hepatic encephalopathy (HE) differs from that seen in chronic liver disease, since the former type is associated with cerebral edema much more frequently. In fact, cerebral edema is the leading cause of death in patients with ALF in whom grade 3 or 4 HE develops. Mortality rates of 50% to 85% are not uncommon in these patients.[92] Consequently, the severity of HE is a critical element in judging the timing for liver transplantation. Outcome is improved if transplantation is performed well before development of grade 4 HE.[93] Attention to HE is also of the utmost importance, since although most patients fully recover from ALF, they are often left with neurologic sequelae as a result of anoxic brain damage from intracranial hypertension related to cerebral edema. In patients who have altered mental status, other causes, such as hypoglycemia, hypoxia, sepsis, electrolyte or acid base disturbances, drug toxicity, or intracranial hemorrhage must be ruled out.

Patients with ALF should be cared for in a quiet area of the ICU to avoid unnecessary stimuli, which might worsen cerebral edema and trigger uncal herniation. The head of the bed should be elevated only 10 to 20 degrees, despite traditional thinking to the contrary.[94] Sedatives of any kind should be avoided, especially benzodiazepines because of their longer half-life in patients with liver dysfunction, which makes the assessment of mental status more difficult. Patients with grade 3 or 4 HE should undergo elective endotracheal intubation if they are considered for liver transplantation. If they are not transplant candidates, intubation can be postponed for patients with grade 3 HE as long as they are closely monitored. Care must be taken to avoid a traumatic or stressful intubation since this can lead to a sudden increase in intracranial pressure and possibly trigger uncal herniation. Sedation with propofol and/or fentanyl is best. Paralysis with *cis*-atracurium may also be helpful to prevent surges in ICP related to psychomotor activity.

Most aspects of treating acute HE are similar to those used in the management of chronic HE in end-stage liver disease. Lactulose is a mainstay, despite the lack of firm evidence to support its efficacy in acute HE. Initially, lactulose is given via nasogastric tube (30 mL every 2 to 4 hours) at the first sign of encephalopathy, with the dose titrated to achieve 2 to 3 semiformed bowel movements a day. Lactulose can also be given as a retention enema (300 mL in 1 L of tap water rectally every 4 hours). It is customary to monitor serum ammonia levels to follow the course of HE. Even though these levels do not correlate with the grade of encephalopathy, they do help to establish trends. Arterial levels appear to be more accurate than venous samples, as a result of the variable degree to which peripheral muscles metabolize ammonia. The benzodiazepine antagonist flumazenil has been used for acute HE, but it only transiently increases the level of consciousness.

Cerebral edema is a common complication in patients with ALF. However, it is often difficult to determine the onset of cerebral edema on the basis of clinical examination alone. A specific coma scale may be used to follow the patient's course, but papilledema is usually absent and head CT scan results are often normal. The first clinical sign may be deteriorating brain stem function, with sluggish pupils and slow oculovestibular reflexes, but these findings are rather insensitive markers of increased ICP. Consequently, the use of ICP monitors is now recommended for patients in grade 3 or 4 HE to detect and aggressively manage any significant rise in ICP which might indicate the onset of cerebral edema. Mean arterial pressure minus ICP should be kept at a level of more than 50 mm Hg. Although ICP monitoring has not been shown to improve survival in patients with ALF,[95] it is helpful nonetheless in improving outcome for those being considered for liver transplantation. In these patients, ICP monitoring has been found to increase patient survival, from onset of grade 4 HE until death, from a mean of 10 hours without ICP monitoring to a mean of 60 hours with it.[95]

Mannitol is the pharmacologic treatment of choice for patients in whom developing cerebral edema is suspected. Given by repeated boluses of 0.5 to 1.0 mg/kg, mannitol has been shown to increase the survival of patients with grade 4 HE in a randomized controlled clinical trial.[96] Mannitol should be administered whenever ICP rises to a level of more than 25 mm Hg or the patient develops signs of neurologic deterioration (e.g., unequally sized pupils, altered breathing pattern, decerebrate posturing). Barbiturates, particularly thiopental, are an effective alternative to treat elevated ICP when mannitol fails.[97] Corticosteroids for prophylaxis or as active treatment have not been shown to be of any benefit. Hyperventilation is also not an effective method for reducing ICP.[98] Patients with cerebral edema that is not responsive to medical therapy may ultimately require a decompressive craniotomy, although even with this the prognosis often remains dismal.

LIVER TRANSPLANTATION Given the high mortality rates of ALF, liver transplantation can be life-saving in selected cases. Early selection of patients who might benefit from transplantation is critical. The main reasons for listing a patient for liver transplantation are: worsening encephalopathy, evidence of cerebral edema, and marked prolongation of the PT. Contraindications to transplantation include: active infection, irreversible brain damage, and multiorgan system failure.

Another option is heterotopic auxiliary liver transplantation in cases in which there is significant potential for the patient's damaged liver to regain normal function. This procedure involves the transplantation of a donor liver to another site within the recipient's abdomen without removing the recipient's liver. It allows for the withdrawal of immunosuppression at a future point in time when the patient's own liver has fully recovered, such that rejection of the transplanted organ eventually ensues.

LIVER SUPPORT DEVICES Because of the severe shortage of liver donors, many patients with ALF are unable to receive the necessary transplantation. Two bioartificial liver models are under evaluation in clinical trials and others are at various stages of development.[99] The Bioartificial Liver (BAL) uses cells that are porcine derived while the Extracorpeal Liver Assist Device (ELAD) uses cells derived from a hepatoblastoma line. Well-designed controlled trials of these devices are currently underway, however clinical experience so far has been favorable.[100–103] The use of these liver-support devices as bridges to transplantation will likely play an important role in the future management of acute liver failure.

CIRRHOSIS AND ITS COMPLICATIONS

Cirrhosis is the end result of a wide variety of chronic, progressive liver diseases, which lead to diffuse destruction of the hepatic parenchyma with subsequent replacement by collagenous scar tissue and regenerating nodules. Proper management of patients with cirrhosis in the ICU requires an in-depth knowledge of its important sequelae, all of which occur independently of the cause of the underlying chronic liver disease. These complications include portal hypertension with variceal bleeding, ascites, SBP, HE, and hepatorenal syndrome.

Although the diagnosis of cirrhosis remains a histomorphologic one, a thorough history, physical examination, and laboratory tests often suggest it. At history-taking, patients often complain of fatigue and malaise. Other symptoms relate to the complications of cirrhosis, such as weight gain and increased abdominal girth from ascites or hematemesis from variceal bleeding. Findings of chronic liver disease on physical examination include palmar erythema, Dupuytren's contracture, spider angiomata, gynecomastia, testicular atrophy, ascites, caput medusae, splenomegaly, and asterixis. Hepatomegaly is often present. The left lobe of the liver is often firm and extends below the xiphoid process. Laboratory tests may reveal anemia and thrombocytopenia, a prolonged PT, an elevated serum bilirubin level, and a decreased serum albumin level. The severity of a patient's liver disease can be classified using the Child-Turcotte-Pugh scoring system (Table 11–12).

Ascites

Cirrhosis is the most common cause of ascites, accounting for about 80% of cases.[104] Other causes include infection, malignancy, Budd-Chiari syndrome, CHF, nephrotic syndrome, and pancreatitis. The development of ascites is a pivotal event in the natural history of cirrhosis; 50% of patients with ascites die within 2 years.[104] This makes ascites an indication for liver transplantation.

Several factors are involved in the development of ascites in patients with chronic liver disease. Portal hypertension plays an important role by increasing hydrostatic pressure within the splanchnic capillary bed. Hypoalbuminemia also

TABLE 11–12 Child-Turcotte-Pugh Scoring System for Severity of Liver Disease

	Points		
	1	2	3
Encephalopathy	None	Easily controlled	Difficult to control
or Grade	None	1–2	3–4
Ascites	Absent	Slight, easily controlled with diuretics	Moderate to severe, despite diuretics
Total bilirubin level (mg/dL)	< 2	2–3	> 3
Total bilirubin level (mg/dL) in PBC or PSC or other cholestatic liver diseases	< 4	4–10	> 10
Albumin level (mg/dL)	> 3.5	2.5–3.5	< 2.8
Prolongation of PT (sec)	1–3	4–6	>6
or INR	< 1.7	1.7–2.3	> 2.3

SCORING:
Child's A = 5–7 points
Child's B = 8–11 points
Child's C = > 11 points
ABBREVIATIONS: PT, prothrombin time; INR, international normalization ratio; PBC, primary biliary cirrhosis; PSC, primary sclerosing cholangitis.

leads to decreased oncotic pressure, which favors extravasation of fluid from the vasculature into the peritoneal cavity. Furthermore, increased hepatic sinusoidal pressure causes lymphatic leaking, which contributes to the formation of ascites. Altered renal function also leads to increased retention of sodium and water in patients with ascites.

One theory for the development of ascites hypothesizes that sequestration of blood into the splanchnic vascular bed leads to decreased effective circulating blood volume, which results in enhanced central sympathetic outflow and activation of the renin-angiotensin system, increased ADH release, and decreased release of atrial natriuretic peptide. Another theory is that the impaired clearance of vasoactive substances, such as nitric oxide, endotoxins, and prostacyclins, leads to decreased effective circulating blood volume, which then causes sodium and water retention.

Most complications related to moderate-to-severe ascites result from the effects of increased abdominal pressure. They include dyspnea, reflux esophagitis, anorexia, nausea, vomiting, and escape of ascitic fluid along tissue planes into the chest and scrotum. The severity of these complications is proportional to the volume and rate of ascitic fluid accumulation. The hepatorenal syndrome and spontaneous bacterial peritonitis are also seen only in patients with ascites.

DIAGNOSIS Although ascites is an easy enough diagnosis on physical examination when more than 2 L is present, detecting ascites when there is less than this amount can be challenging. The classic physical findings of ascites include bulging flanks, flank dullness, shifting dullness, positive fluid wave, and the "puddle sign." If bulging flanks are noted, percussion of the patient's flanks should be performed, since the lack of flank dullness indicates the absence of any ascites with an accuracy of more than 90%.[105] However, flank dullness is also the least specific finding because it is found in close to 70% of patients without ascites. Although a positive fluid wave is the most specific (82%) test for ascites, it is the least sensitive of all (less than 50%).[105] The "puddle sign" can detect as little as 120 mL of ascites, but this test is difficult to perform because patients must be examined while on their hands and knees. It also has a sensitivity and specificity of only 50%.[105]

Patients suspected of having ascites should undergo abdominal ultrasonography, which can detect as little as 100 mL of fluid.[104] Plain abdominal x-ray films may demonstrate a generalized haziness with loss of the psoas shadow, but they are generally insensitive. CT scanning of the abdomen can detect small amounts of ascites and, at the same time, give valuable information regarding the liver and other intra-abdominal structures.

DIAGNOSTIC PARACENTESIS The first step in evaluating patients with ascites is a careful analysis of the ascitic fluid. All patients with new onset ascites, those with known ascites who are hospitalized, and those who develop a deterioration in clinical status (e.g., confusion, fever, abdominal pain, or hepatorenal syndrome) should have diagnostic paracentesis to rule out SBP. This recommendation derives from the fact that the usual signs and symptoms of peritonitis are unreliable in patients with ascites and 10% to 27% of patients with ascites who are admitted to the hospital have an unsuspected infection.[106]

A diagnostic paracentesis is performed under sterile conditions using a 20- to 23-gauge angiocatheter and a 50-mL syringe. The safest site of puncture is along the linea alba between the umbilicus and symphysis pubis in the area of maximum dullness to percussion. Areas of scarring should be avoided. To avoid an enlarged spleen, an alternative site for paracentesis is in the right flank, about 1 1/2 inches above and medial to the superior iliac crest. Approximately 50 mL of ascitic fluid should be removed for immediate analysis.

Despite the fact that most patients with ascites related to cirrhosis have a coagulopathy, this should not preclude a diagnostic paracentesis unless the patient has evidence of DIC or fibrinolysis. Furthermore, prophylactic transfusions of FFP and platelets are not necessary in most cases. Abdominal-wall hematomas have been reported in only 1% of these patients, despite the fact that over two-thirds of patients in one study had a prolonged PT.[107] Runyon[104] states that, with such a low risk, approximately 140 U of FFP or platelets, or both, would have to be administered to prevent the transfusion of 2 U of packed RBCs. Hemoperitoneum and bowel-wall perforation are even less likely to occur.

Although there are a multitude of tests that can be ordered on ascitic fluid, most of these are not cost-effective (Table 11–13). When a paracentesis is performed for the first time, routine tests on the ascitic fluid should include a CBC count and differential, bacterial culture and sensitivity, and an albumin level to determine the serum-ascites albumin gradient (SAAG), as described later. A polymorphonucleocyte (PMN) count of 250 cells/µL or more denotes presumptive evidence of infected ascites and mandates empiric therapy with intravenous broad-spectrum antibiotics. Prospective trials have shown that inoculating ascitic fluid into blood culture bottles at the bedside has a greater sensitivity for detect-

TABLE 11–13 Laboratory Tests on Ascitic Fluid

Required	Optional	Rarely necessary
CBC count	Total protein level	AFB smear
Culture[a]	LDH level	TB culture
Albumin[b] level	Glucose level	Cytology
	Amylase level	
	Triglyceride level	
	Gram's stain	

[a]Inoculated in blood culture bottles at the bedside.
[b]Obtain serum albumin level at time of paracentesis.
ABBREVIATIONS: CBC, complete blood cell; AFB, acid-fast bacteria; LDH, lactate dehydrogenase; TB, tuberculosis.

ing bacterial growth than inoculating agar plates and broth in the laboratory (80% versus 50%, respectively).[108,109]

If the ascitic fluid is bloody, a "corrected" PMN count should be calculated. This can be done by subtracting one PMN from the absolute PMN count for every 250 RBCs seen in the ascitic fluid (this is the maximum expected ratio of PMNs to RBCs present in peripheral blood[110]) or determining the ratio of PMNs to RBCs in the patient's peripheral blood and adjusting the ascitic count accordingly. Gross blood usually suggests trauma during the tap, although in selected cases, it may also suggest underlying malignancy or an infection with tuberculosis or fungi.

The SAAG is calculated by subtracting the ascitic albumin concentration from a simultaneous serum level. A SAAG of 1.1 g/dL or more indicates the presence of portal hypertension or a cardiac cause, whereas a SAAG of less than 1.1 g/dL suggests other causes, such as neoplastic or inflammatory disease. The SAAG establishes the diagnosis of portal hypertension and cirrhosis with an accuracy of 97%.[111]

Optional tests on ascitic fluid include total protein level, lactate dehydrogenase (LDH) level, and glucose level. The results can assist in differentiating SBP from secondary bacterial peritonitis. The ascitic total protein level is also useful, since levels of less than 1.0 g/dL correlate with an increased risk of SBP as a result of the decreased concentration of opsonins.[112] A Gram's stain may help to identify patients with intestinal perforation, but this test has only a 10% sensitivity in detecting any bacteria in documented cases of SBP.[113] Cultures for mycobacteria and fungi or cytologic examination should only be done in patients with a high pretest probability (i.e., clinical suspicion and low SAAG with a predominance of lymphocytes on differential), given the very low sensitivity of each test. An elevated amylase level in patients with ascites suggests pancreatic disease, whereas elevated levels of triglycerides indicates chylous ascites caused by lymphatic obstruction from lymphoma, tumor, infection, or trauma.

SPONTANEOUS BACTERIAL PERITONITIS One should always consider the possibility of SBP in patients with ascites admitted to the hospital, in those in whom an infection is suspected, or in those who are presenting with abdominal pain, encephalopathy, or worsening renal function. Whenever SBP is a consideration, patients should have ascitic fluid analyzed. The definitive diagnosis of SBP requires a positive ascitic fluid culture without evidence of an intra-abdominal surgically correctable source. An initial ascitic fluid PMN count of 250 cells/μL or more is considered presumptive evidence of SBP, and intravenous broad-spectrum antibiotics should be started while awaiting culture results.[104] Empiric antibiotic therapy is also recommended in patients with a PMN count of less than 250 cells/μL, if there are signs or symptoms of infection, because this may represent an early stage of SBP before an appropriate neutrophil response is mounted. Withholding antibiotics could result in sepsis and death from overwhelming infection.

Antibiotic coverage for SBP should be relatively broad in spectrum, until the results of cultures and sensitivities become available. Cefotaxime or a similar third-generation cephalosporin remain the treatment of choice for SBP, since they cover the most common pathogens, *Escherichia coli, Klebsiella pneumoniae,* and pneumococci.[104] Anaerobic organisms are rarely identified as a cause of SBP. Recently, a randomized, controlled trial has shown that 5 days of antibiotic therapy is as effective as 10 days of such therapy in well-characterized SBP, with or without bacteremia.[114] A repeated paracentesis in 2 or 3 days is usually not necessary, although it may be useful when a patient fails to improve or secondary bacterial peritonitis is a consideration.

Risk factors for developing SBP include low opsonin levels in conjunction with ascitic total protein levels of less than 1.0 g/dL, recent variceal bleeding (especially if hypotension occurs), and a previous episode of SBP.[104] The use of norfloxacin (400 mg/day orally) has been shown to prevent SBP in patients with low ascitic total protein levels (i.e., low opsonins) and a previous history of SBP.[115,116] However, oral antibiotics do not prolong survival and can select for resistant gut flora. In fact, the long-term use of ciprofloxacin was identified in a recent report as an important risk factor for developing fungal infections.[117] Intermittent doses of ciprofloxacin (750 mg/week) and using norfloxacin only for inpatients may prevent SBP without selecting for resistant flora.[118,119]

Until randomized trials can document cost savings or survival benefits, the use of long-term antibiotic prophylaxis should only be considered in those with risk factors for developing SBP and in those awaiting liver transplantation. Diuresis may actually help prevent SBP by increasing ascitic fluid opsonins, complement, and antibody levels, whereas repeated large-volume paracentesis (LVP) may remove opsonins and thereby increase the risk of developing SBP.

The use of intravenous albumin in addition to antibiotic therapy has been shown to reduce the incidence of renal impairment and death in patients with cirrhosis and SBP.[120] This large study was not blinded and used substantial amounts of albumin. The data suggests that albumin infusion in a subgroup of patients with more advanced liver disease or more severely impaired renal function may be beneficial. Whether smaller doses of albumin would be just as effective should be addressed.

SECONDARY BACTERIAL PERITONITIS Secondary bacterial peritonitis is an infection of the ascitic fluid caused by a surgically treatable condition. It can either result from a perforated viscus (duodenal ulcer) or loculated abscess (perinephric abscess). Secondary bacterial peritonitis can masquerade as SBP, and it is important to differentiate the two, since the latter only requires antibiotic treatment, whereas the former requires surgical intervention. Typically, signs and symptoms do not help in differentiating SBP from secondary peritonitis.

One of the best methods is to analyze in detail the initial ascitic fluid and to carefully monitor the response to therapy. Characteristically, in the setting of free perforation, the PMN count is considerably more than 250 cells/μL (usually in the thousands of cells) and multiple organisms are identified on Gram's stain and culture. In addition, two or three of the following ascitic fluid criteria are present:

1. Total protein level of 1.0 g/dL or more
2. LDH level of more than the upper limit of normal for serum
3. Glucose level of less than 50 mg/dL

The sensitivity of these criteria is reported to be 100%, but the specificity is only 45%.[121]

Patients with ascitic fluid analysis that fulfill these criteria should undergo upright plain films of the abdomen, water-soluble contrast studies of the GI tract, and an abdominal CT scan to detect evidence of a perforation or abscess formation. In patients suspected of having secondary peritonitis, anaerobic coverage should be added to the initial antibiotic regimen and a surgical consultation obtained. With SBP, repeat ascitic PMN count results at 48 hours are invariably below pretreatment levels when appropriate antibiotics are used, whereas in secondary peritonitis the PMN count continues to rise despite broad-spectrum antibiotic therapy.

TREATMENT OF UNCOMPLICATED ASCITES
Dietary Sodium Restriction

The initial treatment of uncomplicated cirrhotic ascites is directed at improving hepatic function by withholding hepatotoxic drugs (especially alcohol) and by maximizing nutritional status. However, the mainstay of treatment primarily involves the restriction of dietary sodium intake and the use of diuretics to induce a natriuresis. Dietary sodium intake should be restricted to 2000 mg/day (88 mmol/day). Fluid restriction, although often used, is not necessary unless the serum sodium concentration drops to less than 120 mmol/L, since natriuresis usually results in the passive loss of excess body water as well.

Diuretic Therapy

Simply waiting for patients with ascites to develop a natriuresis spontaneously on sodium restriction alone is not justified, since only 15% of patients lose weight and note an improvement in their ascites with this form of therapy.[113] Diuretics are therefore required in most patients. The best approach is to begin with a combination of spironolactone and furosemide. This also helps to maintain a stable level of serum potassium, by balancing the effects of a potassium-sparing diuretic (i.e., spironolactone) with a potassium-losing diuretic (i.e., furosemide).

Therapy is initiated with 100 mg of spironolactone plus 40 mg of furosemide, given together orally each morning. Close monitoring of serum electrolyte levels, renal function tests, and blood pressure is necessary during the initiation phase of diuretic therapy. After 3 to 4 days, if the patient's body weight and sodium excretion remain unchanged, the dose of each diuretic should be doubled to 200 mg/day and 80 mg/day, respectively. To enhance diuresis further, the doses can be increased incrementally every 3 to 4 days to a maximum of 400 mg/day of spironolactone and 160 mg/day of furosemide, maintaining the 100:40 ratio in doses. Dietary sodium restriction and dual diuretics are effective in well over 90% of patients.[122]

A common misconception is that urinary sodium concentrations are of no use in managing patients on diuretics. Since the main problem with cirrhotic ascites is renal sodium retention, determining sodium excretion can prove helpful in deciding upon the efficacy of medical treatment. The goal is to achieve a sodium loss in excess of intake. The total daily excretion of sodium via nonurinary mechanisms is about 10 mmol/day in afebrile cirrhotic patients.[104] Thus, with a maximum dietary sodium intake of 88 mmol/day (i.e., 2,000 mg/day), the goal of diuretic therapy should be to achieve a urinary sodium of more than 78 mmol/day. Patients who excrete more than 78 mmol/day of sodium but who do not lose weight are most probably consuming more dietary sodium than the recommended 88 mmol/day, whereas those with a urinary sodium excretion of less than 78 mmol/day who do not lose weight should have the dosages of their diuretics increased.

There is no clearly defined amount of weight that patients should lose when they have moderate to severe ascites, as long as peripheral edema is present. However, once peripheral edema resolves, patients should lose no more than 0.5 kg/day. This usually prevents prerenal azotemia, hyperkalemia, and other related problems. Indications to withhold diuretics temporarily include a serum sodium of less than 120 mmol/L despite fluid restriction, a serum creatinine level of more than 2.0 mg/dL, or the onset of orthostatic symptoms or HE.

Large-Volume Paracentesis

Compared to diuretics, LVP provides a rapid method of removing several liters of ascitic fluid with a large-bore needle connected to vacuum bottles. This results in shorter hospital stays and avoids many of the side effects of diuretics. However, in terms of readmission rates to the hospital, survival rates, or cause of death, LVP has been found to be no better than diuretics.[123,124] In addition, LVP does little to correct the underlying cause of ascites, namely renal sodium retention. For this reason, LVP should not be used as first-line therapy for patients with ascites. However, in patients with tense ascites, a single LVP that removes 4 to 6 L of fluid can be done rapidly and safely without any colloid infusion.[125–127]

TREATMENT OF REFRACTORY ASCITES Ascites is defined as "refractory" when it is unresponsive to a sodium-restricted diet and maximum doses of spironolactone (400 mg/day) and furosemide (160 mg/day), in the absence of any potentially reversible factors, such as prostaglandin inhibitors (e.g., NSAID ingestion).[128] Patients should not be labeled as having refractory ascites unless they have first been found to be compliant with their diet by measuring 24-hour urine sodium excretion. In addition, they should have a urine sodium concentration of less than 78 mmol/day, despite maximum doses of diuretics. The term "refractory ascites" can also be applied in patients who have developed clinically significant complications during diuretic therapy. Consequently, fewer than 10% of patients with cirrhosis and ascites truly fit the definition of being refractory.[104] Further options for these patients include serial LVP, peritoneovenous shunts (rarely performed nowadays), TIPS, or liver transplantation.

Serial Large-Volume Paracenteses

Serial LVPs, done approximately every 2 weeks, are an effective way of removing ascites for patient comfort or other reasons. The sodium concentration of ascitic fluid is close to 130 mmol/L, so the amount of sodium removed with each LVP can easily be calculated. Runyon[104] states that if a patient is complying with an 88 mmol/day sodium diet and loses 10 mmol/day via nonurinary mechanisms but excretes no measurable sodium in the urine, a 6-L LVP would remove 780 mmol of sodium (i.e., 130 mmol/L × 6 L = 780 mmol), which is equivalent to 10 days' worth of retained sodium (780 mmol/day = 78 mol per 10 days). Patients with urinary sodium losses can be expected to require serial LVPs even less frequently. On the other hand, if patients go less than 10 days before needing another LVP, they are clearly not compliant with their dietary sodium restriction. Serial LVPs are not without complications, such as iatrogenic SBP and abdominal-wall infections or hematomas. In addition, frequent LVPs can deplete ascitic total protein levels and lead to malnutrition and lower opsonin levels, predisposing the patient to SBP.

Peritoneovenous Shunts

Peritoneovenous (LeVeen or Denver) shunts were once popular surgical options for refractory ascites. A small-bore catheter was tunneled under the skin from the peritoneal cavity to the internal jugular vein to permit the return of ascitic fluid directly to the systemic circulation. Some of these shunts included a single-way valve and/or pump to maintain unidirectional flow (e.g., Denver shunt). However, DIC was a common complication of these shunts, and most became occluded within a few weeks. Furthermore, no survival benefit was shown compared with medical therapy.[129,130] These shunts may also make liver transplantation more difficult. As a result, peritoneovenous shunts are no longer performed at most centers.

Transjugular Intrahepatic Portacaval Shunt

A procedure recently introduced for selected cases of variceal bleeding, TIPS has also been shown to be effective for patients with refractory ascites, resulting in better control of ascites, an increase in lean body mass, and improvements in the Child-Pugh score.[131] However, prospective studies are needed to determine if these short-term clinical benefits are accompanied by prolonged survival. Furthermore, TIPS may lead to an exacerbation of HE and result in decompensated liver function, prompting an urgent liver transplant. Moreover, TIPS dysfunction and frequent revisions are not uncommon.

COLLOID REPLACEMENT DURING LVP The use of colloid replacement to prevent fluid shifts with LVP remains a controversial issue. Ginés et al[132] have shown that patients who do not receive intravenous albumin after LVP may develop more perturbations in serum electrolytes, plasma renin, and serum creatinine, compared with those given intravenous albumin. However, no patients developed any symptoms and the changes detected did not appear to be clinically significant. There were also no differences in morbidity or mortality between the two groups.

One problem with this and similar studies is that they included patients who did not have clear-cut refractory ascites. For example, in the Ginés et al study, 40% of patients had tense ascites from "inadequate sodium restriction or insufficient diuretic dosage (or both)" and 31% did not even receive diuretics before hospitalization. By contrast, in another study of patients with well-documented diuretic-resistant ascites, there was no rise in plasma renin activity, central blood volume, or GFR after a 5-L LVP was performed without giving intravenous albumin.[126] This may be because patients with advanced cirrhosis and diuretic-resistant ascites have some degree of "circulatory hyporeactivity," whereas patients with less advanced liver disease and diuretic-sensitive ascites are more sensitive to intravascular volume depletion with LVP.[133]

There are other concerns associated with the routine use of intravenous albumin. First of all, no study to date has demonstrated any survival advantage using colloid replacement for patients undergoing LVP. Furthermore, albumin, when given exogenously, has been shown to increase its own degradation[134] and to decrease its own synthesis in vitro.[135] Albumin is also expensive, at close to $1250 per LVP.[104] Given this, it is difficult to justify its routine use. However, if intravenous albumin is used, 10 g should be infused per liter of ascites removed, not to exceed 50 g. Recent studies recommend giving half the intravenous albumin infusion immediately after LVP and the other half 6 hours later.[104]

Several colloid agents other than albumin are available for plasma expansion after LVP. Dextran-70 (given in a proportion of 6 g per liter of ascites removed) has been shown to prevent the hypovolemic changes associated with a 5-L LVP[136] and to be equivalent to albumin in preventing any hemodynamic complications.[137] However, another study suggests that dextran-70 is not as effective as albumin, although no difference in survival was noted between the two.[138] The main advantage of using intravenous dextran is that it costs 30 times less than intravenous albumin. Hemaccel has also shown no significant differences in hemodynamics, complications, or survival rates compared to albumin in patients with refractory ascites.[139] These plasma expanders may prove to be useful alternatives to albumin. However, further studies are needed before their widespread use is recommended.

To summarize, an LVP should be avoided in patients with diuretic-sensitive ascites, unless they present with tense ascites. Instead, better compliance of the patient with diuretic therapy and strict dietary sodium restriction should be emphasized. Serial LVP should be reserved for the 10% of patients with truly refractory ascites who actually may be less sensitive to LVP-related intravascular volume changes than diuretic-sensitive patients. Thus, these patients likely do not require intravenous albumin or other colloid replacement in the first place.

Hepatic Encephalopathy

Hepatic encephalopathy (HE) is a potentially reversible neuropsychiatric syndrome that is seen in both acute and chronic liver disease. In chronic liver disease, HE helps to define a patient's prognosis as one of the five elements that constitute the Child-Turcotte-Pugh classification of liver disease severity (Table 11–12). Present in 50% to 70% of patients with cirrhosis,[140] HE may be either overt or subclinical. Overt HE is characterized by disorientation, lethargy, somnolence, asterixis, and hyperflexia. Patients with subclinical HE may present with irritability, poor short-term memory, problems in concentrating, or altered sleep-wake cycles. Several grading systems have been developed, which use specific features, such as the level of consciousness, perturbations in personality and intellect, neurologic signs, or EEG changes. The most useful is the West Haven set of criteria (Table 11–9).

The pathogenesis of HE remains unclear, although a variety of mechanisms have been proposed, including alterations in the blood-brain barrier, changes in cerebral energy metabolism, the presence of false neurotransmitters, and elevated gut-derived brain ammonia levels. None of the manifestations of HE are specific to this disorder, and it is imperative to rule out other causes of altered mental status in patients with chronic liver disease (Table 11–14).

TREATMENT
Precipitating Causes

The treatment of acute episodes of HE involves a multifaceted approach. Any precipitating factors should be identified and corrected (Table 11–15). When specific precipitating factors cannot be identified, Doppler ultrasonography should be done to search for large portosystemic shunts, which can be corrected angiographically or surgically. A nonabsorbable disaccharide, such as lactulose, should also be administered to clear the gut of ammonia and other substances that may cause HE.

Dietary Protein Intake

A major goal in the management of HE is to reduce the production and absorption of ammonia. This can be done by restricting the dietary intake of protein and by inhibiting urease-producing colonic bacteria. Patients should initially be placed on a

TABLE 11–14 Causes of Abnormal Mental Status in Chronic Liver Disease

Electrolyte disturbances
Hypoglycemia
Hypoxia
Infection
Bleeding (both gsatrointestinal and intracranial)
Alcohol withdrawal
Drug intoxication (narcotics and benzodiazepines)

limited protein diet (i.e., less than 20 g/day). When the clinical status improves, protein intake can be increased by 10 to 20 g/day every 3 to 5 days until the patient's protein tolerance has been established. Patients with cirrhosis require a minimal daily protein intake of 0.8 to 1.0 g/kg to maintain nitrogen balance.

Lactulose

The nonabsorbable disaccharide lactulose acts as a cathartic to remove ammoniagenic substrates from the GI tract. In addition, lactulose acidifies the intestinal contents to create an environment hostile to urease-producing lactobacilli, thereby further decreasing the luminal production of ammonia. Lactulose also reduces the absorption of ammonia by nonionic diffusion and results in a net movement of ammonia from the bloodstream into the GI tract. Initially, patients should be started on large doses of lactulose (30 to 50 mL every 1 to 2 hours) until catharsis begins, then the daily dose of lactulose should be titrated (typically 15 to 30 mL, 3 to 4 times a day) to achieve 3 to 4 semi-formed stools daily. Lactulose enemas (300 mL in 1 L of water) may also be used if oral or nasogastric administration is not feasible. Lactulose is effective not only in controlling acute exacerbations of HE but also in maintaining chronic HE in remission.

TABLE 11–15 Precipitating Factors for Hepatic Encephalopathy

Excessive dietary protein
Gastrointestinal bleeding
Exacerbation of underlying liver disease
Infection (including SBP)
Dehydration
Hypoxia
Hypokalemia
Azotemia
Constipation
Portosystemic shunts (spontaneous, surgical, or transjugular intrahepatic)

ABBREVIATION: SBP, spontaneous bacterial peritonitis.

Antibiotics

Antibiotics directed against urease-producing bacteria have also proven to be effective in treating HE, but they are rarely used as first-line agents because of their potential side effects when used in the long term. These agents are usually reserved for patients who are refractory to lactulose alone. Neomycin in doses of 6 g/day, in divided doses, is similar in efficacy to lactulose.[139] Since small amounts of neomycin are absorbed, ototoxicity and nephrotoxicity may be a problem, especially with continuous use. Metronidazole at doses of 800 mg/day has benefits similar to neomycin.[139]

New Treatments

Several innovative treatments for HE have shown promise. One involves increasing the tissue metabolism of ammonia by infusing substrates, such as ornithine aspartate[141] or sodium benzoate.[142] These substrates were of some benefit in small controlled trials, but their role in clinical practice remains unclear. The use of flumazenil can only be recommended for HE that has been precipitated by the use of benzodiazepines. Parenteral or enteral formulas enriched with branched-chain amino acids may also improve HE by reducing brain concentrations of aromatic amino acids, thought to act as false neurotransmitters. Since most patients with HE tolerate standard synthetic amino-acid preparations reasonably well, branched-chain amino acids should be reserved for those with malnutrition who are intolerant to routine protein supplementation.[143] Zinc may also play an important role in HE. Two of the five enzymes responsible for the metabolism of ammonia to urea require zinc as a co-factor. In one study, overt HE was reversed after zinc supplementation in patients with cirrhosis who were zinc-deficient.[144] Ultimately, liver transplantation is the only treatment that permanently reverses HE by restoring normal liver function and correcting portosystemic shunts.

Hepatorenal Syndrome

PATHOGENESIS Cirrhosis is associated with a wide spectrum of renal abnormalities, and the kidney is central to the development of ascites and its complications. The most severe form of functional renal failure is the hepatorenal syndrome. Although the exact pathogenesis of hepatorenal syndrome is unknown, it is characterized by renal hypoperfusion caused by increased vascular resistance that leads to a low GFR. Anatomically and histologically, the kidneys are normal and remain capable of proper function if transplanted into an individual without liver disease. Furthermore, normal renal function returns rapidly after liver transplantation is performed for hepatorenal syndrome.

The hepatorenal syndrome has been reported in 7% to 15% of patients with cirrhosis admitted to the hospital.[145] In a large series of nonazotemic patients with cirrhosis and ascites who were followed prospectively for 5 years,[146] the probability of developing hepatorenal syndrome was 20% at 1 year and 40% at 5 years. Patients with marked sodium retention who were unable to excrete a water load had an increased risk of developing hepatorenal syndrome, as were those with abnormal systemic hemodynamics characterized by low arterial pressure, high plasma renin activity, and increased plasma norepinephrine levels. Finally, poor nutritional status, the presence of esophageal varices, and the absence of hepatomegaly all suggested an increased risk of developing hepatorenal syndrome. The Child-Turcotte-Pugh classification of liver disease severity did not correlate with the risk of developing hepatorenal syndrome.[146]

DIFFERENTIAL DIAGNOSIS Other causes of acute renal failure in patients with cirrhosis include nephrotoxicity from drugs (particularly NSAIDs or aminoglycosides), acute tubular necrosis from hypotension and radiographic contrast material, obstructive uropathy, and prerenal azotemia from bleeding, vomiting, diarrhea, or renal fluid losses from overly aggressive diuresis. Unfortunately, there is no specific diagnostic test for hepatorenal syndrome. One must first rule out other causes of acute renal failure and identify any reversible factors. The International Ascites Club has recently proposed specific criteria to help in the diagnosis of hepatorenal syndrome (Table 11–16).[128]

MANAGEMENT The management of patients with hepatorenal syndrome remains difficult, since the mechanisms responsible for it are poorly defined. There is no effective treatment, despite several trials assessing drugs intended to reverse renal vasoconstriction. Thus, much of the treatment for hepatorenal syndrome involves supportive therapy, especially the identification, removal, and treatment of any factors known to precipitate acute renal failure. All drugs with potential renal toxicity should be stopped, low blood pressure from hemorrhage or dehydration returned toward baseline, electrolyte levels corrected, and all infections identified and treated. Dialysis or continuous hemofiltration should be considered in patients recovering from ALF or awaiting liver transplantation, with the hope that renal function will return once liver failure improves. The use of TIPS has been shown to improve renal function in patients with hepatorenal syndrome,[147] although more information is needed before further recommendations can be made.

TABLE 11–16 **Diagnostic Criteria of Hepatorenal Syndrome**

1. Absence of shock, infection, bleeding or current use of nephrotoxic drugs
2. Serum creatinine > 1.5 mg/dL, or 24-hour creatinine clearance < 40 mL/min
3. No improvement with withdrawal of diuretics and plasma volume expansion with 1.5 L of isotonic saline
4. No evidence of obstruction or renal parenchymal disease on ultrasound
5. Proteinuria of < 500 mg/day

Liver transplantation is currently the only definitive therapy for hepatorenal syndrome. Although patients with hepatorenal syndrome who undergo liver transplantation may develop more complications, the probability of survival 3 years after transplant is 60%, only slightly reduced from the 70% to 80% rate noted for patients without hepatorenal syndrome.[148]

ACUTE COLONIC PSEUDO-OBSTRUCTION

Pathogenesis

Acute colonic pseudo-obstruction is characterized by acute dilation of the large intestine without any evidence of mechanical obstruction. The pathogenesis of acute pseudo-obstruction is not known, but a major factor is thought to be an imbalance in the enteric autonomic nervous system. Acute colonic pseudo-obstruction usually accompanies serious medical conditions, such as intra-abdominal inflammation, metabolic derangements (hyponatremia, hypokalemia, hypermagnesemia, and hypomagnesemia), neurologic disorders, respiratory failure requiring intubation, MI, sepsis, and the excessive use of narcotics and sedatives.

Clinical Presentation

Patients usually present with abdominal pain, distention or constipation, or a combination of these. More often, the patient is already in the ICU as a result of another serious illness. On examination, the abdomen is distended and tympanitic, with reduced or absent bowel sounds. In some cases, a tender dilated cecum may be palpable. Abdominal radiographs reveal dilation of the colon and possibly the small bowel as well. The cecum is typically enlarged to a significant degree. Since acute pseudo-obstruction and mechanical obstruction present with similar clinical features, a water-soluble enema or colonoscopy may be required to differentiate the two.

MANAGEMENT   In general, the management of acute pseudo-obstruction is conservative. Patients should be placed on bowel rest and the upper GI tract decompressed with a nasogastric tube at intermittent suction. Frequent turning of the patient may help release intestinal gas, but a rectal tube is of limited benefit. Electrolyte and fluid abnormalities should be corrected, and drugs that depress colonic motility should be withdrawn. With treatment of the underlying medical condition, colonic function usually returns to normal. A few patients who do not improve with conservative treatment may go on to sustain a cecal perforation. However, the risk of this does not correlate well with the absolute cecal diameter, but rather with the duration of cecal distention.[149]

If the cecal diameter fails to improve after 2 to 3 days of conservative management, more aggressive intervention is required. Treatment with neostigmine has been shown to be an effective way to decompress the colon in patients with acute pseudo-obstruction.[150] Mechanical obstruction must be ruled out before the use of neostigmine. Finding air throughout all colonic segments, including the rectosigmoid, on plain radiographs can rule out mechanical obstruction. If air is not seen in the rectosigmoid colon, a radiocontrast enema must be used to ensure a mechanical obstruction does not exist. Exclusion criteria for the use of neostigmine include a baseline heart rate of less than 60 beats/min or systolic blood pressure of less than 90 mm Hg; active bronchospasm requiring medication; treatment with a prokinetic drug, such as metoclopramide, in the preceding 24 hours; history of colon cancer or partial colon resection; active GI bleeding; or a creatinine level of more than 3 mg/dL. The dose of neostigmine is 2.0 mg, given intravenously over 3 to 5 minutes. Patients should be monitored by ECG, and frequent blood pressure recordings should be obtained for at least the first 30 minutes after administration. The patient should remain supine for at least 60 minutes after injection. Atropine, 1.0 mg, should be available at the bedside as needed for symptomatic bradycardia. If the patient fails to respond, a second dose can be given similarly 3 hours later.

If conservative measures fail to relieve acute colonic distention, a cecostomy or other surgical approaches are indicated. Colonoscopy is often used, and success rates range from 73% to 91%.[151] As the colonoscope is withdrawn, a small decompression tube may be left in the cecum, but the benefit of this approach is unproven.

SUMMARY

Gastrointestinal problems are commonly seen in the intensive care unit either as the primary reason for admission or the consequence of critical illness. A careful and systematic approach to these patients, as outlined in this chapter, is of the utmost importance. Much of the success in managing these patients has arisen from improvements in critical care medicine as is covered in this intensive care manual.

REFERENCES

1. Goggs JS. Gastroesophageal varices: Pathogenesis and therapy of acute bleeding. *Gastroenterol Clin North Am* 1993;4:22.
2. Talbot-Stern JK. Gastrointestinal bleeding. *Emerg Med Clin North Am* 1996;14:173.
3. Steffes C, Fromm D. The current diagnosis and management of upper gastrointestinal bleeding. *Adv Surg* 1992;25:331.
4. Laine L, Peterson W. Bleeding peptic ulcer. *N Eng J Med* 1994;331:717.

5. Sugawa C, Steffes CP, Nakamura R, et al. Upper gastrointestinal bleeding in an urban hospital. *Ann Surg* 1990;212:521.
6. Rockall TA, Logan RF, Devlin HB, et al. Incidence of and mortality from acute upper gastrointestinal haemorrhage in the United Kingdom. *Br Med J* 1995;311:222.
7. Friedman LF, Martin P. The problem of gastrointestinal bleeding. *Gastroenterol Clin North Amer* 1993;22:717.
8. Terdiman JP, Ostroff JW. Gastrointestinal bleeding in the hospitalized patient: A case-control study to assess risk factors, causes, and outcome. *Am J Med* 1998; 104:349.
9. Cook DJ, Fuller HD, Guyatt GH, et al. Risk factors for gastrointestinal bleeding in critically ill patients. *N Engl J Med* 1994;330:377.
10. Bobek BM, Alejandro CA. Stress ulcer prophylaxis: The case for a selective approach. *Cleveland Clin J Med* 1997;64:533.
11. Loperfido S, Monica F, Maireni L, et al. Bleeding peptic ulcer occurring in the hospitalized patients: Analysis of predictive and risk factors and comparison with out of hospital onset of hemorrhage. *Dig Dis Sci* 1994;39:698.
12. Zimmerman J, Meroz Y, Arnon R, et al. Predictors of mortality in hospitalized patients with secondary upper gastrointestinal haemorrhage. *Gastrointest Endosc* 1992; 38:235.
13. NIH Consensus Conference. Therapeutic endoscopy and bleeding ulcers. *JAMA* 1989;262:1369.
14. Chung SS, Lau JY, Sung JJ, et al. Randomised comparison between adrenaline injection alone and adrenaline injection plus heat probe treatment for actively bleeding peptic ulcers. *Br Med J* 1997;314:1307.
15. Jensen DM, Kovacs TOG, Jutabha R, et al. CURE multicenter, randomized, prospective trial of gold probe vs. injection and gold probe for hemostasis of bleeding peptic ulcers. *Gastrointest Endosc* 1997;45:AB92.
16. Woods KL. Acute upper GI bleeding: Pitfalls and pearls in a board review and update in clinical gastroenterology. American College of Gastroenterology, Arlington, VA, 1998: IB-83.
17. Lau JY, Sung JY, Chan ACW, et al. Repeat endoscopic treatment or surgery in the management of patients with rebleeding peptic ulcers after initial endoscopic hemostasis: A prospective randomized controlled trial. *Gastrointest Endosc* 1998;47: AB87.
18. Lau JYW, Sung JJY, Lam Y-H, et al. Endoscopic retreatment compared with surgery in patients with recurrent bleeding after initial endoscopic control of bleeding ulcers. *N Engl J Med* 1999;340:751.
19. Shuman RB, Schuster DP, Zuckerman GR. Prophylactic therapy for stress ulcer bleeding: A reappraisal. *Ann Intern Med* 1987;106:562.
20. Wilcox CM, Spenney JG. Stress ulcer prophylaxis in medical patients: Who, what and how much? *Am J Gastroenterol* 1988;83:1199.
21. Cook DH, Guyatt GH, Marshall J, et al. A comparison of sucralfate and ranitidine for the prevention of upper gastrointestinal bleeding in patients requiring mechanical ventilation. *N Eng J Med* 1998;338:791.
22. Pingleton SK, Hadzima SK. Enteral alimentation and gastrointestinal bleeding in mechanically ventilated patients. *Crit Care Med* 1983;11:13.
23. Ben-Menachem T, Fogel R, Patel RV, et al. Prophylaxis for stress-related gastric hemorrhage in the medical ICU. A randomized, controlled, single-blinded study. *Ann Intern Med* 1994;121:568.

24. Cello JP. Endoscopic management of esophageal variceal hemorrhage: Injection, banding, glue, octreotide, or a combination? *Semin Gastrointest Dis* 1997;8:179.
25. Gostout CJ, Viggiano TR, Balm RK. Acute gastrointestinal bleeding from portal hypertensive gastropathy: Prevalence and clinical features. *Am J Gastroenterol* 1993;88: 2030.
26. Grace ND. Diagnosis and treatment of gastrointestinal bleeding secondary to portal hypertension. *Am J Gastroenterol* 1997;92:1081.
27. Graham DY, Smith JL. The course of patients after variceal hemorrhage. *Gastroenterology* 1981;80:800.
28. Terdiman JP. The importance of accurate diagnosis and vigorous care of the patient with liver disease and gastrointestinal hemorrhage. *Semin Gastrointest Dis* 1997;8:166.
29. Make R. A study of octreotide in esophageal varices. *Digestion* 1990;(suppl) 45:60.
30. Planas R, Quer JC, Boix J, et al. A prospective randomized trial comparing somatostatin and sclerotherapy in the treatment of acute variceal bleeding. *Hepatology* 1994;20:370.
31. Shields R, Jenkins SA, Baxter JN, et al. A prospective randomized controlled trial comparing the efficacy of somatostatin with injection sclerotherapy in the control of bleeding esophageal varices. *J Hepatol* 1992;15:128.
32. Sung JJ, Chung SC, Lai CW, et al. Octreotide infusion or emergency sclerotherapy for variceal hemorrhage. *Lancet* 1993;342:6307.
33. Besson I, Ingrand P, Person B, et al. Sclerotherapy with or without octreotide for acute variceal bleeding. *N Eng J Med* 1995;335:555.
34. Gimson AES, Ramage JK, Panos MZ, et al. Randomized trial of variceal banding ligation versus injection sclerotherapy for bleeding esophageal varices. *Lancet* 1993; 342:391.
35. Hou MC, Liu HC, Kuo BIT, et al. Comparison of endoscopic variceal injection sclerotherapy and ligation for the treatment of esophageal variceal hemorrhage: A prospective randomized trial. *Hepatology* 1995;21:1517.
36. Laine L, Cook D. Endoscopic ligation compared with sclerotherapy for treatment of esophageal variceal bleeding. A meta-analysis. *Ann Int Med* 1995;123:280.
37. Laine L, El-Newihi HM, Migikovsky B, et al. Endoscopic ligation compared with sclerotherapy for the treatment of bleeding esophageal varices. *Ann Intern Med* 1993;119:1.
38. Lo GH, Lai KH, Cheng JS, et al. A prospective randomized trial of sclerotherapy versus ligation in the management of bleeding esophageal varices. *Hepatology* 1995;22: 466.
39. Stiegmann GV, Goff JS, Michaletz-Onody PA, et al. Endoscopic sclerotherapy as compared with endoscopic ligation for bleeding esophageal varices. *N Engl J Med* 1992;326:1527.
40. Laine L, Stein C, Sharma V. Randomized comparison of ligation versus ligation plus sclerotherapy in patients with bleeding esophageal varices. *Gastroenterology* 1996; 111:529.
41. Sung JJ, Chung SC, Yung MY, et al. Prospective randomized study of effect of octreotide on rebleeding from oesophageal varices after endoscopic ligation. *Lancet* 1995;346:1666.
42. Lay CS, Tsai YT, Teg CY, et al. Endoscopic variceal ligation in prophylaxis of first variceal bleeding in cirrhotic patients with high-risk esophageal varices. *Hepatology* 1997;25:1346.

43. Sarin SK, Lamba GS, Kumar M, et al. Comparison of endoscopic ligation and propranolol for the primary prevention of variceal bleeding. *N Engl J Med* 1999;340:988.

44. Zimmerman HM, Curfman KL. Acute gastrointestinal bleeding. *AACN Clinical Issues* 1997;8:449.

45. DeMarkles MP, Murphy JR. Acute lower gastrointestinal bleeding. *Med Clin North Am* 1993;77:1085.

46. Banks PA. Practice guidelines in acute pancreatitis. *Am J Gastroenterol* 1997;92:377.

47. Banorjee AK, Kaul A, Bache E, et al. An audit of fatal acute pancreatitis. *Postgrad Med* 1995;71:472.

48. Gumaste VV, Roditis N, Mehta D, et al. Serum lipase levels in nonpancreatitic abdominal pain versus acute pancreatitis. *Am J Gastroenterol* 1993;88:2051.

49. Gorelick FS. Acute pancreatitis. In Yamada T (ed.) *Textbook of gastroenterology*, 2nd ed. Philadelphia: Lipincott, 1995:2064.

50. Kemppainen EA, Hendstrom J, Puolakkainen PA, et al. Rapid measurement of urinary trypsinogen-2 as a screening test for acute pancreatitis. *N Engl J Med* 1997;336:1788.

51. Tenner S, Dubner H, Steinber W. Predicting gallstone pancreatitis with laboratory parameters: A meta-analysis. *Am J Gastroenterol* 1994;89:1863.

52. Liu CL, Lo CM, Fan ST. Acute biliary pancreatitis: Diagnosis and management. *World J Surg* 1997;21:149.

53. Toskes PP, Greenberger NJ. Approach to the patient with pancreatic disease. In Isselbacher KJ, Braunwald E, Wilson JD, et al. (eds.) *Harrison's principles of internal medicine*, 13th ed. New York: McGraw-Hill, 1994:1516.

54. Bradley III EL. A clinically based classification system for acute pancreatitis. *Arch Surg* 1993;128:586.

55. Ranson JH, Rifkind KM, Roses DF, et al. Prognostic signs and the role of operative management in acute pancreatitis. *Surg Gynecol Obstet* 1974;139:69.

56. Demmy TL, Burch JM, Feliciano DV, et al. Comparison of multiple parameter prognostic systems in acute pancreatitis. *Am J Surg* 1988;156:492.

57. Agarwal N, Pitchumoni CS. Assessment of severity in acute pancreatitis. *Am J Gastroenterol* 1991;86:1385.

58. Dominguez-Munoz JE, Carballo F, Garcia MJ, et al. Evaluation of the clinical usefulness of APACHE II and SAPS systems in the initial prognostic classification of acute pancreatitis: A multicenter study. *Pancreas* 1993;8:682.

59. Wilson C, Heath DI, Imrie CW. Prediction of outcome in acute pancreatitis: A comparative study of APACHE-II, clinical assessment and multiple factor scoring systems. *Br J Surg* 1990;77:1260.

60. Balthazar EJ, Freeny PC, van Sonnenberg E. Imaging and intervention in acute pancreatitis. *Radiology* 1994;193:297.

61. Levant JA, Secrist DM, Resin H, et al. Nasogastric suction in the treatment of alcoholic pancreatitis: A controlled study. *JAMA* 1974;51:229.

62. Loiudice TA, Lang J, Mehta H. Treatment of acute alcoholic pancreatitis: The role of cimetidine and nasogastric suction. *Am J Gastroenterol* 1984;79:553.

63. Luiten EJT, Hop WCJ, Lange JF, et al. Controlled clinical trials of selective decontamination for treatment of severe pancreatitis. *Ann Surg* 1995;222:57.

64. D'Amico D, Favia G, Biasiator, et al. The use of somatostatin in acute pancreatitis: Results of a multicenter trial. *Hepatogastroenterol* 1990;37:92.

65. Neoptolemos JP, Carr-Locke DL, London NJ, et al. Controlled trial of urgent retrograde cholangiopancreatography and endoscopic sphincterotomy versus conservative treatment for acute pancreatitis due to gallstones. *Lancet* 1988;2:979.

66. Fan ST, Lai ECS, Mok FPT, et al. Early treatment of acute biliary pancreatitis by endoscopic papillotomy. *N Eng J Med* 1993;328:228.

67. Fölsch UR, Nitsche R, Lüdtke R, et al. Early ERCP and papillotomy compared with conservative treatment for acute biliary pancreatitis. *N Eng J Med* 1997;336:237.

68. Kamath PS. Clinical approach to the patient with abnormal liver test results. *Mayo Clinic Proc* 1996;71:1089.

69. Schaffner JA, Schaffner F. Assessment of the status of liver. In Henry JB (ed.). *Clinical diagnosis and management by laboratory methods*, 18th ed. Philadelphia: W.B. Saunders, 1991:229.

70. Yee HF, Lidofsky SD. Fulminant hepatic failure. In Feldman M, Scharschmidt BF, Sleisenger MH (eds.) *Sleisenger and Fordtran's gastrointestinal and liver disease: pathophysiology/diagnosis/management*, 6th ed. Philadelphia: W.B. Saunders, 1998: 1355.

71. McCashland TM, Shaw BW Jr., Tape E. The American experience with transplantation for acute liver failure. *Semin Liver Dis* 1996;16:427.

72. Bismuth H, Samuel D, Castaing D, et al. Liver transplantation in Europe for patients with acute liver failure. *Semin Liver Dis* 1996;16:415.

73. Spooner JB, Harvey JG. Paracetamol overdose:Facts not misconceptions. *Pharmaceut J* 1993;252:707.

74. Lee WM. Medical progress: Acute liver failure. *N Eng J Med* 1993;329:1862.

75. Lee WM. Medical progress: Hepatitis B virus infection. *N Eng J Med* 1997;337:1733.

76. Saracco G, Macagno S, Rosina F, et al. Serologic markers with fulminant hepatitis in persons positive for hepatitis B surface antigen; a worldwide epidemiologic and clinical survey. *Ann Intern Med* 1988;108:380.

77. Bernuau J, Goudeau A, Poynard T, et al. Multivariate analysis of prognostic factors in fulminant hepatitis B. *Hepatology* 1986;6:648.

78. Yoshiba M, Dehara K, Inoue K, et al. Contribution of hepatitis C virus to non-A, non-B fulminant hepatitis in Japan. *Hepatology* 1994;19:829.

79. Yanagi M, Kaneko S, Unoura M, et al. Hepatitis C virus in fulminant hepatic failure. *N Engl J Med* 1995;324:1895.

80. Asher LVSS, Innis BL, Shrestha MP, et al. Virus-like particles in the liver of a patient with fulminant hepatitis and antibody to hepatitis E virus. *J Med Virol* 1990;31:229.

81. O'Grady JG, Schalm SW, Williams R. Acute liver failure: redefining the syndromes. *Lancet* 1993;342:273.

82. O'Grady JG, Alexander GJM, Hayllar KM, et al. Early indicators of prognosis in fulminant hepatic failure. *Gastroenterology* 1989;97:439.

83. Shakil AO, Kramer D, Mazariegos A et al. Acute liver failure: Clinical features, outcome, analysis, and applicability of prognostic criteria. *Liver Transplantation* 2000;6:163.

84. Harrison PM, Keays R, Bray GP, et al. Late N-acetylcysteine administration improves outcome for patients developing paracetamol-induced fulminant hepatic failure. *Lancet* 1990;335:1026.

85. Harrison PM, Wendon JA, Gimson AES, et al. Improvement by acetylcysteine of hemodynamics and oxygen transport in fulminant hepatic failure. *N Engl J Med* 1991; 324:1852.

86. Baudouin SV, Howdle P, O'Grady JG, et al. Acute lung injury in fulminant hepatic failure following paracetamol poisoning. *Thorax* 1995;50:399.
87. Rolando N, Harvey F, Brahm J, et al. Prospective study of bacterial infection in acute liver failure: An analysis of fifty patients. *Hepatology* 1990;11:49.
88. Rolando N, Wade JJ, Stangou A, et al. Prospective study comparing the efficacy of prophylactic parenteral antimicrobials, with or without enteral decontamination, in patients with acute liver failure. *Liver Transplant and Surgery* 1996;2:8.
89. Rolando N, Philpott-Howard J, Williams R. Bacterial and fungal infection in acute liver failure. *Semin Liver Dis* 1996;16:389.
90. Rolando N, Gimson A, Wade J, et al. Prospective controlled trial of selective parenteral and enteral antimicrobial regimen in fulminant liver failure. *Hepatology* 1993;17:196.
91. Gazzard BG, Henderson JM, Williams R. Early changes in coagulation following a paracetamol overdose and a controlled trial of fresh frozen plasma therapy. *Gut* 1975;16:617.
92. Caraceni P, Van Thiel DH. Acute liver failure. *Lancet* 1995;345:163.
93. Daas M, Plevak DJ, Wijdicks EF, et al. Acute liver failure: Results of a 5-year clinical protocol. *Liver Transplant and Surgery* 1995;1:210.
94. Davenport A, Will EJ, Davison AM. Effect of posture on intracranial pressure and cerebral perfusion pressure in patients with fulminant hepatic and renal failure after acetaminophen self poisoning. *Crit Care Med* 1990;18:286.
95. Keays TR, Alexander GJM, Williams R. The safety and the value of extradural intracranial pressure monitors in fulminant hepatic failure. *J Hepatol* 1993;18:205.
96. Canalese J, Gimson AES, Davis C, et al. Controlled trial of dexamethasone and mannitol for the cerebral edema of fulminant hepatic failure. *Gut* 1982;23:625.
97. Forbes A, Alexander GJM, O'Grady JG, et al. Thiopental infusion in the treatment of intracranial hypertension complicating fulminant hepatic failure. *Hepatology* 1989;10:306.
98. Ede R, Gimson AES, Bihari D, et al. Controlled hyperventilation in the prevention of cerebral edema in fulminant hepatic failure. *J Hepatol* 1986;2:43.
99. Maddrey WC. Bioartificial liver in the treatment of hepatic failure. *Liver Transplantation* 2000;6(Suppl 1):S27.
100. Chen SC, Hewitt WR, Watanabe FD, et al. Clinical experience with procine hepatocyte-based liver system. *Int J Artif Organs* 1996;19:664.
101. Watanabe FD, Mullon Claudy J-P, Hewitt WR. Clinical experience with a bioartificial liver in fulminant hepatic failure? *Ann Surg* 1997;225:484.
102. Bismuth H, Figuerio J, Samuel D. What should we expect from a bioartificial liver in fulminant hepatic failure? *Artif Organs* 1998; 22:26.
103. Ellias AJ, Hughes RD, Wendon JA, et al. Pilot-controlled trial of the extracorporeal liver assist device in acute liver failure. *Hepatology* 1996;24:1446.
104. Runyon BA. AASLD practice guidelines. Management of adult patients with ascites caused by cirrhosis. *Hepatology* 1999;27:264.
105. Cattau E, Benjamin SB, Knuff TE, et al. The accuracy of the physical exam in the diagnosis of suspected ascites. *JAMA* 1982;247:1164.
106. Guarner C, Runyon BA. Spontaneous bacterial peritonitis: pathogenesis, diagnosis, and treatment. *Gastroenterologist* 1995;3:311.
107. Runyon BA. Paracentesis of ascitic fluid: A safe procedure. *Arch Intern Med* 1986; 14:2259.
108. Runyon BA, Canawati HN, Akriviadis EA. Optimization of ascitic fluid culture technique. *Gastroenterology* 1988;95:1351.

109. Castellote J, Xiol X, Verdaguer R. Comparison of two ascitic fluid culture methods in cirrhotic patients with spontaneous bacterial peritonitis. *Am J Gastroenterol* 1990; 85:1605.
110. Hoefs JC. Increase in ascites WBC and protein concentration during diuresis in patients with chronic liver disease. *Hepatology* 1981;1:249.
111. Runyon BA, Montano AA, Akriviadis EA, et al. The serum-ascites albumin gradient is superior to the exudate-transudate concept in the differential diagnosis of ascites. *Ann Intern Med* 1992;117:215.
112. Runyon BA. Low-protein-concentration ascitic fluid is predisposed to spontaneous bacterial peritonitis. *Gastroenterology* 1986;91:1343.
113. Runyon BA. Care of patients with ascites. *N Engl J Med* 1994;338:337.
114. Runyon BA, McHutchison JG, Antillon MR, et al. Short-course vs. long-course antibiotic treatment of spontaneous bacterial peritonitis: A randomized controlled trial of 100 patients. *Gastroenterology* 1991;100:1737.
115. Soriano G, Teixedo M, Guarner C, et al. Selective intestinal decontamination prevents spontaneous bacterial peritonitis. *Gastroenterology* 1991;100:477.
116. Ginès P, Rimola A, Planas R, et al. Norfloxacin prevents spontaneous bacterial peritonitis recurrence in cirrhosis: results of a double-blind placebo-controlled trial. *Hepatology* 1990;12:716.
117. Wade JJ, Rolando N, Hayllar K, et al. Bacterial and fungal infections after liver transplantation. *Hepatology* 1995;21:1328.
118. Novella M, Sola R, Soriana G, et al. Continuous versus inpatient prophylaxis of the first episode of spontaneous bacterial peritonitis with norfloxacin. *Hepatology* 1997;25:532.
119. Rolachon A, Cordier L, Bacq Y, et al. Ciprofloxacin and long-term prevention of spontaneous bacterial peritonitis: Results of a prospective controlled trial. *Hepatology* 1995;22:1171.
120. Sort P, Navasa M, Arroyo V, et al. Effect of intravenous albumin in renal impairment and mortality in patients with cirrhosis and spontaneous bacterial peritonitis. *N Engl J Med* 1999;341:403.
121. Akriviadis EA, Runyon BA. The value of an algorithm in differentiating spontaneous from secondary bacterial peritonitis. *Gastroenterology* 1990;98:127.
122. Stanley MM, Ochi S, Lee KK, et al. Peritoneovenous shunting as compared with medical treatment in patients with alcoholic cirrhosis and massive ascites. *N Engl J Med* 1989;321:1632.
123. Ginès P, Arroyo V, Quintero E, et al. Comparison of paracentesis and diuretics in the treatment of patients with cirrhosis with tense ascites: Results of a randomized controlled study. *Gastroenterology* 1987;93:234.
124. Salerno F, Badalamenti S, Incerti P, et al. Repeated paracentesis and IV albumin infusion to treat "tense" ascites in cirrhotic patients: A safe and alternative therapy. *J Hepatol* 1987;93:234.
125. Guazzi M, Polese A, Magini F, et al. Negative function of ascites on the cardiac function of cirrhotic patients. *Am J Med* 1995;59:165.
126. Peltekian KM, Wong F, Liu PP, et al. Cardiovascular, renal, and neurohumoral response to single large-volume paracentesis in cirrhotic patients with diuretic-resistant ascites. *Am J Gastroenterol* 1997;92:394.
127. Runyon BA. Patient selection is important in studying the impact of large-volume paracentesis on intravascular volume. *Am J Gastroenterol* 1997;92:371.
128. Arroyo V, Ginès P, Gerbes AL, et al. Definition and diagnostic criteria of refractory ascites and hepatorenal syndrome in cirrhosis. *Hepatology* 1996;23:164.

129. Stanley MM, Ochi S, Lee KK, et al. Peritoneovenous shunting as compared with medical treatment in patients with alcoholic cirrhosis and massive ascites. *N Engl J Med* 1989;321:1632.

130. Ginés P, Arroyo V, Vargas V, et al. Paracentesis with intravenous infusions of albumin as compared with peritoneovenous shunting in cirrhosis with refractory ascites. *N Engl J Med* 1991;325:829.

131. Trotter JF, Suhocki PV, Rockey DC. Transjugular intrahepatic portosystemic shunt (TIPS) in patients with refractory ascites: Effect on body weight and Child-Pugh score. *Am J Gastroenterol* 1998;92:1891.

132. Ginés P, Tito L, Arroyo V, et al. Randomized study of therapeutic paracentesis with and without intravenous albumin in cirrhosis. *Gastroenterology* 1988;94:1493.

133. Moller S, Bendtsen F, Henriksen JH. Effect of volume expansion on systemic hemodynamics and central and arterial blood volume in cirrhosis. *Gastroenterology* 1995;109:1917.

134. Rothschild M, Oratz M, Evans C, et al. Alterations in albumin metabolism after serum and albumin infusions. *J Clin Invest* 1964;43:1874.

135. Pietrangelo A, Panduro A, Chowdury JR, et al. Albumin gene expression is downregulated by albumin or macromolecule infusion in the rat. *J Clin Invest* 1992;89:1775.

136. Terg R, Berreta J, Abecasis R, et al. Dextran administration avoids hemodynamic changes following paracentesis in cirrhotic patients: A safe and inexpensive option. *Dig Dis Sci* 1992;37:79.

137. Fassio E, Tery R, Landeira G, et al. Paracentesis with dextran 70 vs. paracentesis with albumin in cirrhosis with tense ascites. *J Hepatol* 1992;14:310.

138. Planas R, Ginès P, Arroyo V, et al. Dextran-70 versus albumin as plasma expanders in cirrhotic patients with tense ascites treated with total paracentesis. Results of a randomized trial. *Gastroenterology* 1990;90:1736.

139. Salerno F, Badalamenti S, Lorenzano, et al. Randomized comparative study of hemaccel vs. albumin infusion after total paracentesis in cirrhotic patients with refractory ascites. *Hepatology* 1991;13:707.

140. Riordan SM, Williams R. Treatment of hepatic encephalopathy. *N Engl J Med* 1997;337:473.

141. Kircheis G, Nilius R, Held C, et al. Therapeutic efficacy of L-ornithine-L-aspartate infusions in patients with cirrhosis and hepatic encephalopathy; results of a placebo-controlled, double-blind study. *Hepatology* 1997;25:1351.

142. Sushma S, Dasarathy S, Tanden RK, et al. Sodium benzoate in the treatment of acute hepatic encephalopathy: a double-blind randomized trial. *Hepatology* 1992;16:138.

143. Nompleggi DJ, Bonkovsky HL. Nutritional supplementation in chronic liver disease; an analytical review. *Hepatology* 1994;19:518.

144. Van der Rijt CC, Schalm SW, Schat H, et al. Overt hepatic encephalopathy precipitated by zinc deficiency. *Gastroenterology* 1991;100:1114.

145. Bataller R, Ginés P, Guevara M, et al. Hepatorenal syndrome. *Semin Liver Dis* 1997;17:233.

146. Ginés A, Escorsell A, Ginés P, et al. Incidence, predictive factors, and prognosis of the hepatorenal syndrome in cirrhosis with ascites. *Gastroenterology* 1992;105:229.

147. Guevara M, Ginés P, Bandi JC, et al. Transjugular intrahepatic portosystemic shunt in hepatorenal syndrome: Effects on renal function and vasoactive systems. *Hepatology* 1998;28:416.
148. Bataller R, Ginés P, Guevara M, et al. Hepatorenal syndrome. *Semin Liver Dis* 1997;17:233.
149. Johnson CD, Rice RP, Kelvin FM, et al. The radiological evaluation of gross cecal distention: Emphasis on cecal ileus. *Am J Radiology* 1985;145:1211.
150. Ponec RJ, Saunders MD, Kimmey MB. Neostigmine for the treatment of acute colonic pseudo-obstruction. *N Engl J Med* 1999;341:137.
151. Lopez-Kostner F, Hool GR, Lavery IC. Management and causes of acute large-bowel obstruction. *Surg Clin North Am* 1997;77:1265.

CHAPTER 12

Approach to Hematologic Disorders

Janice L. Zimmerman

INTRODUCTION

An adequate number of functional platelets, a sufficient quantity of clotting factors, and intact vasculature are necessary to maintain hemostasis. In the critically ill patient, defects in these components are common and often result in bleeding. An organized approach to the diagnosis of a bleeding disorder and appropriate management are necessary to ensure optimal patient outcome. The history and physical examination along with laboratory tests usually allow the identification of platelet abnormalities, coagulation cascade abnormalities, and fibrinolytic defects. The most commonly used laboratory tests to evaluate abnormal bleeding are the prothrombin time (PT), activated partial thromboplastin time (aPTT), and platelet count. In the appropriate clinical setting, tests of fibrinolysis and fibrinogen levels may be indicated. The results of laboratory tests for common bleeding disorders in critically ill patients are presented in Table 12–1.

Platelet Abnormality

Petechiae on the skin and mucus membranes or spontaneous gingival and nasal mucosal bleeding suggest an abnormality in platelet number or function. Immediate bleeding after surgery or trauma also suggests a platelet abnormality. Information regarding use of medications such as aspirin or NSAIDs should be sought. A platelet count should be determined and a low count should be confirmed by examination of the peripheral smear to assess platelet size or the presence of clumping. The bleeding time is used to assess platelet function but is

TABLE 12–1 Laboratory Studies in Bleeding Disorders

Abnormality	Platelet count	Bleeding time	PTT	PT	TT	FDP	D-Dimer
Thrombocytopenia	A	A[a]	N	N	N	N	N
von Willebrand's disease	N	A	A	N	N	N	N
TTP	A	A	N	N	N	N	N
Platelet dysfunction	N	A	N	N	N	N	N
DIC	A	A	A	A	A	A	A
Hepatic failure	N-A	N	A	A	A	N-A	N[b]
Hemophilia A or B	N	N	A	N	N	N	N
Thrombolytic agent	N	N	A	A	A	A	A
Heparin	N	N	A	N-A	A	N	N
Coumadin	N	N	N-A	A	N	N	N

[a]Abnormal if < 100,000/μL.
[b]May have mild elevation.
ABBREVIATIONS: PTT, partial thromboplastin time; PT, prothrombin time; FDP, fibrin degradation products; TTP, Thrombotic thrombocytopenic purpura; DIC, disseminated intravascular coagulopathy; A, abnormal; N-A, normal or abnormal; N, normal.

infrequently used in critically ill patients. The bleeding time is prolonged if: the platelet count is less than 100,000/μL (100×10^9/L), aspirin or NSAIDS have been used, or severe hypofibrinogenemia is present.

Coagulation Cascade Abnormality

A defect in the coagulation cascade (Figure 12–1) is suggested by hemorrhage into joints, subcutaneous tissue, or muscle; bleeding that responds poorly to local pressure; and delayed bleeding after trauma or surgery. The primary laboratory studies used to assess the intrinsic and extrinsic coagulation systems are the PT and aPTT. Abnormalities of factors II (prothrombin), V, X, or fibrinogen prolong the result of both tests. The International Normalized Ratio (INR) adjusts the PT for differences in sensitivity of test reagent and is used to monitor oral

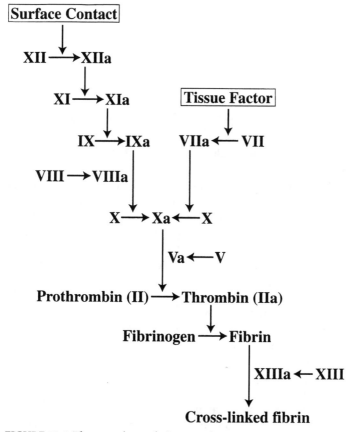

FIGURE 12–1 The normal coagulation cascade

anticoagulation. The addition of normal plasma to the test reagents when the PT or aPTT is abnormal can be used to screen for the presence of inhibitors or factor deficiencies. In general, correction of the PT or aPTT with normal plasma suggests factor deficiencies while lack of correction indicates the presence of an inhibitor. The thrombin time is sensitive to low levels of fibrinogen or abnormal fibrinogen and inhibitors of thrombin (i.e., heparin, FDPs). Specific factor assays are also available but should be used selectively, after results of more common tests are noted to be abnormal.

Fibrinolytic Abnormality

Fibrinolysis is activated by the same factors that activate the coagulation cascade. Laboratory studies include measurement of fibrin degradation products (FDP), which are produced from the degradation of fibrin and fibrinogen and D-dimers, which result from the degradation of cross-linked fibrin, not fibrinogen.

PLATELET DISORDERS

Acquired Thrombocytopenia

Thrombocytopenia exists when the platelet count is less than 150,000/μL (150 × 10^9/L). Thrombocytopenia may result from impaired production, enhanced destruction, or sequestration of platelets. Increased destruction of platelets may be caused by immune or nonimmune mechanisms (Table 12–2).

Management of thrombocytopenia in critically ill patients should begin with confirmation of the platelet count by examination of the peripheral smear. The presence of large platelets on the smear may suggest increased platelet destruction. Effective treatment of the underlying disorder is critical to successful resolution of thrombocytopenia. If thrombocytopenia results from defective production or nonimmune destruction, intervention relies on supportive platelet transfusions until the underlying disorder is corrected. Recombinant human interleukin-11, a thrombopoietic growth factor, may reduce the need for platelet transfusion after chemotherapy, but experience is limited in other clinical situations. Immune-mediated thrombocytopenias require specific interventions, but platelet transfusions are generally avoided except in life-threatening hemorrhage. The decision to transfuse platelets should take into account the underlying disorder, presence of active bleeding, plans for invasive procedures, and the risk of spontaneous bleeding. The risk of spontaneous bleeding increases with platelet counts of less than 10,000/μL (10 × 10^9/L). However, invasive procedures or trauma may necessitate the use of platelet transfusions at higher threshold counts. An automatic transfusion trigger for platelets is not warranted.

TABLE 12–2 **Causes of Thrombocytopenia**

Impaired production

Drugs or toxins (i.e., chemotherapy, radiation)
Myelophthisis (i.e., neoplasm, infection, fibrosis)
Aplastic disorders
Vitamin B_{12}, folate deficiency
Myeloproliferative disorders
Viral illness

Enhanced destruction

Immune-mediated
  Autoantibody (idiopathic thrombocytopenic purpura)
  Isoantibody (post-transfusion purpura)
  Drug-induced (heparin, quinidine, sulfas)
  Immune complex disorders
Nonimmune
  Disseminated intravascular coagulation
  Thrombotic thrombocytopenic purpura or hemolytic
    uremic syndrome
  Mechanical (i.e., intravascular devices, cardiopulmonary bypass)
  Dilutional
Sequestration
  Hypersplenism
Hypothermia

Idiopathic Thrombocytopenic Purpura

Patients with immune mediated idiopathic thrombocytopenic purpura (ITP) usually do not have serious bleeding. Treatment is initiated with corticosteroids (prednisone, 1 to 2 mg/kg daily). In the presence of life-threatening hemorrhage or planned invasive procedures, intravenous immunoglobulin G (IgG) may be used (in a dosage of 0.4 to 0.5 g/kg daily for 4 to 5 days) to obtain a transient elevation in platelet count. Patients who are nonresponsive to corticosteroids may require splenectomy. Other agents, such as vincristine, cyclophosphamide, and danazol, have been used for ITP refractory to other interventions. In addition, dexamethasone 40 mg/day for 4 days has been used with some success. Platelets should be transfused only for severe hemorrhage.

Post-Transfusion Purpura

Post-transfusion purpura is a rare syndrome that develops 5 to 12 days after transfusion. It occurs in women who lack the platelet antigen PL-A1 who were previously sensitized during pregnancy. Thrombocytopenia can develop after use of any blood product containing platelet material in such patients. There is a rapid decrease in the platelet count to less than 10,000/µL (10×10^9/L) in 12 to 24 hours. Treatment includes high-dose intravenous IgG (1 g/day for 2 to 3 days). Plasmapheresis may also be warranted in severe cases, and corticosteroids may be considered. In general, platelet transfusion should be avoided.

Thrombotic Thrombocytopenic Purpura

Thrombotic thrombocytopenic purpura (TTP) is characterized by an inherited or acquired deficiency of von Willebrand's factor–cleaving protease. The diagnostic pentad includes fever, thrombocytopenia, microangiopathic hemolysis, renal dysfunction, and fluctuating neurologic abnormalities. However, all findings may not be present initially. This syndrome can be distinguished from DIC by normal fibrinogen levels and normal coagulation tests. The treatment of choice is plasma exchange, using plasmapheresis with infusion of fresh frozen plasma (FFP). If plasmapheresis is delayed for several hours, FFP transfusion should be initiated. In addition, corticosteroids (such as prednisone, 1 mg/kg daily) are often used. RBC transfusions should be used only as needed and platelets should be withheld, unless life-threatening hemorrhage occurs. Plasma exchange is usually continued for at least 5 days or for 2 days after normalization of the platelet count. The platelet count, hemoglobin level, and LDH level are followed as markers of effective therapy.

Heparin-Induced Thrombocytopenia

Heparin-induced thrombocytopenia (HIT) is the result of an IgG-to-heparin–platelet factor 4 complex. This syndrome can develop with heparin made from beef or pork in all doses and all routes of administration. HIT is less common with low-molecular-weight heparin products. Patients receiving heparin should have their platelet count monitored and heparin discontinued if the platelet count drops to less than 50,000/μL (50 × 10⁹/L) or bleeding develops. Although assays are available for the platelet antibody, they are costly and not routinely performed. Up to 20% of patients with HIT develop arterial or venous thrombosis, which may occur even after discontinuation of heparin. Warfarin administration can be considered for continued anticoagulation therapy, but more immediate therapy may be necessary because of the delayed onset of warfarin effects. Alternatives for anticoagulation include danaparoid sodium and other experimental agents that may be available, including ancrod, hirudin, and argatroban. Low-molecular-weight heparins should not be used if HIT develops.

Extracorporeal Circulation

Extracorporeal circulation can result in a decreased platelet number from aggregation on membranes. Platelet function is also impaired but usually returns to normal within 3 days after cardiopulmonary bypass. Microvascular bleeding is the typical post-bypass finding. Any coexistent coagulation abnormalities should be identified and treated. Platelet transfusion should be considered when the platelet count is less than 100,000/μL (100 × 10^9/L) or the bleeding time is increased. Use of aprotinin to decrease platelet dysfunction and inhibit fibrinolysis has been characterized by decreased bleeding after bypass.

Platelet Dysfunction

In the critically ill patient, platelet dysfunction most commonly results from uremia or use of antibiotics. Uremia-related platelet dysfunction may result in hemorrhage. Dialysis is the treatment of choice but requires time to initiate. In the short term, desmopressin (0.3 μg/kg IV every 12 hrs) can be used to increase von Willebrand's Factor (vWF) levels and improve platelet aggregation, but tachyphylaxis develops rapidly. Conjugated estrogens (0.6 mg/kg IV every day for 5 days) are also effective, but the full effect on platelets takes several days.

COAGULATION DISORDERS

Disseminated Intravascular Coagulation

DIC is an acquired coagulopathy that occurs in the clinical settings including obstetrical disasters, shock, severe sepsis, burns, trauma, transfusion reactions, malignancy, inflammatory diseases, and anaphylaxis. Manifestations range from mild to severe. Activation of coagulation, which results in consumption of clotting factors and platelets, and plasmin generation with resultant fibrinolysis contribute to bleeding. Evidence of excessive clotting and fibrinolysis by laboratory evaluation are necessary to confirm the diagnosis (Table 12–1). Up to 10% of patients may present with thrombosis rather than bleeding. Intravascular thrombosis results in microangiopathic hemolysis, with schistocytes evident on the peripheral smear. Fibrinogen levels are decreased from consumption, but the level must be interpreted in the context of the clinical setting. Fibrinogen is an acute-phase reactant, and levels may be normal even when fibrinogen use is increased. Antithrombin III levels are also decreased in DIC but are not routinely measured. Platelets are consumed as a result of diffuse aggregation. The elevation of D-dimers is the most useful and specific test for fibrinolysis.

Treatment relies on correction of the underlying disorder and the use of blood products for significant morbidity (i.e., bleeding, organ dysfunction). A nonbleeding patient with laboratory evidence of DIC may not require any blood products unless invasive procedures are planned. Coagulation factors can be replaced with FFP. Cryoprecipitate is indicated if fibrinogen levels are less than 100 mg/dL (1.0 g/L). Repeated transfusions of platelets may be needed.

The use and dosage of heparin in DIC is controversial. Heparin inhibition of thrombin may theoretically inhibit formation of microvascular thrombi, which fuel DIC. Potential indications for use of heparin include amniotic fluid embolism, chronic DIC, DIC with thromboses, and severe persistent DIC. Routine use of heparin during induction therapy for promyelocytic leukemia is no longer recommended. A loading dose of heparin is usually not recommended. Uncontrolled trials using low-molecular-weight heparins in DIC have also been reported. The goal of heparin use is to suppress coagulation, increase fibrinogen levels, and decrease D-dimer levels. Fibrinolytic inhibitors, such as epsilon-aminocaproic or tranexamic acid, are not recommended. Topical use may be appropriate in patients with mucous membrane bleeding. Antithrombin III is a natural inhibitor of coagulation that inactivates thrombin and factor Xa. Levels are decreased in DIC, and use of antithrombin III has been proposed in clinical situations. Few randomized trials have been performed, and improvement in laboratory tests has not led to clinically relevant benefits.

Hepatic Insufficiency

Impaired coagulation in patients with liver disease may be causd by decreased factor production, platelet sequestration, or marrow suppression of platelet production by toxins (alcohol). The laboratory evaluation may mimic DIC. FDPs are elevated as a result of poor hepatic clearance, but D-dimer levels are normal or only mildly elevated. Levels of factor VIII, which is not produced in the liver, are normal, in contrast to low levels in DIC. Intervention is indicated only for active bleeding or invasive procedures. Vitamin K should be given to correct any deficiency, and FFP used to replace factor deficiencies when indicated. Prophylactic administration of FFP before liver biopsy or paracentesis is not recommended unless the PT exceeds 16 to 18 seconds or the PTT exceeds 55 to 60 seconds. Cryoprecipitate is rarely needed, since fibrinogen levels are usually maintained at adequate levels.

Massive Transfusion

Bleeding in massive transfusion is a multifactorial hemostatic process, which may be caused by dilutional "washout" of platelets and coagulation factors, development of DIC, hypothermia, or rarely, citrate toxicity that leads to hypocalcemia. Decreased or dysfunctional platelet levels are usually the initial defect. Empiric therapy with transfusion of platelets may be considered when 150% of the normal blood volume is lost, if platelet counts are not readily available. Coagulation factor depletion occurs later than platelet loss, and replacement with FFP should be guided by measurement of PT and PTT. Empiric replacement formulas are not recommended. Cell-saver devices should be considered, when feasible, to decrease transfusion of RBC products.

Congenital Coagulation Disorders

The clinical manifestations of hemophilia A (factor VIII deficiency) and hemophilia B (factor IX deficiency) are indistinguishable. Both disorders require factor replacement in minor trauma or major surgery. Factor levels of 10% to 20% are usually sufficient for minor trauma, 30% for minor bleeding, and 50% for major surgery or bleeding. A variety of specific factor concentrates are available, and the hematologist should be consulted for appropriate doses, frequency of administration, and duration of treatment. Increased amounts of transfused factors may be necessary during active bleeding.

The most common inherited coagulation disorder is von Willebrand's disease (vWD), which may be caused by quantitative or qualitative abnormalities in vWF. Impaired platelet adhesion may result in bleeding at the site of injury during elective surgery. vWD may also be diagnosed incidentally by finding a prolonged PTT in an otherwise asymptomatic patient. The diagnosis is confirmed by test results showing decreased levels of vWF activity, vWF antigen, factor VIII, or a prolonged bleeding time. Desmopressin can be used to increase production of vWF in patients with quantitative abnormalities. Intravenous administration of desmopressin (0.2 to 0.3 µg/kg over 30 minutes) is preferred in seriously ill patients, but the subcutaneous route can also be used. Desmopressin is generally ineffective in patients with qualitative defects of vWF. Some factor VIII concentrates (e.g., Humate-P, manufactured by Armour, Inc., Kankakee, IL) may also provide adequate levels and types of vWF. Cryoprecipitate contains vWF but also carries an increased risk of disease transmission. However, cryoprecipitate may be indicated in patients with qualitative defects of vWF when no other source is readily available.

Vitamin K Deficiency

Acquired vitamin K deficiency may be present in ICU patients, particularly those with inadequate dietary intake treated with antibiotics that alter bacterial flora in the gut. High-risk patients include the elderly, homeless persons, alcoholics and those with malabsorption syndromes. Vitamin K, 5 to 10 mg, can be administered subcutaneously or intravenously, depending on the urgency; additional doses are given every 2 to 3 days. Intravenous administration requires monitoring for possible allergic reactions. Effects on the PT should be seen in 8 to 12 hours with correction to normal by 24 to 48 hours. Severe bleeding requires use of FFP to provide coagulation factors.

Thrombolytic Agents

Thrombolytic agents are used in many critical illnesses. Despite benefit, serious hemorrhage can occur from clot dissolution and inhibition of clotting. Significant hemorrhage is treated with volume (crystalloid or colloid) and RBC transfusion, as indicated. Local measures may be applied, if possible, to stop bleeding. Cryoprecipitate or FFP can be used to replace coagulation factors. A drop in fibrinogen occurs with streptokinase administration, and cryoprecipitate should be considered for empiric treatment when serious bleeding occurs. If heparin has been administered, protamine can be used to reverse its effects in severe bleeding.

Warfarin

Excessive anticoagulation with warfarin may occur inadvertently or as a result of drug interactions. Characteristically, the PT is prolonged but the PTT may also be abnormal because of depletion of factors common to the intrinsic and extrinsic coagulation pathways. In acute hemorrhage, FFP administration is warranted to replace factors. Vitamin K administration can be considered, taking into account the underlying reasons for chronic anticoagulation.

Heparin

Heparin should be discontinued in patients with significant bleeding. Protamine can reverse heparin effects in severe hemorrhage but is less effective with low-molecular-weight heparins. One milligram of protamine reverses the effect of about 100 U of heparin.

BLOOD COMPONENTS FOR HEMOSTASIS

The following recommendations are based on several practice guidelines developed by professional organizations. The critical care physician should be familiar with the products and guidelines of their institution.

Fresh Frozen Plasma

FFP contains all coagulation factors. FFP is available as a single unit of 200 to 250 mL or as a single-donor pheresis unit of 400 to 600 mL, which is equivalent to two standard units of FFP. FFP is indicated in coagulopathy caused by a documented deficiency of coagulation factors in the presence of active bleeding and before operative or other invasive procedures. Significant factor deficiencies are usually documented by a PT of more than 18 seconds, PTT of more than 55 to 60 seconds, or a coagulation factor assay result of less than 25% activity. FFP can be considered in massive blood transfusion when evidence of coagulation factor deficiencies exist or there is continued bleeding. Use of FFP is warranted for reversal of warfarin's effect if immediate hemostasis is required and for deficiencies of antithrombin III (if concentrate of the factor is not available), heparin cofactor II, protein C, or protein S. FFP is also used in plasma exchange for TTP and hemolytic uremic syndrome (HUS), but it is not indicated for volume expansion or nutritional support.

The usual starting dose of FFP is one plasmapheresis unit. The goal is to achieve 30% concentration levels for most coagulation factors. Doses of 10 to 15 mL/kg of body weight may be required, with lesser amounts (5 to 8 mL/kg) indicated for reversal of warfarin effects. Smaller doses or no additional FFP may be needed if platelets are also transfused. For every five to six units of random donor platelets, the patient receives the equivalent of one unit of FFP. Coagulation tests should be repeated after infusion is completed to assess the need for further FFP, using goals of PT of less than 18 seconds or PTT of less than 60 seconds. The half-life of factor VII is approximately 6 hours, so FFP may have to be infused every 6 to 8 hours. Rapid infusion, rather than continuous infusion, is needed to achieve adequate factor levels. The need for FFP must be anticipated, since 30 to 45 minutes are required for thawing.

Platelets

A random donor unit of platelets contains 5.5 to 10×10^{10} platelets. A single donor pheresis unit contains approximately 4×10^{11} platelets. Filtration and ultraviolet radiation are used to reduce alloimmunization. The most common reason for platelet transfusion is decreased bone marrow production (i.e., leukemias, chemotherapy). Platelet administration is indicated when counts are 5000/μL (5×10^9/L) or less, or when counts are 5000 to 30,000/μL (5 to 30×10^9/L) and significant bleeding risk exists. Scattered petechiae and small amounts of blood in urine or stool do not necessarily suggest a high risk of bleeding. Surgery or life-threatening bleeding may require platelet transfusion when platelet counts are less than 50,000/μL (50×10^9/L). Automatic prophylactic platelet transfusions at a threshold of 20,000/μL (20×10^9/L) in stable nonbleeding patients are no longer advocated. Platelets may be used with enhanced platelet destruction only if clinically significant bleeding occurs with platelet counts of 20,000 to 50,000/μL (20 to 50×10^9/L). In ITP, platelets should be reserved for life-threatening hemorrhage. Platelet transfusion is contraindicated in TTP and HUS, except for major surgery or life-threatening bleeding. Transfusion of platelets may be warranted in life-threatening hemorrhage resulting from platelet dysfunction, if other interventions are unsuccessful.

A random donor unit increases the platelet count by 5,000 to 10,000/μL (5 to 10×10^9/L). Bleeding, fever, infection, alloimmunization, splenomegaly, and intravascular consumption can decrease the expected platelet increment. The suggested dose is one unit of random donor platelets per 10 kg of body weight, or one pheresis unit if weight is 90 kg or less. A platelet count should be obtained 1 hour after transfusion to assess the effect of transfusion. Patients who receive multiple platelet transfusions may develop suboptimal increments from alloimmunization. Single-donor HLA-matched or ABO cross-matched platelet units may be effective in these patients.

Cryoprecipitate

Cryoprecipitate contains factors VIII and XIII, fibrinogen, and vWF. Indications for use include hypofibrinogenemia with clinical bleeding or a bleeding risk from invasive procedures. Levels of fibrinogen of more than 100 mg/dL (1 g/L) are generally adequate for hemostasis. In patients with hypofibrinogenemia, one unit of cryoprecipitate per 5 kg of body weight is the empiric dose; in vWD, one unit per 10 kg of body weight can be used.

ANEMIA

Anemia is defined as a decrease in circulating RBC mass, but in the clinical setting, measurements of hemoglobin concentration and hematocrit are readily available and more commonly used criteria. Physiologically, anemia results in a decrease in oxygen-carrying capacity of the blood. Since hemoglobin level and hematocrit result are influenced by variations in plasma volume, changes in these variables may not necessarily reflect a change in oxygen-carrying capacity. Anemia is a common finding in critically ill patients and may result from an acute illness or a chronic underlying condition. Anemia is usually well tolerated if adequate blood volume is maintained. The need for volume must be separated from oxygen-carrying capacity needs when making decisions regarding intervention. Hypovolemia is best treated with crystalloids and colloids, while RBC transfusion is reserved for significant decreases in oxygen-carrying capacity.

Causes

1. Decreased RBC production: Anemia caused by decreased RBC production is often the result of underlying chronic illness or acute critical illness. Anemia of chronic disease often develops in patients with inflammatory disease, cancer, immune disorders, and chronic infection. In patients with chronic renal insufficiency, anemia results from a primary decrease in erythropoietin production. An abnormally low reticulocyte count implicates a bone-marrow production problem. More specific causes of decreased RBC production include the following:
   A. Iron deficiency: Low mean corpuscular volume (MCV), low ferritin and serum iron levels
   B. Vitamin B_{12} and folate deficiency: high MCV
   C. Infection: Particularly *Mycobacterium avium* complex (in HIV-infected patients), disseminated fungal infections, parvovirus B19.
   D. Exogenous toxins: Chemotherapeutic agents, radiation, ethanol, therapeutic drugs (i.e., zidovudine)
   E. Disseminated cancers
   F. Myeloproliferative syndromes
   G. Hemoglobinopathies
2. Increased RBC destruction: Anemia results from increased destruction of RBCs when hemolysis exceeds the capacity of bone marrow to increase erythropoiesis. Hemolysis of RBCs may occur by an immune or nonimmune mechanism, but both types of mechanisms are characterized by an elevated reticulocyte count. Intravascular hemolysis results in increases of LDH and bilirubin levels. Plasma haptoglobin levels decrease as hemoglobin is bound and removed from the plasma. However, it

is not necessary to routinely measure haptoglobin. In the presence of severe hemolysis, free hemoglobin may be measured in the plasma or urine. Extravascular hemolysis is characterized by RBC destruction in the reticuloendothelial system, primarily in the spleen. Characteristic findings are jaundice and splenomegaly. Haptoglobin levels are normal or only slightly reduced in this situation.

A. Immune destruction: Immune destruction of RBCs is usually caused by a warm-reacting IgG antibody. An immune hemolytic anemia may be seen in conjunction with vasculitic conditions, infection, cancer (particularly lymphoproliferative disorders), and drugs. Some drugs to be considered in critically ill patients as a cause of immune hemolysis include cephalosporins, protamine, penicillin, isoniazid, quinidine, rifampin, and sulfonamide agents. Microspherocytes, in addition to fragmented cells, are seen on the peripheral blood smear.

Therapy for immune hemolytic anemia resulting from warm-reactive antibodies is corticosteroid administration (prednisone, 60 to 80 mg/day). In unresponsive patients, splenectomy, high-dose IgG, or immunosuppressive drugs may be considered. Corticosteroids are less effective in immune hemolysis caused by cold-reactive antibodies (IgM). Warming acral parts of the body may be sufficient to alleviate symptoms, but plasmapheresis may be necessary to reduce the concentration of IgM antibodies. In patients with drug-induced immune hemolysis, discontinuation of the drug is usually the only necessary treatment.

RBC transfusion in patients with immune hemolysis optimally requires identification of the antibody and selection of compatible units. In some cases, the blood bank may only be able to provide the least incompatible blood type. Blood should be warmed to body temperature for patients with cold-reacting antibodies. Transfusion should be undertaken only when necessary and then with close monitoring.

B. Nonimmune destruction: Nonimmune destruction of RBCs may be caused by mechanical mechanisms or endogenous RBC abnormalities. Fragmentation and destruction of RBCs in the circulation may result from increased sheer stresses caused by turbulent blood flood, as in arteriovenous malformations. Hemolysis may occur with malfunction of intravascular prosthetic devices and disorders affecting blood vessels, producing a microangiopathic hemolytic process (e.g., DIC, TTP). A blood smear will show RBC fragmentation. Direct parasitization of RBCs by malaria organisms or bacterial products (i.e., *Clostridia* species toxins) may result in hemolysis.

Homozygous sickle cell disease is a chronic hemolytic condition, resulting from abnormal hemoglobin, that is usually well compensated. Increased hemolysis should prompt a search for a second disorder. Hereditary RBC enzyme deficiencies can also result in hemolysis. The most common deficiency is glucose-6-phosphate dehydrogenase (G6PD) deficiency. Episodic hemolytic episodes in G6PD deficiency can be precipitated by fever, infection, and drugs, such as nitrofurantoin, primaquine, and sulfonamides.

3. Anemia from RBC loss: Blood loss is a common cause of anemia in the critically ill patient. Blood loss may be acute or chronic and occur from GI lesions or vascular abnormalities. The existence of a coagulopathy exacerbates accompanying blood loss. The measured hemoglobin level in acute blood loss may not accurately reflect the RBC volume lost. Phlebotomy for laboratory tests is an important source of blood loss in the ICU, particularly in patients with arterial lines. The blood volume removed should be minimized in the critically ill patient to prevent a significant nosocomial contribution to worsening anemia. Human erythropoietin has been used in the preoperative setting to increase autologous blood donation but has not been evaluated in the critically ill patient with blood loss.

Consequences

As oxygen-carrying capacity decreases in anemia, compensatory mechanisms are initiated. Decreased blood viscosity and an increase in heart rate result in increased cardiac output, which is an attempt by the body to maintain oxygen delivery to the tissues. Additional compensation occurs at the tissue level, where an increase in oxygen extraction (despite decreased oxygen delivery) maintains tissue oxygen uptake. The lower limit of hemoglobin level tolerated in humans is not known. The multiple concomitant factors that exist in the critically ill patient make it even more difficult to determine a threshold below which tissue oxygenation is impaired. Factors that must be considered include volume status, cardiopulmonary reserve, and metabolic demands. The optimum hemoglobin level in the critically ill has not been defined. Increases in hemoglobin from transfusion may not result in improved oxygen delivery or improved oxygen consumption by tissue. Increases in hemoglobin level alter blood viscosity, which may be detrimental.

The clinical manifestations of anemia vary with the cause and severity, the rapidity of onset, and the presence of concomitant disorders. Inadequate oxygen delivery may result in tachypnea, mental confusion, angina, and evidence of anaerobic metabolism (lactic acidosis). In the critically ill patient, the ability to communicate symptoms is impaired. Tachycardia and hypotension are often signs of hypovolemia, although they may also be seen in conjunction with impaired oxygen delivery. Pallor, overt blood loss, or jaundice resulting from a hemolytic process may be noted.

Management

Laboratory evaluation of anemia in the critically ill patient should be tailored to the individual. Tests that are important to obtain before transfusion include a CBC count (hemoglobin level, hematocrit, RBC indices), reticulocyte count, peripheral blood smear, and RBC folate level (if indicated). If a hemoglobinopathy is suspected, a blood sample should be obtained before transfusion for hemoglobin electrophoresis. Evidence of hemolysis can be determined by measurement of serum bilirubin and LDH levels. Vitamin B_{12} and serum iron levels can be obtained if warranted, but deficiencies can be determined even after RBC transfusion. If immune hemolysis is considered, blood should be sent to the blood bank for direct and indirect Coombs' tests. Stool guiac test for fecal occult blood should be performed and urine assessed for presence of blood. Other tests should be used to assess the impact of anemia by assessing evidence of ischemia. Lactate levels may be elevated in the setting of anaerobic metabolism, or ischemic changes may be noted on ECG.

The optimum management of anemia requires identification of the underlying cause and appropriate intervention, which may include control of bleeding, volume replacement, treatment of infection, or removal of bone-marrow toxins or immunosuppressive therapies. Transfusion of RBC products should also be considered in the management of anemia.

The decision to transfuse blood products for anemia must take into account risks and benefits to the individual patient. The only indication for transfusion of RBCs is increase of oxygen-carrying capacity to support adequate oxygen consumption at the tissue level. Arbitrary transfusion thresholds based on hemoglobin concentration are not recommended for use. Rather, physiologic markers of impaired tissue oxygenation should be used to guide decisions on transfusion. In the critically ill patient, the following indicators, if available, may suggest tissue hypoxia: mixed venous PO_2 of less than 25 mm Hg, oxygen extraction ratio of more than 50%, oxygen consumption less than 50% of baseline measurement, and elevated lactate levels. The presence of ongoing blood loss, the patient's cardiopulmonary reserve, presence of concomitant disease, effects of hypovolemia, presence of acute or chronic anemia, and metabolic oxygen demands should be evaluated.

Current guidelines do not specifically address transfusion in critically ill patients and few studies are available to provide guidance. The effects of RBC transfusion on tissue oxygen consumption are variable, even if oxygen delivery is increased. In general, a hemoglobin of 7 to 9 g/dL is adequate for most patients. A higher hemoglobin level may be warranted in critically ill patients with cardiac disease. Patients with chronic anemia may tolerate a hemoglobin value at the lower end of the range. Authors of most transfusion guidelines propose that transfusion is rarely indicated when the hemoglobin is more than 10 g/dL and is almost always indicated for hemoglobin levels of less than 6 g/dL. Transfusion is not acceptable for volume expansion or promotion of wound healing. Transfusion should be avoided, if possible, in patients with severe aplastic anemia who may be candidates for bone marrow transplantation.

TRANSFUSION THERAPY FOR ANEMIA

Whole Blood

Whole blood is rarely available because of the multiple advantages of component therapy (Table 12–3). Therefore, most whole blood donations are separated into components. Whole blood contains RBCs, platelets, WBCs, and plasma, which

TABLE 12–3 **Blood Products for Transfusion in Adults**

Blood Component	Content	Volume (mL)	Indications
Whole blood	RBCs (HCT 40%–45%) Plasma WBCs Platelets (nonviable)	500–515	Rarely available ± Massive hemorrhage
RBCs	RBCs (HCT 60%–80%) Plasma WBCs Platelets (nonviable)	250–350	Improve oxygen-carrying capacity
Leukocyte-reduced RBCs	RBCs (HCT ≈ 90%) Plasma (minimal) WBCs (85%–95% depleted, $< 5 \times 10^6$/U)	200	Prevention of severe febrile transfusion reactions Prevention of alloimmuniza-tion in patients requiring multiple transfusions
Washed RBCs	RBCs (HCT ≈ 60%) WBCs (minimal)	340	Prevention of severe allergic reactions Prevention of anaphylaxis in IgA-deficient patients
Irradiated RBCs	RBCs	250–350	Prevention of graft versus host disease in immuno-compromised patients
Frozen RBCs	RBCs WBCs (minimal)	170–190	Autologous transfusion Rare blood types
Platelets	Platelets Plasma WBCs RBCs		Enhanced platelet destruction: Life-threatening bleed in ITP Platelets 20,000–50,000/μl + excessive bleeding Contraindicated in TTP
Single donor Random donor	$3–8 \times 10^{11}$ platelets $5.5–10 \times 10^{10}$ platelets	200–400 50	Decreased platelet production ± enhanced destruction: Platelets < 5000/μL Platelets 5000–30,000/μL + significant bleeding risk Platelets < 50,000/μL + inva-sive procedures or life-threatening bleed
Fresh frozen plasma	All coagulation factors (1 U/mL) Complement Fibrinogen (1–2 mg/mL)		Bleeding or risk of bleeding with congenital or acquired deficiency of clotting factors Reversal of warfarin effect Plasma exchange for TTP/HUS
Random donor Single donor		200–250 400–600	Massive blood transfusion with deficiency of clotting factors

(continued)

TABLE 12–3 **Blood Products for Transfusion in Adults (continued)**

Blood Component	Content	Volume (mL)	Indications
Cryoprecipitate	Factor VIII (80–120 U)	10	Fibrinogen deficiency (< 100 mg/dL) with bleeding or risk for bleeding
	Factor XIII (40–60 U)		
	Fibrinogen (200–300 mg) vWF (80 U) Plasma		von Willebrand's disease (unresponsive to desmopressin) Factor XIII deficiency Hemophilia A (if factor VIII concentrate not available)

ABBREVIATIONS: RBC, red blood cell; HCT, hematocrit; WBC, white blood cell; TTP, thrombotic thrombocytopenic purpura; HUS, hemolytic uremic syndrome; IgA, immunoglobin A; ITP, idiopathic thrombocytopenic purpura; vWF, von Willebrand factor.

contains coagulation factors. However, platelet function and function of factors V and VIII are rapidly lost during storage (within 24 to 48 hours). The indication for use of whole blood is correction of a simultaneous deficit of oxygen-carrying capacity and blood volume, such as might occur in massive hemorrhage. In general, RBC concentrates with crystalloid or colloid volume replacement are preferred in these situations.

Packed Red Blood Cells

Whole blood is fractionated into RBCs and platelet-rich plasma. A solution of citrate-phosphate-dextrose (CPD) or CPD plus adenine, glucose, mannitol, and sodium chloride is added as a preservative and anticoagulant. A unit of RBCs typically has a hematocrit of about 70% and an approximate volume of 250 mL. A unit of RBCs contains some residual plasma, platelets, and WBCs. One unit of RBCs increases the hemoglobin by approximately 1 g/dL and the hematocrit by 3% in a stable, nonbleeding average-sized adult.

Leukocyte-Reduced Red Blood Cells

A centrifuge and filter procedure in the blood bank can reduce WBCs by 85%, with recovery of 90% of RBCs. In-line leukocyte reduction filters can remove up to 98% of WBCs in a unit of blood and can be used at the bedside. This blood product can be used in patients who experience febrile transfusion reactions and to avoid antigen sensitization (alloimmunization) in patients who have received multiple blood transfusions (i.e., patients with leukemia, transplant recipients).

Washed Red Blood Cells

Washed RBCs undergo resuspension in saline to remove further plasma and WBCs. This product is used to prevent severe febrile transfusion reactions and anaphylaxis. The procedure reduces RBC count of the product by 10% to 20%, WBC count by approximately 85%, and plasma by 99%.

Irradiated Red Blood Cells

Gamma irradiation eliminates immunologically competent lymphocytes. This blood product is used to prevent graft versus host disease in immunocompromised recipients. Patients with AIDS do not routinely require irradiated RBCs.

Frozen Red Blood Cells

Red blood cells are frozen in glycerol or dimethylsulfoxide. This product can be stored at -30°C for up to 10 years. This method is used for storage of rare blood units.

Administration of Blood Products

When feasible, consent for transfusion of blood products should be obtained before administration, from the patient or the patient's surrogate decision maker, after explanation of risks and benefits. Administration of blood requires careful patient and blood product identification to avoid mishandling and errors. The intravenous catheter should be at least 18-gauge to allow adequate flow. Only isotonic saline should be used as a diluent with blood components.

Patients should be observed for the first 5 to 10 minutes of each transfusion for immediate adverse side effects and at regular intervals thereafter. Each unit of blood should be administered within 4 hours of its arrival to the floor to minimize the risk of bacterial contamination. Premedication with acetaminophen and diphenhydramine can be used in patients with previous febrile transfusion reactions. Administration of multiple units of blood may be appropriate with major hemorrhage. In less urgent situations, physicians should consider transfusing one unit at a time, followed by clinical assessment to avoid unnecessary transfusions.

RISKS OF TRANSFUSION

The following list is an abbreviated summary of risks and adverse reactions associated with transfusion of blood products. Risks must be taken into account when deciding to administer a transfusion to an individual patient.

1. Disease transmission: Currently, blood units are tested for HIV-1, HIV-2, human T-cell lymphotropic viruses (HTLV-I and HTLV-II), hepatitis B virus, and hepatitis C virus. In immunocompromised patients, testing for the presence of CMV is recommended. The risk of disease transmission for a unit of blood varies from 1 in 30,000 to 1 in 2,000,000 patients, depending on the infectious agent. Bacterial contamination of blood units is rare, and the most common organism is *Yersinia enterocolitica.*

2. Hemolytic reactions: Acute hemolytic reactions are caused by preformed antibodies in the blood recipient and can result in death. This type of reaction is usually the result of identification errors, leading to transfusion of incompatible blood products. Symptoms develop shortly after administration of incompatible blood and include fever, chills, back pain, chest pain, nausea, vomiting, and hypotension. In the critically ill patient, these symptoms may be attributed to other factors or masked by sedation and alteration of consciousness. Acute renal failure from hemoglobinuria, DIC, and ARDS may occur. If an acute hemolytic reaction is suspected, the transfusion should be stopped immediately, the intravenous tubing replaced, and appropriate samples obtained for investigation by the blood bank. Further management includes maintenance of intravascular volume and protection of renal function. Delayed hemolytic reactions may occur 3 or 4 weeks after transfusion, as a result of primary and anamnestic antibody responses to RBC antigens.

3. Febrile nonhemolytic reactions: These reactions are characterized by fever, chills, anxiety, pruritus, and occasionally, respiratory distress all of which occur 1 to 6 hrs after the start of transfusion. The reaction results from antibodies against donor plasma proteins or WBC antigens. Bacterial contamination of blood products may cause similar manifestations but rarely occurs. Premedication is usually sufficient to avert febrile reactions. Methods to remove WBCs (leukocyte-reduced RBCs) may also reduce the risk of febrile reactions.

4. Anaphylactic reactions: Anaphylaxis may be seen in patients who are IgA-deficient and receive blood products containing IgA. Washed RBCs should be used in these individuals to maximally reduce plasma content.

5. Volume overload: The volume of blood products used (Table 12–3) and the cardiovascular status of the patient must be assessed on a continual basis during transfusion to avoid precipitating pulmonary edema. Routine administration of diuretics during transfusion is not appropriate in critically ill patients.

6. Noncardiogenic pulmonary edema: Acute lung injury may be caused by donor antibodies to recipient neutrophils or reactive lipid products from donor blood cell membranes. Typically the reaction occurs within 24 hours after receiving a blood product, with the onset or worsening of dyspnea, hypoxemia, and diffuse pulmonary infiltrates. Appropriate supportive care should be instituted and resolution can be expected within a week.

7. Graft versus host disease: A graft versus host reaction may occur in immunocompromised recipients of transfused functional lymphocytes. Fever, rash, and liver function abnormalities occur 2 to 6 weeks after transfusion.

8. Post-transfusion purpura: See section on coagulation disorders.
9. Hypothermia: A decrease in core temperature may be seen with rapid infusion of large volumes of chilled blood. Blood-warming devices can prevent this problem.
10. Metabolic complications: Rapid infusion of citrated blood products (more than 100 mL/min) may, rarely, cause citrate toxicity in conjunction with acute hypocalcemia. The QT interval or ionized calcium level can be monitored and calcium administered, when indicated. During storage, potassium leaks from RBCs and infusion of large quantities of blood may result in transient hyperkalemia.
11. Immunosuppression: The relationship of exposure to blood products and immunosuppression has not been fully clarified. However, several studies suggest blood transfusion may increase the risk for postoperative infection and recurrence of cancer.

SUMMARY

A thorough knowledge of common blood disorders seen in intensive care is essential for all intensivists. This chapter has summarized these common abnormalities, their work-up, and treatment.

SUGGESTED READING

American College of Physicians. Practice strategies for elective red blood cell transfusion. *Ann Intern Med* 1992;116:403.

American Society of Anesthesiologists. Practice guidelines for blood component therapy. *Anesthesiology* 1996;84:732.

American Society of Hematology ITP Practice Guideline Panel. Diagnosis and treatment of idiopathic thrombocytopenic purpura: Recommendations of the American Society of Hematology. *Ann Intern Med* 1997;126:319.

Bick RL. Disseminated intravascular coagulation. *Med Clin North Am* 1994;78:511.

Cicek S, Demirkilic U, Kuralay E, et al. Postoperative aprotinin: effect on blood loss and transfusion requirements in cardiac operations. *Ann Thorac Surg* 1996;61:1372.

College of American Pathologists. Practice parameter for the use of fresh–frozen plasma, cryoprecipitate, and platelets. *JAMA* 1994;271:777.

Goodnough LT, Brecher ME, Kanter MH, AuBuchon JP. Blood transfusion. *N Engl J Med* 1999;340:438.

Guidelines for red blood cell and plasma transfusion for adults and children. *Can Med Assoc J* 1997;156:S1.

Hèbert PC, Wells G, Blajchman MA, et al. A multicenter, randomized, controlled clinical trial of transfusion requirements in critical care. *N Engl J Med* 1999;340:409.

Hèbert PC, Wells G, Tweeddale M, et al. Does transfusion practice affect mortality in critically ill patients? *Am J Respir Crit Care Med* 1997;155:1618.

Humphries JE. Transfusion therapy in acquired coagulopathies. *Hemat Onc Clinics N Am* 1994;8:1181.

Isaacs C, Robert NJ, Bailey FA, et al. Randomized placebo-controlled study of recombinant human interleukin-11 to prevent chemotherapy-induced thrombocytopenia in patients with breast cancer receiving dose-intensive cyclophosphamide and doxorubicin. *J Clin Onc* 1997;15:3368.

Lechner K, Kyrle PA. Antithrombin III concentrates—are they clinically useful? *Thromb Haemostasis* 1995;73:340.

Levy JH, Pifarre R, Schaff HV et al. A multicenter, double-blind, placebo-controlled trial of aprotinin for reducing blood loss and the requirement for donor-blood transfusion in patients undergoing repeat coronary artery bypass grafting. *Circulation* 1995;92:2236.

Marik PE, Sibbald WJ. Effect of stored-blood transfusion on oxygen delivery in patients with sepsis. *JAMA* 1993;269:3024.

Price TH, Goodnough LT, Vogler WR, et al. The effect of recombinant human erythropoietin on the efficacy of autologous blood donation in patients with low hematocrits: a multicenter, randomized, double-blind, controlled trial. *Transfusion* 1996;36:29.

Rebulla P, Finazzi G, Marangoni F, et al. The threshold for prophylactic platelet transfusions in adults with myeloid leukemia. *N Engl J Med* 1995;337:1870.

Rintels PB, Kenney RM, Crowley JP. Therapeutic support of the patient with thrombocytopenia. *Hemat Onc Clinics N Am* 1994;8:1131.

Rutherford CJ, Frenkel EP. Thrombocytopenia: Issues in diagnosis and therapy. *Med Clin North Am* 1994;78:555.

Simon TL, Alverson DC, AuBuchon J, et al. Practice parameter for the use of red blood cell transfusions. *Arch Pathol Lab Med* 1998;122:130.

Warkentin TE, Kelton JB. A 14-year study of heparin-induced thrombocytopenia. *Am J Med* 1996;101:502.

Warkentin TE, Levine MN, Hirsh J, et al. Heparin-induced thrombocytopenia in patients treated with low-molecular-weight heparin or unfractionated heparin. *N Eng J Med* 1995;332:1330.

Welch HG, Meehan KR, Goodnough LT. Prudent strategies for elective red blood cell transfusion. *Ann Intern Med* 1992;116:393.

Approach to Coma

CURTIS BENESCH

INTRODUCTION

Caring for a comatose patient requires a basic understanding of consciousness and the pathophysiologic processes that lead to its derangement. This chapter discusses current definitions of coma and related states of consciousness, provides a systematic approach to the evaluation of a patient in coma, and describes current treatment recommendations for common causes of coma.

DEFINITION OF CONSCIOUSNESS

Consciousness can be defined broadly as the state of awareness of self and surroundings.[1] More specific definitions of consciousness have included three distinct components: wakefulness, the capacity to detect and encode internal and external stimuli, and the capacity to formulate goal-directed behavior.[2] In this definition, self-awareness is not a prerequisite for consciousness, e.g., an individual with advanced dementia. In general, disorders of consciousness are the result of impairment in either one or both of the critical elements of consciousness: arousal and content.[1] Disorders of arousal (coma) are the focus of this chapter. Disorders of content, such as dementia or confusional states, typically do not require intensive care and therefore are excluded from this discussion.

Disorders of Arousal

Disorders of arousal are often characterized by terms ranging from alert to comatose. Coma has been described as the state of unarousable unresponsiveness in which an individual lies with eyes closed, lacking awareness of self and the environment.[3] Patients in coma do not exhibit normal sleep-wake cycles. Stupor refers to a state of unresponsiveness from which the individual can be aroused only by vigorous and repeated stimuli. Obtundation refers to a less severe state of unresponsiveness that requires touch or voice to maintain arousal. Lethargic patients appear somnolent but may be able to maintain arousal spontaneously or with repeated light stimulation.

Although these terms suggest discrete levels of consciousness, disorders of arousal exist along a continuum and often fluctuate over time. Documentation of impaired arousal should include precise recordings of responses by the patient to varying external stimuli.

Anatomy of Consciousness

The anatomic substrate for consciousness consists of a diffuse, interdependent network of brainstem, thalamic, and cortical neurons. The brainstem reticular formation (RF), however, is often considered the neurophysiologic seat of consciousness.[4] Experimental work has shown that stimulation of the brainstem tegmentum results in activation of the cortical and behavioral signs of arousal, even in the absence of auditory and somatosensory input to the cortex.[5,6] Similarly, lesions of the RF result in electroencephalographic slowing and impaired arousal despite otherwise normal sensory input.

The RF arises in the lower medulla and extends rostrally into the pons and midbrain. The most rostral portions of the RF include the nucleus reticularis and intralaminar nuclei of the thalamus. Diffuse cortical projections from the ascending reticular activating system (ARAS) travel via these thalamic connections or from brainstem nuclei directly, such as the raphe nucleus and the locus ceruleus. Basal forebrain structures, including the limbic system, receive projections from the ARAS through hypothalamic pathways. Corticoreticular fibers arise from cingulate, orbito-frontal, superior temporal, and occipital cortices and provide feedback to the brainstem RF. Altered or reduced levels of consciousness are the result of either diffuse and bilateral impairment of cerebral hemispheric function or failure of the brainstem ARAS or both.

DIAGNOSIS OF COMA AND RELATED CONDITIONS

The diagnosis of coma requires careful clinical evaluation of the unresponsive patient and familiarity with the terms that describe related states of decreased arousal. Rates of misdiagnosis of coma and vegetative states have ranged from 15% to 43% in the United States and Great Britain.[7,8] Leading factors contributing to misdiagnosis were traumatic cause, severe visual impairment, and duration of 3 months or more between time of injury and admission to a rehabilitation facility.[7,9]

Coma

Patients in coma lie with their eyes closed and are unable to interact meaningfully with the environment. These patients do not communicate or perform intentional movements. Specific diagnostic criteria for coma have been offered by the American Congress of Rehabilitation Medicine[10] (Table 13–1). Coma is a time-limited condition; by 4 weeks after onset, surviving individuals have either emerged into more responsive states or have begun exhibiting signs of the vegetative state (VS).

Vegetative State

The vegetative state (VS) is characterized by the capability for eye opening and long periods of wakefulness, along with continued absence of meaningful interaction with the environment. Patients in VS may open their eyes spontaneously or in response to stimuli, but reproducible visual pursuit is lacking. These patients cannot communicate, follow commands, or demonstrate intentional movements. Some reflex movements, such as blinking, yawning, or orienting to

TABLE 13–1 **Neurobehavioral Criteria for the Diagnosis of Coma**

1. Eyes do not open spontaneously or to stimulation
2. Patient does not follow commands
3. Patient does not mouth or utter recognizable words
4. Patient does not demonstrate intentional movements
5. Patient cannot sustain visual pursuit movements when eyes are manually held open
6. Criteria 1 through 5 are not secondary to use of paralytic agents

SOURCE: Modified with permission from American Congress of Rehabilitation Medicine. Recommendations for use of uniform nomenclature pertinent to patients with severe alterations in consciousness. *Arch Phys Med Rehab* 1995;76:205–209.

sound, may be preserved. Diagnostic criteria for the vegetative state are provided in Table 13–2. This state is defined as "persistent" vegetative state (PVS) if signs are present at 1 month after traumatic or nontraumatic causes or if present for 1 month in patients with degenerative disorders or developmental malformations. This condition becomes "permanent" when the diagnosis of irreversibility can be established with reasonable clinical certainty.

Minimally-Conscious State

Patients with brain injuries may exhibit features of both coma and VS as well as intermittent periods of self-awareness and meaningful interaction with the environment. This condition has been defined as the "minimally-conscious state" (MCS).[11] In MCS, consciousness is severely altered but behavioral awareness of self or environment can be demonstrated. Patients in MCS, at times, may exhibit any one of the following[11]:

1. The ability to follow commands
2. Gestural yes and no responses
3. Intelligible verbalizations
4. Environmentally contingent movements or affective responses

TABLE 13–2 **Neurobehavioral Criteria for the Diagnosis of the Vegetative State**

1. Eyes do not open spontaneously or to stimulation
2. Patient does not follow commands
3. Patient does not mouth or utter recognizable words
4. Patient does not demonstrate intentional movements
5. Patient cannot sustain visual pursuit movements when eyes are manually held open
6. Criteria 1 through 5 are not secondary to use of paralytic agents

SOURCE: Modified with permission from American Congress of Rehabilitation Medicine. Recommendations for use of uniform nomenclature pertinent to patients with severe alterations in consciousness. *Arch Phys Med Rehab* 1995;76:205–209.

Coma, PVS, and MCS can be considered time-dependent behavioral states along a similar continuum. Approximately 10% of patients with traumatic coma and up to 15% of patients with nontraumatic coma evolve into PVS.[12] Similarly, MCS can be considered a transitional state indicative of either an improving or deteriorating level of consciousness.[11] MCS may also be a permanent outcome after a traumatic brain injury.

Conditions that Mimic Coma

Numerous behavioral conditions that resemble coma exist. Clinical differentiation of these behavioral states is important because of the wide range of underlying causative factors and the variable prognosis of these conditions. Akinetic mutism (AM) is characterized by severe apathy and the absence of spontaneous speech and movement. Although patients appear unresponsive, they remain alert and fully aware of their environment. Spontaneous visual tracking is present and helps distinguish this condition from VS. The term "abulia" describes less severe cases.[13] AM is associated with lesions in the mesial and basal frontal lobes, septum, cingulate cortex, and bilateral mesencephalon.[3] Common causes of AM include obstructive hydrocephalus and craniopharyngioma, both of which may be reversible with treatment.

The locked-in syndrome, or de-efferented state, occurs with lesions involving the ventral pons bilaterally, resulting in quadriplegia and loss of lower cranial nerve function; wakefulness and awareness of the environment are normal as a result of preservation of the pontine tegmentum along with the cerebral cortex. Electroencephalography reveals normal cortical activity in this syndrome. Vertical eye movements and blinking are often preserved and may be the only way for the patient to communicate with the outside world.

Psychogenic unresponsiveness is an uncommon cause of coma. Psychiatric causes of coma include conversion disorder, malingering, fugue state, catatonic schizophrenia and severe depression. Patients with suspected psychogenic unresponsiveness may appear to be unable to respond to their environment, despite the fact that normal function of the hemispheres and the ARAS can usually be demonstrated on neurologic examination.

CAUSES OF COMA

The metabolic and toxic causes of coma are legion and account for a majority of unresponsive patients. In one study of 500 patients presenting with coma, 326 were found to have diffuse and metabolic brain dysfunction.[3] Drug overdose and toxic effects of prescription medications accounted for over half of the patients with coma caused by diffuse cerebral dysfunction. Many metabolic and toxic causes of coma are reversible and are often preceded by a gradual decline in the level of consciousness. Fever, sepsis, and metabolic perturbations are more likely to cause coma in patients with previous brain injury. Some conditions with mul-tifocal involvement of the CNS, such as cerebral vasculitis, encephalitis, sub-arachnoid hemorrhage or adrenoleukodystrophy, may resemble a metabolic encephalopathy more than focal structural disease. Nonconvulsive status epilep-ticus and sagittal sinus thrombosis may present with nonfocal findings and are often unrecognized causes of coma.

Structural lesions causing coma are often grouped on the basis of whether they occur above or below the tentorium. Supratentorial lesions cause coma by either directly encroaching on diencephalic structures, such as the thalamus, or by indirectly compressing those structures during transtentorial herniation. Rapidly expanding mass lesions, such as malignant tumors, abcesses, hema-tomas, and infarctions with edema, are common examples of supratentorial le-sions causing coma. Infratentorial lesions cause coma by similar mechanisms, either by direct involvement of the ARAS or by compression of the brainstem from nearby structures, such as the cerebellum. Destructive lesions of the brain-stem causing coma primarily consist of infarction and hemorrhage, but demyeli-nation, infection, neoplastic invasion, and central pontine myelinolysis may also result in coma. Mass lesions in the posterior fossa often lead to direct compres-sion of the brainstem ARAS.

ASSESSMENT OF THE COMATOSE PATIENT

The approach to the comatose patient begins with ascertaining as much histori-cal information as possible in a timely manner. Sources may include family, emergency medical personnel, or other witnesses. The patient's personal belong-ings may yield clues to the cause of coma as well. After stabilization of the pa-tient, phone calls and interviews may prove especially helpful.

The initial physical assessment of the unresponsive patient consists of simulta-neously establishing stable vital signs, administering urgent therapy for poten-tially reversible causes of coma, and surveying the patient for readily identifiable causes. Patients in coma often require endotracheal intubation to ensure ade-quate oxygenation and to protect the airway. In cases of possible trauma, the neck should be stabilized and indications for emergent surgical intervention must be evaluated. Empirical treatment with glucose, thiamine, naloxone, and flumazenil should be considered in all patients. Any patient who receives glucose should first receive thiamine (at least 100 mg) to avoid precipitating Wernicke's disease (polioencephalitis hemorrhagica superior), especially in the alcoholic or malnourished patient. For those patients with suspected drug overdose, nalox-one, an opiate antagonist, may be used; opioid-dependent individuals, however, may experience symptoms of acute withdrawal. Flumazenil is a competitive an-tagonist of benzodiazepines and reverses the anxiolytic, sedative, muscle relaxant, and respiratory depressant properties of all of the currently available benzodi-azepines. It also reverses anticonvulsant effects and should therefore be avoided in patients who present with seizures and coma and in those taking benzodi-azepines for seizure control.

General Examination

Unresponsive patients should undergo a brief but systematic general examina-tion with specific attention to the following components.

TEMPERATURE Hypothermia results in decreased cerebral metabolism and im-paired arousal. The most common cause is prolonged exposure to the cold, per-haps following an accident or cerebral infarction. Other causes of hypothermia include shock, hypothyroidism, and some drug overdoses (e.g., phenobarbital). Hyperthermia is most commonly seen in conjunction with infection; central le-sions causing fever are rare but may include subarachnoid hemorrhage or hypo-thalamic structural abnormalities. Hyperthermia may also occur along with heat stroke and other related conditions. Anticholinergic overdose may produce fever in the absence of diaphoresis.

RESPIRATION Slow, shallow breathing is often indicative of drug ingestion, espe-cially CNS depressants, whereas rapid or irregular respirations suggest hypoxia, acidosis, obstruction, structural brainstem disease, fever, or sepsis. Specific pat-terns of abnormal respiration suggest varying levels of brain injury, but mechanical ventilation often precludes their assessment (Figure 13–1). Cheyne-Stokes respira-tions are characterized by long cycles of alternating hyperpnea and hypopnea. This pattern of respiration is typically seen with bihemispheric or high pontine lesions but may occur in metabolic encephalopathies and CHF. Cheyne-Stokes respiration generally carries a more favorable prognosis than other abnormal respiratory pat-terns.

Rapid-cycle periodic breathing, with one to two waxing breaths, followed by two to four rapid breaths, and then one to two waning breaths, is associated with increased ICP and lower pontine lesions. Since the rapid-cycle breathing progno-sis is much poorer than the prognosis for Cheyne-Stokes respiration, the two pat-terns must be distinguished.

Central neurogenic hyperventilation is a rare form of hyperpnea with respira-tory rates as high as 70/min. Lesions of the pontine tegmentum have accompanied this pattern but recognition and localization of this disorder remain controver-sial.[3,14] Similar patterns of hyperpnea can result from pulmonary processes and in-creased ICP from CNS mass lesions. Apneustic breathing is characterized by a prolonged pause after inspiration and is usually seen in patients with middle to caudal pontine lesions involving the dorsolateral tegmentum. Ataxic breathing de-scribes an irregular pattern of rate and rhythm indicative of a medullary lesion. Ataxic respirations often immediately precede respiratory arrest.

HEART RATE Bradycardia may be a sign of increased ICP, and when combined with hypertension and respiratory irregularities, constitutes the Cushing reflex.

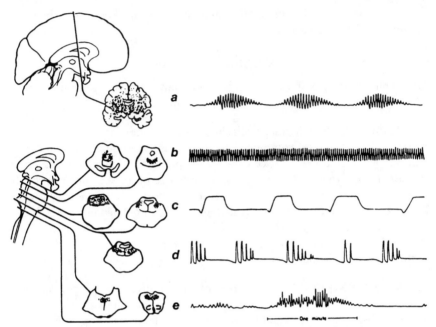

FIGURE 13–1 *Respiratory patterns in comatose patients. Abnormal respiratory patterns characteristic of pathologic lesions* (shaded areas) *at various levels of the brain. Tracings by chest-abdomen pneumograph, inspiration reads up. a, Cheyne-Stokes respiration; b, central neurogenic hyperventilation; c, apneusis; d, cluster breathing; e, ataxic breathing.*
SOURCE: *Used with permission from Plum F, Posner J.* The diagnosis of stupor and coma, *3rd ed. Philadelphia, PA: F.A. Davis, 1982.*

Heart block, MI, and overdose with certain drugs, such as beta blockers, may also lead to bradycardia. Tachycardia accompanies fever, anemia, hypovolemia, hyperthyroidism, and ingestion of anticholinergic drugs.

BLOOD PRESSURE Patients in coma may develop hypertension as the direct result of CNS injury, such as subarachnoid or intracerebral hemorrhage. In hypertensive encephalopathy, blood pressure elevation is the cause of impaired consciousness. Hypotension is often the result of sepsis, MI, aortic dissection, shock, intoxication, or Addison's disease.

SKIN A brief examination of the skin can aid significantly in the diagnosis of coma (Table 13–3). The presence of a petechial rash suggests meningococcemia or other infection, hemorrhagic disorder, or drug ingestion.

HEAD AND NECK The cranium should be examined for signs of trauma, such as skull depressions or hemotympanum. Ecchymosis near the orbits or over the

TABLE 13–3 Skin Rashes in Comatose Patients

Lesions or Rash	Possible Cause
Antecubital needle marks	Injected opiate drug abuse
Pale skin	Anemia or hemorrhage
Sallow, puffy appearance	Hypopituitarism
Hypermelanosis (increased pigment)	Porphyria, Addison's disease, chronic nutritional deficiency, disseminated malignant melanoma, chemotherapy
Generalized cyanosis	Hypoxemia or carbon monoxide poisoning
Grayish-blue cyanosis	Methemoglobin (aniline or nitrobenzene) intoxication
Localized cyanosis	Arterial emboli or vasculitis
Cherry-red skin	Carbon monoxide poisoning
Icterus	Hepatic dsyfunction or hemolytic anemia
Petechiae	Disseminated intravascular coagulation, thrombotic thrombocytopenic purpura, drugs
Ecchymosis	Trauma, corticosteroid use, abnormal coagulation from liver disease or anticoagulants
Telangiectasia	Chronic alcoholism, occasionally vascular malformations of the brain
Vesicular rash	Herpes simplex
	Varicella
	Behçet's disease
	Drugs
Petechial-purpuric rash	Meningococcemia
	Other bacterial sepsis (rarely)
	Gonococcemia
	Staphylococcemia
	Pseudomonas species
	Subacute bacterial endocarditis
	Allergic vasculitis
	Purpura fulminans
	Rocky Mountain spotted fever
	Typhus
	Fat emboli
Macular-papular rash	Typhus
	Candida species
	Cryptococcus species
	Toxoplasmosis
	Subacute bacterial endocarditis
	Staphylococcal toxic shock
	Typhoid
	Leptospirosis
	Pseudomonas species sepsis
	Immunological disorders
	Systemic lupus erythematosus
	Dermatomyositis
	Serum sickness
Other skin lesions	
Ecthyma gangrenosum	Necrotic eschar often seen in the anogenital or axillary area in *Pseudomonas* species sepsis

(continued)

TABLE 13–3 Skin Rashes in Comatose Patients (continued)

Lesions or Rash	Possible Cause
Splinter hemorrhages	Linear hemorrhages under the nail, seen in subacute bacterial endocarditis, anemia, leukemia, and sepsis
Osler's nodes	Purplish or erythematous painful, tender nodules on palms and soles, seen in subacute bacterial endocarditis
Gangrene of digits' extremities	Emboli to larger peripheral arteries

SOURCE: Reprinted with permission from Berger JR. Clinical approach to stupor and coma. In: Bradley WG, Daroff RB, Fenichel GM, Marsden CD, eds. Neurology in clinical practice, 2nd ed. Boston: Butterworth-Heineman, 1996:39–59.

mastoid suggests skull fracture, but these findings may be delayed for 2 to 3 days after trauma. Lacerations on the tongue and buccal mucosa suggest generalized convulsions. Neck stiffness may be the result of infection or subarachnoid hemorrhage.

FUNDUSCOPY Visualization of the fundi may reveal papilledema, indicating increased ICP; the absence of papilledema, however, does not mean that the ICP is normal. Papilledema also occurs in hypertensive encephalopathy. Subhyaloid hemorrhages are strongly diagnostic of subarachnoid hemorrhage or shaken baby syndrome in the comatose patient.

ABDOMEN The acute abdomen suggests infection or traumatic injury to internal organs. Organomegaly may provide clues to underlying conditions leading to coma, such as CHF, portal hypertension, carcinoma, or hematologic malignancies.

Neurologic Examination

The purpose of the neurologic examination is to aid in the diagnosis, treatment, and prognosis of patients in coma. Careful neurologic evaluation helps in localizing the lesion or lesions causing coma, which is a necessary prelude to initiating definitive treatment. Serial neurologic assessments capture fluctuations over time and help to document any effects of treatment. Finally, the neurologic examination still provides the most salient information about prognosis.

The neurologic examination may vary, depending on hemodynamic status, body temperature, presence of infection, and intrinsic sleep-wake cycles. Sedatives, hypnotics, and other psychoactive medications commonly obscure findings of neurologic examination, especially states of arousal; the dosages of these medications at the time of the examination must be noted. The neurologic examination should focus on the following three components: state of consciousness, brainstem function, and motor system.

STATE OF CONSCIOUSNESS The neurologic examination begins with assessing the state of consciousness. Observation from the bedside should precede active stimulation, with close attention to spontaneous motor activity, eye movements, patterns of respiration, ventilator settings, infusion rates of intravenous medications, and monitor readings. For example, determining the level of arousal in a patient with relative hypotension and increased ICP may be misleading because of transient decreases in the cerebral perfusion pressure. If the patient fails to exhibit any signs of spontaneous arousal, several forms of stimulation (e.g., visual, auditory, tactile, and noxious) may be required to fully assess arousal. The examiner should begin with normal volume speech or light touch, before progressing to more forceful or noxious stimuli. Supraorbital pressure and nasal tickle are usually sufficiently noxious; pinching soft tissues and applying nailbed pressure with reflex hammers are rarely necessary. Specific responses must be recorded for each type of stimulus.

The Glasgow Coma Scale (GCS) is a widely recognized standardized instrument used to measure the severity of traumatic brain injury.[13] This scale consists of three subscales: eye opening to stimulation, best verbal response, and best motor response (Table 13–4). The combined final score ranges from 3 to 15 and serves as a measure of overall level of consciousness. The GCS has been used in predictive models of outcome in head injury, intracerebral hemorrhage, and hypoxic-ischemic coma. Despite its widespread use and acceptance, the GCS may not capture important clinical changes and should not be viewed as a substitute for careful neurologic assessment.

TABLE 13–4 Glasgow Coma Scale

Best Motor Response	Score
Obeys	6
Localizes	5
Withdraws	4
Abnormal flexion	3
Extensor response	2
Nil	1

Best Verbal Response	Score
Oriented	5
Confused conversation	4
Inappropriate words	3
Incomprehensible sounds	2
Nil	1

Eye Opening	Score
Spontaneous	4
To speech	3
To pain	2
Nil	1

NOTE: Total score is normally between 3 and 15. See Table 13–5.

BRAINSTEM EXAMINATION Evaluation of brainstem function facilitates localization and may identify possible causes of coma. The brainstem examination should focus on the following components: pupillary size and reactivity, ocular motility, and the corneal reflex.

Pupillary Size and Reactivity

Pupillary size is determined by the level of afferent input from the optic nerves, chiasm, and tracts, and the balance of efferent input via the sympathetic and parasympathetic nervous systems. Interruption at any point in these pathways may lead to abnormal or asymmetric pupillary size (Figure 13–2). Metabolic or toxic conditions may result in small, reactive pupils (diencephalic pupils). Pontine lesions, particularly hemorrhage, cause pinpoint pupils. Despite their extremely small size, these pupils usually remain reactive if viewed with a magnifying glass. Asymmetric pupils suggest Horner's syndrome on the side of the smaller pupil (miosis), caused by interruption of sympathetic fibers, or third-nerve palsy on the contralateral side, accounting for dilation (mydriasis) and oculomotor abnormalities. A fixed and di-

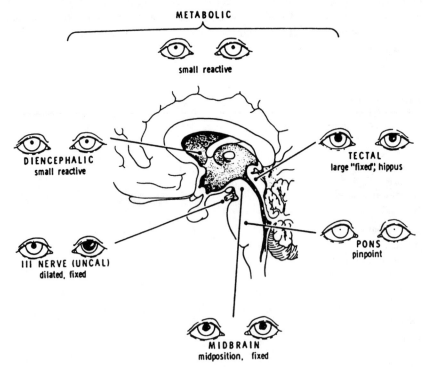

FIGURE 13–2 *Pupillary size in comatose patients. Pupils in comatose patients.*
SOURCE: *Used with permission from Plum F, Posner J. The diagnosis of stupor and coma, 3rd ed. Philadelphia, PA: F.A. Davis, 1982.*

lated pupil may signal herniation of the temporal lobe (uncal herniation) from a supratentorial mass lesion; oculomotor abnormalities due to compression of the third cranial nerve, usually occur subsequent to pupillary dilation.

Ocular Motility

Evaluation of ocular motility consists of first examining the eyes in resting position and noting any deviation or spontaneous movements, and second, performing reflex testing using either head rotation or caloric testing. Horizontal disconjugate gaze in the resting position in a sleeping or lightly comatose patient may indicate a latent strabismus. Other causes include lesions of the abducens nerve, oculomotor nerve, or medial longitudinal fasciculus, causing internuclear ophthalmoplegia. These abnormalities may not be evident unless oculocephalic or caloric testing is performed. Disconjugate deviation in the vertical plane (skew deviation) suggests a brainstem lesion.

Conjugate deviation in the horizontal plane suggests either a hemispheric lesion, interrupting supranuclear fibers of gaze control, or a pontine lesion, affecting crossed descending supranuclear pathways or nuclear structures directly. In hemispheric lesions, motor cortex is also frequently involved, causing contralateral weakness; the eyes drift toward the side of normal strength in these patients. Reflex oculomotor testing overcomes the eye deviation (gaze preference). In pontine lesions, involvement of the abducens nerve or adjacent paramedian pontine reticular formation is often accompanied by destruction of the descending corticospinal tract, resulting in contralateral weakness. In this case, eye deviation is toward the side of weakness and cannot be overcome with reflex oculomotor testing (gaze paresis or palsy). Occasionally, focal epileptiform or irritative lesions in the cortex cause temporary conjugate deviation of the eyes away from the lesion.

Spontaneous eye movements include roving eye movements, nystagmus, and conjugate vertical eye movements. Roving eye movements are slow to-and-fro movements in the horizontal plane, the presence of which implies an intact oculomotor system. These movements are difficult to execute voluntarily. Because spontaneous nystagmus reflects an intact interaction between cortical influences and the oculovestibular system, it is rarely seen in patients who are in coma and lack a fully functioning cortex. The presence of nystagmus in the comatose patient raises the possibility of an irritative or epileptiform cortical lesion and may indicate nonconvulsive status epilepticus. Other forms of nystagmus, such as retractory nystagmus and convergence nystagmus, are rare manifestations of mesencephalic lesions. Ocular bobbing is characterized by rapid, conjugate downward jerks of the eye, with a slow return to midposition. It typically reflects a pontine destructive lesion and may be confused with other forms of nystagmus.

Reflex ocular testing is performed using the oculocephalic maneuver (turning the head from side to side) or caloric testing. If the brainstem is intact, the eyes should move conjugately in the direction opposite to the direction of the movement of the head, using the oculocephalic maneuver. Vertical eye movements can be tested in a similar manner.

In caloric testing, the patient is placed in the supine position with the head 30 degrees above the horizontal plane. Cold water (10 to 50 mL of iced water) instilled into the ear canal should produce slow, tonic conjugate movement of the eyes toward the ear infused with cold water; warm water produces the opposite response. Compensatory fast-beating nystagmus is generated by the cortex and, therefore, is not observed in the comatose patient.

Abnormal responses to oculocephalic or caloric testing may be absent, sluggish, or disconjugate; the latter results from cranial nerve palsies, internuclear ophthalmoplegia, or restrictive eye disease. Reflex oculomotor testing must be interpreted with caution in those patients with previous vestibular disease or concurrent use of vestibulotoxic medications (antibiotics such as gentamicin), vestibular suppressants (barbiturates, sedatives), or paralytic agents (succinylcholine).

Corneal Reflex

Light stroking of the cornea with a cotton swab should produce bilateral eyelid closure and upward deviation of the eye (Bell's phenomenon). If present, it implies intact pathways from the mesencephalon to the facial nucleus in the pons. This reflex is usually present unless the patient is deeply comatose.

MOTOR SYSTEM EXAMINATION The remainder of the neurologic examination focuses on the motor system. Patients should be observed for resting posture and spontaneous motor activity. Rhythmic movements of individual or multiple ipsilateral motor groups suggests seizure activity, especially if these movements are stereotypic or tonic-clonic in nature. Nonrhythmic movements of variable muscle groups may represent multifocal myoclonus, commonly seen in anoxic, toxic, and metabolic encephalopathies.

Posturing may occur spontaneously or in response to stimulation. Decerebrate (extensor) posturing is characterized by extension of the lower extremities and adduction and internal rotation of the shoulder and extension of elbows. Decorticate (flexor) posturing consists of flexion at the elbows with shoulder adduction and extension of the lower extremities. Decerebrate posturing is usually the result of midbrain or rostral pontine lesions, bilateral basal forebrain injuries, or severe metabolic encephalopathies, whereas decorticate posturing suggests a lesion above the level of the brainstem. Decorticate posturing and unilateral posturing carry a more favorable prognosis than bilateral decerebrate posturing. Spinal reflexes are mediated at the level of the spinal cord and may be present in patients with absent cortical and brainstem function.

BRAIN HERNIATION Many comatose patients have increased ICP caused by either diffuse cerebral edema or mass lesions and are at risk for cerebral herniation.

Supratentorial forms of herniation include subfalcial ("midline shift"), central (transtentorial), or uncal herniation. Subfalcial herniation refers to displacement of the cingulate gyrus under the falx cerebri, with potential compromise of the anterior cerebral artery and internal cerebral vein. Subfalcial herniation is seen with frontal or parietal lesions and often results in clinical manifestations of depressed levels of arousal and asymmetric motor findings. Central herniation is usually the result of parenchymal lesions of the frontal, parietal, and occipital lobes, leading to compression of diencephalic and midbrain structures and eventual rostrocaudal displacement through the tentorium. Clinical findings include declining levels of arousal and progression from decorticate to decerebrate posturing. Uncal herniation is the result of a lesion of the temporal lobe, which causes medial displacement of the uncus across and eventually over the incisural edge of the tentorium, placing the midbrain, oculomotor nerve, and posterior cerebral artery at risk. Early signs can include ipsilateral pupillary dilation and contralateral motor posturing.

Herniation of posterior fossa contents can also occur, extending rostrally through the tentorium or caudally into the foramen magnum. Unlike the syndromes described earlier, in which clinical manifestations may progress in a rostrocaudal pattern, herniation involving the cerebellum or brainstem directly may result in rapid medullary dysfunction, respiratory failure, and death. In particular, massive intracerebral hemorrhages with intraventricular extension and lumbar punctures in patients with elevated ICP may lead to rapid medullary failure caused by direct compression of the brainstem or downward extension of the medulla into the foramen magnum.

DIAGNOSTIC TESTS

Initial diagnostic tests for the patient in coma should routinely include blood chemistry and hematologic profiles, thyroid studies, an ABG analysis, chest radiograph, ECG, and urinalysis. Additional laboratory studies may include urine toxicology and drug screens, creatine kinase level, serum osmolality study, and serum cortisol level. For those patients with a suspected structural lesion, head imaging studies are often the first diagnostic test obtained. A CT scan of the brain can often be obtained quickly and will identify acute hemorrhage, hydrocephalus, and most mass lesions. The addition of contrast dye improves identification of some tumors and abscesses. MRI is more sensitive for inflammatory and infectious lesions, ischemic changes, demyelinating disease, and lesions affecting posterior fossa structures. Diffusion-weighted imaging can identify ischemic lesions in the hyperacute stage, when CT and conventional MRI results are normal.

Cerebrospinal fluid (CSF) analysis should be performed in patients with suspected meningitis; however, most comatose patients should undergo an imaging study before lumbar puncture to avoid precipitating herniation in a patient with a mass lesion and increased ICP. If the CT scan cannot be obtained immediately, antibiotics can be initiated before obtaining CSF in patients with suspected acute bacterial meningitis.

Electroencephalography (EEG) should be performed immediately in any patient with suspected nonconvulsive status epilepticus. EEGs performed later in the course may suggest specific abnormalities, such as hepatic encephalopathy or herpes encephalitis, and may help delineate other conditions, such as locked-in syndrome, catatonia, and death according to brain criteria.

TREATMENT OF THE COMATOSE PATIENT

Treatment of the comatose patient should focus on reversing identifiable causes of the coma and reducing elevated ICP, when it is present. Several specific causes of coma, such as cerebral infarction, status epilepticus, meningitis, and hypertensive encephalopathy, deserve early consideration for treatment.

Elevated Intracranial Pressure

Elevated ICP may result from either diffuse or focal brain injury. Mass lesions, cerebral edema, and hydrocephalus are the most common causes in the ICU setting. Since the cranium is a rigid compartment, anything that adds volume to its contents—which are brain, blood, and CSF—may exceed intracranial compliance and lead to elevated ICP. Intracranial compliance allows ICP to remain in the normal range (5 to 20 cm H_2O) with small increments in volume. As the intracranial volume increases, however, intracranial compliance falls, and small volume increases can result in dramatic increases in ICP. Direct consequences of elevated ICP include global ischemia from decreased cerebral perfusion pressure (CPP) and herniation of brain tissue.

Clinical manifestations of increased ICP primarily include depressed levels of consciousness and increased blood pressure although changes in blood pressure may be obscured by ongoing antihypertensive therapy in some patients. Other signs of increased ICP include papilledema, headache, vomiting, and palsies of the abducens nerve, but these findings are often unreliable. Comatose patients with suspected elevation of ICP who are being considered for aggressive management should also be considered for invasive ICP monitoring. ICP can be measured by devices placed in the ventricle, subarachnoid space, or brain parenchyma, allowing for determination of the timing and effect of treatments to lower ICP.

The relationship between CPP and ICP is described by the subtracting ICP from mean arterial pressure (MAP), as in the following equation:

$$CPP = MAP - ICP$$

In normal brain, cerebral blood flow (CBF) is maintained over a wide range of CPP by autoregulation. This curve is shifted to the right in patients with chronic hypertension (Figure 13–3). In cases of brain injury, such as tumor, trauma, or infarction, autoregulation is impaired and CBF approaches a linear relationship with CPP. Since CBF is difficult to measure, CPP serves as a useful clinical guide to assessing cerebral perfusion. Thus, as the ICP rises, CPP and CBF fall. Although traditional treatments have focused on lowering ICP, newer approaches have placed greater emphasis on maintaining CPP. Current goals of treatment of ICP should include maintaining ICP at less than 20 cm H_2O and CPP between 70 and 120 mm Hg.

Other determinants of CBF are Pco_2 and Po_2 (Figure 13–4). As Pco_2 increases, CBF increases as well. This relationship underlies the rationale for hyperventilation, since lowering of Pco_2 leads to decreases in CBF and corresponding decreases in ICP because of intracranial volume loss. The effects on CBF of a lower Pco_2 are transient, however, lasting only 12 to 24 hours as CSF bicarbonate concentrations re-equilibrate. Changes in Po_2 have little effect on CBF in the physiologic range, but very low Po_2 leads to large increases in CBF (Figure 12–4).

In treatment of elevated ICP, the first consideration is removal of volume from the intracranial vault, either by surgical resection of a mass lesion or place-

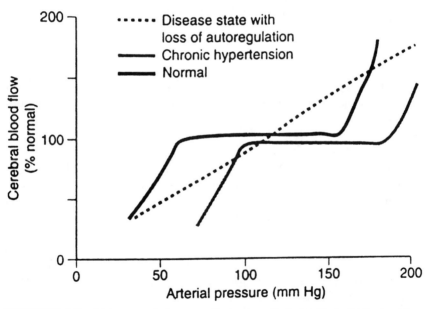

FIGURE 13–3 *Cerebral autoregulation curve. In the normal relationship* (solid line), *with cerebral blood flow held constant across a wide range of cerebral perfusion pressure (50–150 mm Hg). In disease states, (e.g., vasospasm, ischemia, intracranial mass lesion), cerebral blood flow may become pressure–passive* (dotted line). *With chronic hypertension* (gray line), *the auto regulatory curve shifts to the right.* SOURCE: *Used with permission from Marshall R, Mayer S. On call: neurology. 1st ed. Philadelphia: W.B. Saunders, 1997.*

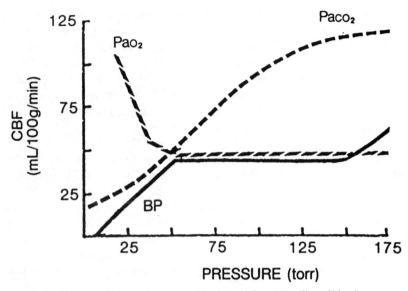

FIGURE 13–4 Effects of P_{CO_2} and P_{O_2} on cerebral blood flow. The effect of blood pressure, P_{CO_2} and P_{O_2} on cerebral blood flow in normal brain. SOURCE: Used with permission from Shapiro H. Intracranial hypertension: Therapeutic and anesthetic considerations. Anesthesiology 1975;43:445.

ment of an intraventricular catheter to remove CSF. Indwelling ventricular catheters can also measure ICP in response to other treatments, such as osmotic diuresis, hyperventilation, and blood pressure management.

OSMOTIC AGENTS Mannitol is the most common osmotic agent used in the treatment of elevated ICP. It is a six-carbon sugar that does not readily cross the blood-brain barrier, thereby creating an osmotic gradient, drawing water from brain parenchyma into the intravascular space.[15] The reduction in extracellular free water results in decreases in intracranial volume and lowering of ICP. This osmotic gradient is further enhanced as mannitol is cleared by the kidneys, with corresponding increases in free water clearance and serum osmolality. Mannitol also decreases blood viscosity by improving erythrocyte flexibility.[16] This change in blood viscosity transiently increases CBF, inducing reflex vasoconstriction and decreased cerebral blood volume.

Mannitol is given in an initial dose of 0.5 to 1.0 g/kg of body weight, followed by 0.25 to 0.5 g/kg every 3 to 5 hours, and may be used in conjunction with diuretics. Maintenance dosing is best tailored to measured changes in ICP. Drawbacks of using osmotic agents include hypotension resulting from volume contraction; exacerbation of CHF by transiently increased intravascular volume; electrolyte abnormalities, particularly disturbances in potassium metabolism;

and hyperosmolality with acute tubular necrosis. Serum osmolality should be maintained at less than 320 mOsm/kg.

HYPERVENTILATION Using hyperventilation to lower P_{CO_2} to 25 to 30 mm Hg reduces ICP within minutes. Hyperventilation produces respiratory alkalosis, which in turn causes cerebral vasoconstriction and decreased CBF; its effects on ICP peak at 30 minutes and may last up to 3 hours. Consequently, hyperventilation is an excellent short-term measure to lower ICP until definitive treatment can be undertaken. Prolonged hyperventilation (more than 24 hours) becomes less effective and should be avoided because it may lead to cerebral ischemia. Lowering the P_{CO_2} below 25 mm Hg may also exacerbate cerebral ischemia by means of severe vasoconstriction, especially in patients with cerebral infarctions.

BLOOD PRESSURE MANAGEMENT Close monitoring of blood pressure is important in the management of ICP. In patients with hypertension and elevated ICP, treatment with a short-acting antihypertensive agent may result in parallel reductions in MAP and ICP. The CPP should not be lowered below 70 mm Hg, because cerebral vasodilation may occur and ICP will increase. Preferred agents for lowering blood pressure include labetolol or nicardipine; sodium nitroprusside is also an effective, short-acting agent, but it leads to cerebral vasodilation and increased ICP.

In those patients with CPP of less than 70 mm Hg and elevated ICP, pressors, such as dopamine, may lead to reflex reductions in ICP by increasing blood pressure and reducing cerebral vasodilation.

SEDATION The controlled environment of the ICU allows the judicious use of sedatives to help control elevated ICP, especially in anxious, fearful, or agitated patients. Sedatives may also facilitate mechanical ventilation in many circumstances, potentially leading to further decreases in ICP. Short-acting agents, such as propofol or midazolam, can be given by intravenous drip and quickly titrated to optimal levels. These agents can be held briefly for serial neurologic examinations, making them preferable to longer-acting neuromuscular blocking agents in critically ill neurologic patients.

In patients with severe, refractory elevated ICP, high-dose pentobarbital may be a reasonable alternative.[17–19] However, pentobarbital can lead to systemic hypotension and thereby reduce CPP, potentially causing further increases in ICP.

GENERAL MANAGEMENT All patients with increased ICP should receive only isotonic fluids (0.9% saline solution), since hypotonic solutions will decrease serum osmolality and lead to further cerebral edema. Hypovolemia should also be avoided, because it may result in decreased CPP and reflex increases in ICP.

Fever increases ICP by increasing cerebral metabolism and blood flow. All fevers in patients with coma should be aggressively treated, using either cooling blankets or antipyretics, as appropriate. Controlled hypothermia (32°C to 34°C) to treat elevated ICP is currently under investigation and may be a useful adjunct in patients with refractory elevations in ICP.

The optimal position of the head in patients with increased ICP is still unknown. Conventional approaches suggest elevating the head of the bed 15 to 30 degrees to promote venous drainage and decrease cerebral blood volume. Recent data suggest that a "head-flat" position may optimize CPP in patients with increased ICP.[20] Until further studies are completed, it is reasonable to raise the head of the bed 15 to 30 degrees, provided the CPP remains more than 70 mm Hg.[15]

Causes of Coma that Require Early Treatment

ACUTE STROKE Acute stroke is now a medical emergency. Recent clinical trials have demonstrated that treatment with intravenous recombinant tissue plasminogen activator (rt-PA) within 3 hours of onset of symptoms in patients with ischemic stroke results in significant functional recovery at 3 months.[21] Consequently, all patients who present with symptoms of stroke of less than 3 hours' duration should be considered for rt-PA treatment, provided no contraindications exist.[22]

In controlled settings, symptomatic intracranial hemorrhage occurs in approximately 6% of patients treated with rt-PA. For those patients with more severe strokes that result in depressed levels of consciousness, the risk of hemorrhage is higher. However, these patients may still benefit from thrombolytic therapy and should be considered for treatment.

Preliminary results with intra-arterial thrombolysis for acute middle cerebral artery occlusion have also been favorable.[23] Coma resulting from acute basilar artery occlusion may also be amenable to intra-arterial thrombolysis.[24] The administration of intra-arterial thrombolytic agents requires rapidly available angiography and considerable technical expertise of the interventionist, thereby limiting its use to highly specialized centers.

Patients with infarction or hemorrhage in the cerebellum may experience an acute deterioration in their level of consciousness caused by direct compression of the brainstem. These patients typically present with symptoms of cerebellar dysfunction (e.g., ataxia, vertigo) and normal mentation. However, they require close monitoring on admission, and neurosurgical consultation should be obtained early in the course of the deficit. If sudden deterioration occurs, decompressive surgery should be strongly considered. Results from several case series of decompressive procedures have demonstrated substantial reductions in mortality and morbidity rates.[25-27]

For patients with massive hemispheric cerebral infarctions or intracerebral hemorrhages, decompressive craniectomy (and possible hematoma evacuation) may also be considered. Several protocols exist; results of this operation have been mixed.[28] Results from the only prospective trial (nonrandomized), however, demonstrated lower mortality rates (without increased morbidity rates) in the surgical group.[25] A large, prospective controlled trial is under way.

STATUS EPILEPTICUS Status epilepticus has been defined as 30 minutes of continuous seizure activity or two or more separate seizures without full recovery of consciousness between them.[29,30] A period of abnormal mentation often follows generalized convulsive seizures, but prolonged unresponsiveness should alert the clinician to the possibility of nonconvulsive status epilepticus. Signs of ongoing seizure activity may be subtle, such as intermittent rhythmic eye movements or brief twitches of facial muscles. Occasionally, the diagnosis can only be made by EEG studies. Treatment for status epilepticus should include a benzodiazepine, followed by a loading dose of phenytoin or fosphenytoin.[29,30] Patients with refractory status epilepticus typically require intubation, barbiturates, and monitoring in an ICU.[29]

MENINGITIS The classic triad of fever, nuchal rigidity, and altered mental status immediately evokes the diagnosis of meningitis, although all three signs are present in only two-thirds of community-acquired cases.[31] All cases of bacterial meningitis in one series had at least one of these findings.[31] In this same series, 51% of patients had abnormal mental status, 22% responded only to painful stimuli, and 6% were unresponsive to all stimuli.

Patients with suspected meningitis should undergo a lumbar puncture to evaluate the CSF. However, the issue of whether or not to obtain a head imaging study before performing a lumbar puncture remains controversial. Most clinicians agree that several clinical features, such as progressive unresponsiveness, seizure, papilledema, or focal neurologic deficits, warrant a CT scan of the head before performing a lumbar puncture.[32] These patients should be treated empirically with broad-coverage antibiotics before undergoing a CT scan. Other studies indicate that the risk of precipitating cerebral herniation by lumbar puncture is low, and therefore patients with suspected meningitis should undergo immediate lumbar puncture, provided the several clinical features mentioned are absent.[32-34]

HYPERTENSIVE ENCEPHALOPATHY Symptoms of malignant hypertension (diastolic blood pressure of more than 130 mm Hg) include headache, seizure, altered mental status, blurred vision, and dyspnea.[35] Papilledema is a defining characteristic and may be accompanied by retinal hemorrhages and "cotton wool" exudates. Up to 12% of patients with malignant hypertension go on to have hypertensive encephalopathy, a syndrome characterized by depressed alertness, impaired intellectual functioning, and seizures.[35] Although the mental status abnormalities may be mild in most cases, some patients have severe impairment of arousal, responding only to vigorous stimulation. In nearly all cases of hypertensive encephalopathy, however, patients show full recovery on reduction of blood pressure.[35] This feature distinguishes these patients from those with malignant hypertension and depressed levels of alertness that result from focal structural disease, such as stroke or hemorrhage.

Reversible posterior leukoencephalopathy is a related condition with clinical features similar to those seen in hypertensive encephalopathy.[36] This syndrome is further characterized by edema in the bilateral parieto-occipital white matter that is detectable on MRI. In addition to hypertension, other precipitating conditions include renal decompensation, fluid retention, and treatment with immunosuppressive drugs.[36]

Treatment of hypertensive encephalopathy requires prompt reduction of blood pressure, usually with a parenteral agent such as labetolol or sodium nitroprusside. Both agents are rapidly effective and easily titrated by intravenous drip. Labetolol is often preferred in patients with elevated ICP, because sodium nitroprusside is a vasodilator and may further increase ICP.[37]

PROGNOSIS

The prognosis of patients in coma depends on the cause and depth of coma and the timing of the assessment. For patients with nontraumatic coma, drug intoxication or metabolic derangements typically have the best prognosis and full recovery is possible; diffuse anoxic injury or focal structural disease, such as intracerebral hemorrhage and subarachnoid hemorrhage, carry a poorer prognosis. Overall, patients with traumatic coma have a more favorable prognosis than patients with nontraumatic coma. Patients with traumatic coma are younger and more likely to regain consciousness after prolonged coma.

Determining the prognosis of patients in coma is a careful but inexact process. Our current knowledge does not allow absolute predictions of recovery or even survival in individual patients. Several studies, however, provide useful guidelines in categorizing the likelihood of recovery or survival based on patients with similar clinical findings.[38, 39] This information helps both families and caregivers provide the most appropriate care for individual patients.

Nontraumatic Coma

Clinical signs provide the most useful predictors of outcome in patients with nontraumatic coma. Levy et al[38] reported outcomes in 500 patients with nontraumatic coma in association with a variety of clinical findings (Figure 13–5). Of those patients with absent corneal responses at 24 hours after the onset of coma, none regained independent function. Patients with preserved brainstem reflexes (i.e., any two of the following: pupillary response, corneal reflex, vestibulo-ocular reflex) and any motor response beyond flaccid at admission regained independence in 17% of cases. If the motor response is withdrawal, the rate of independence reaches 23%.[38]

In another study of patients with nontraumatic coma,[39] death or severe disability at 2 months occurred in 96% of patients with abnormal brainstem responses (defined by the absence of any one of the following findings: pupillary reflex, corneal reflex, conjugate roving eye movements) or absent motor responses to pain at 3 days. Five clinical variables were independent predictors of mortality at

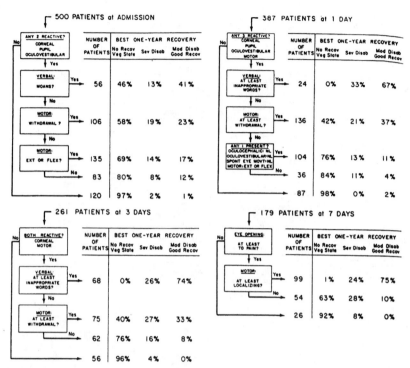

FIGURE 13–5 Prognosis in patients with nontraumatic coma. Estimating prognosis in non-traumatic coma. All patients surviving various early intervals after onset of coma are categorized on basis of sequential criteria relating to clinical examinations. Best levels of recovery within 1 year are given for each of the prognostic groups. Nonreactive motor responses means absence of any motor response to pain. ABBREVIATIONS: No Recov, no recovery; Veg State, vegetative state; Sev Disab, severe disability; Mod Disab, moderate disability; Good Recov, good recovery; Mot, motor response; Ext, extensor; Flex, flexor; Spont Eye Movt, spontaneous eye movements; Nl, normal. SOURCE: Used with permission from Levy DE, Bates D, Caronna JJ, et al. Prognosis in nontraumatic coma. Ann Int Med 1981;94:293–301.

2 months: abnormal brainstem response, absent verbal response, absent withdrawal response to pain, creatinine level of 1.5 mg/dL or more, and age 70 or older.[39]

For patients with hypoxic-ischemic coma (e.g., cardiac arrest), approximately 13% regain independent function within 1 year.[40] In patients with absent pupillary light reflexes at the time of the initial examination, none regained function. Conversely, 41% of patients regained independence if the following were documented on initial examination: pupillary light reflexes, spontaneous eye movements that were roving conjugate , and motor response to pain (extensor, flexor, or withdrawal).[40] Outcomes based on various clinical findings and day of examination are provided in Figure 13–6. These types of simple rules are often very helpful in counseling patients' families.

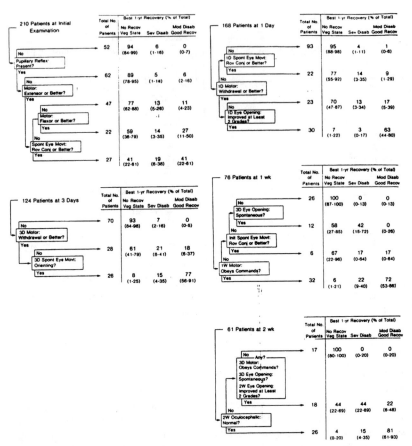

FIGURE 13–6 Prognosis in patients with hypoxic–ischemic coma. Rules based on neurologic examination that classify patients in hypoxic–ischemic coma according to best functional state within first year. Figures in parentheses represent the 95% confidence intervals for percentages given immediately above. Initial examination (top left) was obtained within 6 hours of onset of coma in 55% of patients and within 12 hours in 84%. Modifiers INIT, 1D, 3D, 1W, and 2W refer to initial, 0– to 1–day, 2– to 3–day, 4– to 7–day, and 8– to 14–day examinations, respectively. If no data are available, response to relevant question is considered to be "No." Where changes in clinical signs are used (top right and bottom), difference is between best response of previous time interval and best response of current interval. Physicians applying these rules must exercise caution when residual anesthetics or depressant drugs (including anticonvulsant) are present, should wait until end of each time interval to make certain that best clinical response has been observed, and should not use any rules that require responses that are unavailable for a specific patient. ABBREVIATIONS: recov, recovery; veg, vegetative; disab, disability; sev, severe; mod, moderate; spont eye movt, spontaneous eye movements; rov conj, roving conjugate. SOURCE: Used with permission from Levy DE, Caronna JJ, Singer BH, et al. Predicting outcome from hypoxic–ischemic coma. JAMA 1985;253:1420–1426.

For patients with spontaneous intracerebral hemorrhage, the volume of the hematoma and the score on the GCS are useful predictors of outcome at 30 days after the initial hemorrhage. Using three categories of hematoma volume and two categories of the GCS, the 30-day mortality rate can be predicted with a sensitivity of 96% and a specificity of 98% (Table 13–5).[41] The volume of a hematoma can be measured by a simple ellipsoid method, using conventional CT images.[42]

Traumatic Coma

Patients with traumatic coma have a more favorable prognosis than patients with nontraumatic coma with similar findings on initial examination.[38] In one study of 1000 patients in coma 6 hours after severe head trauma, nearly 50% died, but 17% survived with moderate disability and 22% had a good recovery.[43] Much as in patients with nontraumatic coma, early predictors of outcome in patients with traumatic coma include pupillary response, motor response, eye movements, depth and duration of coma, and age. The cause of injury and presence of skull fracture do not predict outcome.[1]

Vegetative State

Approximately 10% of patients with traumatic coma and 12% of patients with nontraumatic coma evolve into the vegetative state.[12] Of those patients in PVS at 1 month after trauma, 52% regain consciousness within 1 year.[44] The majority of patients recover within the first 6 months. In contrast, only 15% of patients in PVS at 1 month after nontraumatic injury regain consciousness within 1 year. Recovery of function in this group was extremely poor, with only 1% of patients having a good recovery.[44] Outcomes for children in PVS after trauma are more favorable than for adults; outcomes for children are similar to those seen in adults in PVS after nontraumatic coma.

TABLE 13–5 Prognosis in Patients with Spontaneous Intracerebral Hemorrhage

Glasgow Score	ICH Volume (mL)	No. in Risk Group	Prognosis		
			Dead	Expected Dead	Probability of Death by 30 Days
≥ 9	< 30	77	13	15	0.19
≥ 9	30–60	19	11	9	0.46
≥ 9	> 60	17	12	13	0.75
≤ 8	< 30	15	7	7	0.44
≤ 8	30–60	15	11	11	0.74
≤ 8	> 60	19	17	17	0.91

ABBREVIATION: ICH, intracerebral hemorrhage.
SOURCE: Reprinted with permission from Broderick JP, Brott TG, Duldner JE, et al. Volume of intracerebral hemorrhage: a powerful and easy-to-use predictor of 30-day mortality. Stroke 1993;24:987–993.

DETERMINING DEATH ACCORDING TO BRAIN CRITERIA

Determination of death according to brain criteria (i.e., brain death) essentially requires the documentation of absent brainstem and cerebral activity on clinical examination. State laws may vary regarding specific criteria and ancillary diagnostic tests. In most medical settings, death is established by brain criteria when a patient exhibits no meaningful response to external stimuli, initiates no spontaneous respirations, and demonstrates no brainstem reflexes. The assessment of spontaneous respiration requires an apnea test, during which patients are removed from the ventilator and 100% oxygen is provided through a sterile catheter placed in the endotracheal tube. Apnea is defined as no respirations being observed despite high P_{CO_2} pressures (55 to 60 mm Hg) and is confirmed by ABG analysis. Absent brainstem activity is determined by the absence of the following reflexes: pupillary, corneal, gag, and vestibulo-ocular. The vestibulo-ocular reflex is elicited by raising the head 30 degrees and instilling more than 50 mL of ice water into each ear (separated by 5 minutes).

Other ancillary studies for determining brain death include EEG and cerebral blood flow studies. Patients who meet brain death criteria have an isoelectric EEG, but many centers do not require an EEG. Absent cerebral blood flow can be demonstrated with isotope studies or conventional angiography. In all cases of brain death, there must not be other explanations for cerebral inactivity, such as severe hypothermia (32°C or lower), drug intoxication, or severe metabolic derangements. Many centers require two clinical examinations separated by a duration of time (4 to 6 hours) before brain death can be established.

Patients who meet brain criteria for death may be candidates for organ donation. These patients continue to require intensive care, since approximately 50% of them will suffer cardiac arrest within the first 24 hours and nearly all of them will die in 48 to 72 hours.[45,46] Specific protocols exist in most ICUs for the care of potential organ donors to maximize organ viability before harvest.

SUMMARY

Although coma is widely recognized in the intensive care setting, caring for an individual comatose patient often poses a unique set of challenges. However, a systematic approach to the comatose patient, along with close attention to the neurologic examination, will provide the clinician with the most success in the diagnosis, management, and prognosis of this common condition.

REFERENCES

1. Berger JR. Clinical approach to stupor and coma. In: Bradley WG, Daroff RB, Fenichel GM, Marsden CD, eds. *Neurology in clinical practice*, 2nd ed. Boston: Butterworth-Heineman, 1996:39–59.

2. Howsepian AA. The 1994 Multi-Society Task Force consensus statement on the persistent vegetative state: a critical analysis. *Issues Law Med* 1996; 12:3–29.
3. Plum F, Posner J. *The diagnosis of stupor and coma*, 3rd ed. Philadelphia, PA: F.A. Davis, 1982.
4. Giacino JT. Disorders of consciousness: differential diagnosis and neuropathologic features. *Sem Neurol* 1997; 17:105–111.
5. Magoun HW. An ascending reticular activating system in the brain stem. *Arch Neurol Psychiatry* 1951;145–154.
6. Moruzzi G, Magoun HW. Brain stem reticular formation and activation of the EEG. *EEG Clin Neurophysiol* 1949;1:455–473.
7. Childs N, Mercer WN, Childs H. Accuracy of diagnosis of persistent vegetative state. *Neurology* 1993;43:1465–1467.
8. Tresch D, Farrol H, Duthie E, et al. Clinical characteristics of patients in the persistent vegetative state. *Arch Intern Med* 1991;151:930–932.
9. Andrews K, Murphy L, Munday R, et al. Misdiagnosis of the vegetative state: retrospective study in a rehabilitation unit. *Brit Med J* 1996;313:13–16.
10. American Congress of Rehabilitation Medicine. Recommendations for use of uniform nomenclature pertinent to patients with severe alterations in consciousness. *Arch Phys Med Rehab* 1995;76:205–209.
11. Mercer WN, Childs NL. Coma, vegetative state, and the minimally conscious state: diagnosis and management. *Neurologist* 1999;5:186–193.
12. Sorenson S, Kraus J. Occurrence, severity and outcomes of brain injury. *J Head Trauma Rehabil* 1991;6:1–10.
13. Jennet B, Bond M. Assessment of outcome after severe brain damage: a practical scale. *Lancet* 1975;323:480–484.
14. North J, Jennet B. Abnormal breathing patterns associated with acute brain damage. *Arch Neurol* 1974;31:338.
15. Mayer SA, Dennis LJ. Management of increased intracranial pressure. *Neurologist* 1998;4:2–12.
16. Muizelaar J, Wei E, Kontos H, et al. Mannitol causes compensatory cerebral vasoconstriction in response to blood viscosity changes. *J Neurosurg* 1983;59:822–828.
17. Marshall L, Smith R, Shapiro H, et al. The outcome with aggressive treatment in severe head injuries. Part 2. Acute and chronic barbiturate administration in the management of head injury. *J Neurosurg* 1979;50:26–30.
18. Rea G, Rockswold G. Barbiturate therapy in uncontrolled intracranial hypertension. *Neurosurgery* 1983;12:401–404.
19. Eisenberg H, Frankowski R, Contant C, et al. High-dose barbiturate control of elevated intracranial pressure in patients with severe head injury. *J Neurosurg* 1999;1988:15–23.
20. Rosner M, Rosner S, Johnson A. Cerebral perfusion pressure: management protocol and clinical results. *J Neurosurg* 1995;83:949–962.
21. National Institute of Neurological Disorders and Stroke rt-PA Study Group. Tissue plasminogen activator for acute ischemic stroke. *N Engl J Med* 1995;333:1581–1587.
22. Adams H, Brott T, Furlan A, et al. Guidelines for thrombolytic therapy for acute stroke: a supplement to the guidelines for the management of patients with acute stroke. *Circulation* 1996;94:1167–1174.
23. Furlan A, Higashida R, Wechsler L et al. Intra-arterial prourokinase for acute ischemic stroke. The PROACT II study: a randomized controlled trial. Prolyse in Acute Cerebral Thromboembolism. *JAMA* 1999;282:2003–2011.

24. Brandt T, von Kummer R, Muller-Kuppers M, et al. Variables affecting recanalization and outcome. *Stroke* 1996;27:875.
25. Rieke K, Krieger D, Adams H, et al. Therapeutic strategies in space-occupying cerebellar infarction based on clinical, neuroradiological and neurophysiological data. *Cerebrovasc Dis* 1993;3:45–55.
26. Heros R. Surgical treatment of cerebellar infarction. *Stroke* 1992;23:937–938.
27. Klugkist H, McCarthy J. Surgical treatment of space-occupying cerebellar infarctions—4 1/2 years postoperative follow-up. *Neurosurg Rev* 1991;14:17–22.
28. Davis SM, Grotta JC, Donnan GA, et al. Surgical interventions in the treatment of acute ischemic infarction. In:. *Interventional therapy in acute stroke.* Malden, MA: Blackwell Science, 1998:117–130.
29. Willmore LJ. Epilepsy emergencies: the first seizure and status epilepticus. *Neurology* 1998;51(Suppl 4):S34–S38.
30. Working Group on Status Epilepticus. Treatment of convulsive status epilepticus. *JAMA* 1993;270:854–859.
31. Durand ML, Calderwood SB, Weber DJ, et al. Acute bacterial meningitis in adults: a review of 493 episodes. *N Engl J Med* 1993;328:21–28.
32. Lambert HP. Meningitis. *J Neurol Neurosurg Psychiatry* 1994;57:405–415.
33. Archer BD. Computed tomography before lumbar puncture in acute meningitis: a review of the risks and benefits. *Can Med Assoc J* 1993;148:961–965.
34. Stephenson J. Timing of lumbar puncture in severe childhood meningitis. *Brit Med J* 1985;291:1123.
35. Healton E, Brust J, Feinfeld D, et al. Hypertensive encephalopathy and the neurologic manifestations of malignant hypertension. *Neurology* 1982;32:127–132.
36. Hinchey J, Chaves C, Appignani B, et al. A reversible posterior leukoencephalopathy syndrome. *N Engl J Med* 1996;334:494–500.
37. Kaplan NM. Management of hypertensive emergencies. *Lancet* 1994;344:1335–1338.
38. Levy DE, Bates D, Caronna JJ, et al. Prognosis in nontraumatic coma. *Ann Int Med* 1981;94:293–301.
39. Hamel MB, Goldman L, Teno J, et al. Identification of comatose patients at high risk for death or severe disability. *JAMA* 1995;273:1842–1848.
40. Levy DE, Caronna JJ, Singer BH, et al. Predicting outcome from hypoxic-ischemic coma. *JAMA* 1985;253:1420–1426.
41. Broderick JP, Brott TG, Duldner JE, et al. Volume of intracerebral hemorrhage: a powerful and easy-to-use predictor of 30-day mortality. *Stroke* 1993;24:987–993.
42. Kothari RU, Brott TG, Broderick JP, et al. The ABCs of measuring intracerebral hemorrhage volumes. *Stroke* 1996;27:1304–1305.
43. Jennet B, Teasdale G, Braakman R. Prognosis of patients with severe head injury. *Neurosurgery* 1979;4:283–289.
44. Multi-society Task Force on PVS. Medical aspects of the persistent vegetative state. *N Engl J Med* 1994;330:1499–1508,1572–1579.
45. Mackersie R, Bronsther O, Shackford S. Organ procurement in patients with fatal head injuries: The fate of the potential donor. *Ann Surg* 1991;213:143–150.
46. Lindop M. Management of the cadaver donor in the intensive care unit. In: Collins G, Dubernard J, Land W, Persijn G, eds. *Procurement, preservation and allocation of vascularized organs.* Norwell, MA: Kluwer Academic, 1997:55–58.

CHAPTER 14

Approach to Sedation and Airway Management in the ICU

PETER J. PAPADAKOS

INTRODUCTION

Sedation is one of the most important roles of the ICU. Without it, proper therapy becomes difficult in that agitation and pain impart various physiologic changes such as hypertension and tachycardia. The agitated patient also cannot be properly ventilated and monitored. The agitation also affects the nonpatient environment by affecting the way family and friends perceive the ICU care. Agitated patients also affect staffing patterns in the ICU and may increase healthcare costs. A clear knowledge of sedation and pain control and the ability to titrate the many pahrmacological agents is a basic ICU skill. This chapter also reviews the skills of airway management in that they are so interrelated both for medical and legal reasons of scope of practice.

SEDATION AGENTS

Sedation plays a very important role in the management of patients in the ICU. Sedation not only reduces the stress response but also decreases oxygen consumption and allows the patient to be placed on various modes of mechanical ventilation and high levels of PEEP. With properly sedated patients, physicians may be able to reduce complications, improve oxygenation, improve oxygen delivery, facilitate monitoring, and improve outcome.

There are many agents available for sedation, both long- and short-acting. It is imperative that, when using sedation, it be titrated to specific endpoints by using sedation scales, such as the Ramsey scale (Figure 14–1). A good general rule is to have the patient at a sedation level of 2 to 3.

Benzodiazepines

Benzodiazepines are a common group of agents that are used throughout the hospital. They interact with specific receptors throughout the central nervous system (CNS) particularly in the cerebral cortex. Benzodiazepines are commonly administered orally, intramuscularly, and intravenously to provide sedation. The three commonly used agents are diazepam, midazolam, and lorazepam (Figure 14–2). The dosages vary according to individual patient parameters. Benzodiazepines are now more commonly titrated to a sedative effect in a particular pa-

Ramsey Scale	
Level	Clinical Description
1	Anxious and agitated
2	Cooperative, oriented, tranquil
3	Responds only to verbal commands
4	Asleep with brisk response to light stimulation
5	Asleep without response to light stimulation
6	Non-responsive

FIGURE 14–1 The Ramsey sedation scale.

Benzodiazepines			
Agent	Bolus Dosage	Continuous Infusion	P. O. Dosage
Diazepam (Valium)*	0.04 - 0.2 mg/kg IV or IM; 2.5 mg to 5 mg IV or IM q 10 min - Max of 10 mg IV or IM.	N/A	2.5 - 5.0 mg PO
Midazolam (Versed)	0.01 - 0.1 mg/kg; 2.5 - 5 mg IV or IM; Moderate to severe agitation. May repeat every 10 minutes. Max of 20 mg.	0.5 - 8 mg/hr; Titrate by 1 mg/hr every 30 minutes.	N/A
Lorazepam (Ativan)	0.03 - 0.05 mg/kg; 0.5 – 1.0 mg for mild agitation; 1-2 mg q 10 min; May supplement with other agents. Never exceed 4 mg in an hour.	0.5 - 4.0 mg/hr; Should bolus with 1-4 mg to achieve steady state more rapidly.	N/A

- Dosage may be repeated every 3-6 hours.

FIGURE 14–2 Benzodiazepines.

tient rather than to a specific dosage. The shortest-acting commonly used benzodiazepine is midazolam (with a half-life of 1.5 to 3.5 hours). The half-life of benzodiazepines can be markedly prolonged when administered by continuous infusion, especially if the infusion is continued for more than 24 to 48 hours. Continuous infusions saturate the patient's fat stores as a result of the lipid-soluble nature of benzodiazepines. Once fat stores are saturated, there is nowhere for the benzodiazepine to go and its affect is prolonged. This effect can markedly prolong an intubated patient's awakening and limit opportunities for extubation. The current way to choose a benzodiazepine depends on whether the patient is expected to require short-term (i.e., less than 48 hours) or long-term (more than 48 hours) sedation.

Midazolam is commonly used for intermittent sedation or when sedation is required for less than 48 hours. Its short clinical half-life allows the patient to wake up predictably after one-time use. Midazolam also has a nice amnestic effect, which, in a dosage of 2.5 to 5.0 mg, may be ideal for short-term ICU procedures. However, continuous use of midazolam has been characterized by prolonged sedative affects, and therefore, it should be used only for short-term continuous infusion.

Lorazepam is the preferred agent in the ICU for prolonged treatment of anxiety in the critical care patient. Although its clinical half-life is longer than that of midazolam, it has no active metabolites and wake-up times after continuous infusion with lorazepam are the same or less than midazolam. Lorazepam has a significant cost advantage over midazolam. When using lorazepam by continuous infusion, titrating the intravenous drip up and down does not result in immediate increases and decreases in blood levels of the drug because of its long half-life. A bolus of lorazepam should be administered at the time of the dose increase to reach the next steady-state drug level. Therefore, it is recommended that a bolus dose of lorazepam be delivered at a dosage equal to the current hourly rate of the drug before increasing the drip rate. Also, regularly scheduled reductions in

Reversal of Benzodiazepines
Flumazenil is a specific benzodiazepine receptor antagonist that effectively reverses most of the central nervous system effect of benzodiazepines. It should not be used after long term benzodiazepine use. Dosage - 0.2 mg IV over 15 seconds. Titrate over 5-10 minutes for a maximum dosage of 1 mg. For acute benzodiazepine overdose, start with 0.2 mg IV. Titrate up to 5 mg IV. You may repeat dosage every 20 minutes. Never reverse patients who have been on continuous infusions.

FIGURE 14–3 Reversal of benzodiazepines.

hourly drip rates (i.e., decreasing drip rate by 25% every 8 hours) has resulted in faster wake up from sedation.

Diazepam is not commonly used in the ICU because of its long half-life and active metabolites; however, the clinical half-life from one-time dosing is short as a result of the drug's high lipophilic profile. This causes the drug to redistribute quite rapidly into fat stores, limiting its sedative effects.

GENERAL EFFECTS Benzodiazepine agents cause general sedation and respiratory depression. Close monitoring of patients and the use of sedation scales are the keys to appropriate dosing. Also, benzodiazepines are myocardial depressants and vasodilators. Care must be taken in using them in hypovolemic patients; slow titration is important in this patient population.

Midazolam tends to reduce blood pressure and peripheral vascular resistance to the greatest extent.

Benzodiazepines as a group reduce cerebral oxygen consumption and cerebral blood flow and, thereby, decrease ICP.

DRUG INTERACTIONS Ethanol, barbiturates, and other CNS depressants potentiate the sedative effects of benzodiazepines. The sedative effects may be reversed with flumazenil (Figure 14–3). Patients who have been taking benzodiazepines chronically or have been on continuous infusion should not receive flumazenil to reverse the effects of benzodiazepines because this may induce acute withdrawal symptoms, including seizures.

Propofol

The mechanism of action of propofol may involve facilitation of inhibitory neurotransmission mediated by gamma-aminobutyric acid (GABA). Propofol can only be given intravenously and is ideal for use in short-term sedation. Awakening is rapid, owing to a short initial distribution half-life (i.e., 2 to 8 minutes) into fat stores. It is an ideal drug for titration to sedation scales. The normal intravenous dosage range is 0.3 to 130 μg/kg/per minute (average 27 μg/kg/per minute). This dosage range may vary if the patient has a history of heavy use of illicit drugs or ethanol; the patient may require a higher dosage under these circumstances. We do not generally use a loading dose on the patients in the ICU with propofol because of vasodilatory effects and subsequent hypotension; instead, we titrate the drug to sedation scales (i.e., Ramsey scale) and for hemodynamic effect.

EFFECTS ON ORGAN SYSTEMS The major cardiovascular effect of propofol is a decrease in arterial blood pressure, owing to a drop in systemic vascular resistance, cardiac contractility, and preload. The drug should be used carefully in hypovolemic patients and patients with complex medical problems. It has a respiratory depressant effect similar to that of barbiturates, and decreases cerebral blood flow and ICP. A unique characteristic of propofol is its antiemetic and antipruritic effect.

Propofol is felt to be cost-effective in situations where sedation is expected for the short term. It is currently recommended in the ICU only for intubated patients. In short-term use, studies have suggested that the cost of the drug (expensive) can be made up by extubating the patient more quickly (faster awakening) and thus moving the patient out of the ICU sooner and shortening the length of stay. Propofol has been widely used this way in "fast-track" cardiac surgery patients and has decreased the length of stay in critical care units for such patients. Propofol can also be quite useful when rapid sedation and awakening are necessary, such as in neurologic patients who have head injuries or who have had CVAs but are also agitated. The patient may be intermittently awakened to assess mental status and neurologic function and then be rapidly sedated when necessary.

Haloperidol

Haloperidol is a neuroleptic agent with a long track record in treating delirium in critically ill patients and is the drug of choice for this condition.

Haloperidol is initiated at a dose of 3 mg (for mild agitation), 5 mg (for moderate agitation), or 10 mg (for severe agitation) as an intravenous bolus. The dose may be repeated every 15 to 30 minutes, to a maximum of 40 mg per single dose, until adequate sedation is reached. Benzodiazepines work synergistically with haloperidol and may be given simultaneously. Haloperidol effects may take 10 minutes to be seen. Therefore, adding a quick-acting benzodiazepine (i.e., midazolam) to haloperidol therapy in the severely agitated patient is reasonable. Once the patient is sedated, the dosage of haloperidol and the benzodiazepine required to achieve sedation must be calculated and then the dosage must be divided over the following day in a schedule of administering every 6 hours. Reduce the dosage by 50% per day until the patient is off the medications. If the patient becomes agitated again, restart the entire process.

Haloperidol has also been used by continuous infusion in the range of 1 to 40 mg/hr. In cases where the drug has been used for long-term therapy (more than 5 days), tapering over several days may be necessary.

Finally, delirium should be recognized as a symptom and not a diagnosis. Patients who are delirious need their agitation controlled so as to not cause harm to themselves or others, but they also need a complete evaluation for reversible causes of delirium once their agitation is controlled. Such reversible causes may include alcohol withdrawal, infection, hypoxia, and a host of other conditions.

SIDE EFFECTS Extrapyramidal symptoms (such as acute dystonic reactions) are relatively common in patients being treated with neuroleptic agents. These syndromes are characterized by involuntary movements, such as smacking of the lips, lateral jaw movements, and sudden forward thrusts of the tongue. Purposeless movements of all the extremities may occur. This can be treated with diphenhydramine, 50 mg IV, or benztropine, 2 mg IV. The most severe problem is neuroleptic malignant syndrome, which is manifested by a marked elevation in temperature, generalized hypertonicity of skeletal muscles, alterations in blood pressure, tachycardia, cardiac arrhythmias, and fluctuations in the level of consciousness. This is treated with dantrolene, 2.5 mg/kg given intravenously every 5 minutes until the symptoms subside. Rarely does the dosage need to exceed 10 mg/kg. Haloperidol may cause QT prolongation, and the drug should be used cautiously with other drugs that can cause prolongation of the QT interval. If one is using high-dose haloperidol (doses of more than 3 mg), the QT interval should be monitored closely (every 8 to 12 hours), and the drug should be stopped if the QT interval becomes prolonged.

Opioids

Opioids bind to specific receptors distributed throughout the CNS and other tissues. While opioids provide some degree of sedation, they are most effective at producing analgesia. The common opioids used in the ICU are morphine, meperidine, and fentanyl. Figure 14–4 lists their half-lives and usual dosage ranges. Morphine and fentanyl are used intravenously in bolus doses and continuous infusions. Morphine may cause histamine release and has the potential to cause more hemodynamic instability than fentanyl, which does not have this property. The cost of fentanyl is similar to that of morphine. Meperidine is quite expensive and is usually given only in bolus doses. Alfentanil and remifentanil are short-acting narcotic agents, which are not commonly used in the ICU.

SIDE EFFECTS Meperidine has a potential for causing seizures with the accumulation of the meperidine metabolite normeperidine. Many clinicians do not use the drug in patients with decreased renal function. Meperidine should not be

Commonly Used Narcotics in the ICU			
	Bolus IV	**Bolus IM**	**Continuous Infusion**
Morphine	0.05 – 0.1 mg/kg over 10 minutes; Redose q 1-2 hours	2.5-20 mg q 2-6 hours	0.8-10 mg/hr
Fentanyl	0.5 - 2 mcg/kg every 1-2 hours	N/A	1-2 mcg/kg/hr
Meperidine (Demerol)	25-100 mg q 3-4 hours	25-200 mg q 3-4 hours	N/A

Half lives of narcotics: Morphine(I 14-173mins), Fentanyl(155-219mins), and Meperidine(3-4.4hours).

FIGURE 14–4 *Narcotic dosing.*

Reversal of Narcotics
Naloxone is the reversal agent for narcotics. An initial dosage of 0.4 mg to 2 mg may be administered intravenously for acute narcotic overdose. Additional doses may be necessary in 20 to 60 minutes. Alternatively an intravenous loading dosage of 0.4 mg followed by a continuous infusion of 0.1-0.4 mg/hr. Infusion may be titrated by 0.2 mg/hr at two to three-hour intervals.

FIGURE 14–5 Reversal of narcotics.

used in patients who are taking various psychiatric drugs; administration along with monoamine oxide (MAO) inhibitors (e.g., phenelzine, isocarboxazid, L-deprenyl, tranylcypromine) may result in hypertension, coma, hypotension, or potential hyperpyrexia.

All narcotic agents decrease gastrointestinal motility, which may lead to ileus. This can be a major problem in the ICU. Most patients receiving narcotic agents should also be on bowel regimens.

Opioids depress ventilation, especially respiratory rate, so close monitoring is important. The effects of acute overdoses may be reversed with naloxone (Figure 14–5).

GENERAL GUIDELINES All narcotic agents should be titrated to clinical effect. In general, opioids do not seriously impair cardiovascular function, and fentanyl can be used in hemodynamically compromised patients. The effects of combined narcotic and sedative agents may be additive; narcotic agents should be used carefully along with reliance on fixed sedation scales.

Paralytic Agents

Muscle relaxants (chemical paralytics) are sometimes used in the ICU to facilitate mechanical ventilation and to lower oxygen consumption when sedation or analgesia is insufficient. Over the years, chemical paralysis has been used less and less as use of sedative and analgesic agents has improved. Furthermore, the syndrome of persistent paralysis and critical-illness polyneuropathy has been linked with use of paralytic agents and has lessened enthusiasm for their use. Always remember that paralytic agents provide no analgesia or sedation, and sedation must always be provided when they are used.

Paralytic agents are broadly categorized into depolarizing and nondepolarizing agents.

DEPOLARIZING AGENTS Depolarizing agents attach to the alpha subunits of the postjunctional muscle membrane receptor and mimic the action of acetylcholine, thus producing depolarization and subsequent fasciculation. Neuromuscular blockade develops because a depolarized membrane cannot respond to subsequent release of acetylcholine. The primary depolarizing neuromuscular blocking agent is succinylcholine, which is used primarily as an aid to intubation. The usual dosage is 0.6 to 1.5 mg/kg. The agent has a short half-life, with no clinical effect after 5 minutes or so. A small dose of any nondepolarizing drug can be used to block fasciculation from succinylcholine. Use this agent with extreme

Contraindication of Succinylcholine
Succinylcholine can induce a life-threatening hyperkalemia and should be avoided in these patients:
1. Burn patients
2. Denervated patients such a hemiparetics, paraplegics, etc.
3. Patients with closed head injury
4. Patients with intra-abdominal infections
5. Patients with degenerative neuromuscular disease
6. Trauma patients (usually massive soft tissue trauma)

FIGURE 14–6 Contraindications to succinylcholine therapy.

caution in patients with pre-existing spinal cord injury or degenerative neuro-muscular disease, because these patients tend to become extremely hyperkalemic when succinylcholine is given. Contraindications to the use of this agent are listed in Figure 14–6.

NONDEPOLARIZING AGENTS Nondepolarizing agents act by combining with nicotinic cholinergic receptors but do not cause any activation of the receptor; there is no fasciculation with these agents. The commonly used nondepolarizing agents in the ICU are the benzylisoquinolones atracurium and its isomer cisatracurium, as well as the aminosteroids pancuronium and vecuronium. The duration of action and dosages of these agents are listed in Figure 14–7. The ben-zylisoquinolones are intermediate-acting agents that have the potential advan-tage of not relying on renal or hepatic mechanisms for metabolism. These drugs undergo Hoffman elimination and hydrolysis via plasma esterase, which occurs at physiologic pH and temperature. These agents are relatively expensive.

Vecuronium is an intermediate-acting aminosteroid and pancuronium is a long-acting aminosteroid. Pancuronium's action lasts 75 to 90 minutes and is generally given by intermittent injection. The drug builds up in renal and liver failure and also causes tachycardia resulting from its vagolytic properties. Vecuronium is devoid of cardiovascular effects and is generally used in continu-ous infusion form. The drug has prolonged effects in liver failure.

MONITORING Neuromuscular blockade should always be monitored using a train-of-four monitor every 4 to 8 hours, with a goal of two of four twitches. The twitches in a train-of-four monitor are generated by an electric stimulus and progressively fade as relaxation increases. To minimize the amount of the drug used, titrate to two twitches, which denotes 75% block of the neuromuscular junction. Prolonged neu-romuscular blockade with changes in electrolyte levels, i.e., hypophosphaturia, hy-

Non-depolarizing Agents			
	Duration of Action (Minutes)	Loading Dose	Infusion
Atracurium	Intermediate (20-30 min.)	0.23 mg/kg	5 mcg/kg/min
Cisatracurium	Intermediate 20-30 min)	0.1 mg/kg	2-5 mc/kg/min
Vecuronium	Intermediate (20-30 min)	0.05 mg/kg	1 mcg/kg/min
Pancuronium	Long (45-60 min)	0.07 mg/kg	N/A

FIGURE 14–7 Nondepolarizing agents.

pokalemia, and hypermagnesemia, may occur. The muscle strength of the patient and the respiratory function must be evaluated before extubation.

AIRWAY MANAGEMENT

Rapid Sequence Induction

Adept airway management is an essential skill for health care professionals caring for a patient with critical illness. Endotracheal intubation not only protects the airway but also provides a means for positive-pressure ventilation. The majority of emergent intubations should be handled as a full stomach. The technique for rapid sequence induction is shown in Figure 14–8.

Before release of cricoid pressure, check for breath sounds and presence of end-tidal carbon dioxide. This technique can be modified, depending on the patient condition. A patient in cardiopulmonary arrest would not need sedation or paralysis. Thiopental and methohexital are not good sedative agents because they cause hypotension. Ketamine, a phenylcyclidine, can be used as a 1 to 2 mg/kg IV infusion or 3 to 5 mg/kg in an intramuscular injection. Midazolam can also cause hypotension. Baseline ventilator settings are set at a rate of 10 breaths per minute, a tidal volume of 6 to 10 mL/kg, and a FIO_2 of 100% after intubation.

Head Injury

Keep the head in the neutral position during airway management until cervical spine fractures have been ruled out. This can be achieved by in-line immobilization or by use of a hard collar.

- Avoid nasal intubation if a fracture of the base of skull is suspected.
- Avoid aspiration; use rapid sequence induction intubation.
- Sedate patient adequately to prevent hypertensive surges during instrumentation of the airway.

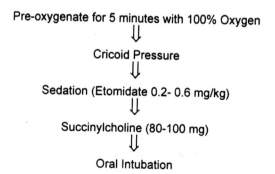

Pre-oxygenate for 5 minutes with 100% Oxygen
⇓
Cricoid Pressure
⇓
Sedation (Etomidate 0.2- 0.6 mg/kg)
⇓
Succinylcholine (80-100 mg)
⇓
Oral Intubation

FIGURE 14–8 Technique for rapid sequence induction of intubation.

During intubation, keep the patient well-sedated to prevent coughing and straining. In the presence of hypovolemia and cardiovascular instability, sedative dosage should be titrated slowly so that blood pressure is not decreased.

• Avoid using succinylcholine.
• Use rocuronium in a dose of 0.9 to 1.2 mg/kg.

Ocular Injury

To prevent an increase in intraocular pressure, avoid succinylcholine; another neuromuscular blocker can be used. Rocuronium, 0.9 to 1.2 mg/kg, is the only nondepolarizing muscle relaxant with an onset of action similar to succinylcholine (60 to 90 seconds).

Burns

Evaluation and knowledge of intravascular volume is critical in burn patients. Sedative agents may need to be titrated to maintain blood pressure. Release of potassium is of concern; therefore, succinylcholine is avoided. Rocuronium may be the best choice of agent. Rapid intubation should be performed on arrival of the patient if airway burns are suspected (i.e., burns to face, around mouth, burned nasal hair and back of mouth, sputum with black carbon particles).

Trauma

Before intubation and sedation, the cervical spine should be evaluated if injuries are suspected. Use in-line traction. Vascular volume is a problem with these patients and sedation may be contraindicated; severe hypotension may develop. If sedation is used, titrate it in slowly. Avoid succinylcholine in massive soft-tissue injuries.

Asthma

If the patient demonstrates increased work of breathing and is fatigued, intubation in a controlled manner is indicated. Sedation with propofol may be useful because of its bronchodilator effect. Avoid prolonged use of neuromuscular blockers because myopathy has been reported.

Elderly Patients

Intravascular volume status must be evaluated in elderly patients. Loose or removable dental work that may be aspirated during intubation should be removed. Evaluate the cervical spine and take care with patients who have severe arthritis that may limit neck motion.

Basic Intubation Criteria

1. Inability to breathe spontaneously
2. Impending loss of airway as a result of swelling or excessive secretions
3. Obtundation
4. Respiratory rate over 40 breaths/minute
5. P_{CO_2} of more than 60 mm Hg
6. P_{O_2} of less than 60 mm Hg on a F_{IO_2} of 1.0
7. Head injury
8. Acute respiratory distress syndrome (ARDS)

Extubation Criteria

These criteria are only guidelines. Weaning and extubation protocols vary from region to region. All data should be collected when the patient is off the ventilator.

1. Patient able to protect airway
2. Decreased secretions
3. Good tidal volumes (5 mL/kg), vital capacity of 10 mL/kg on minimal support, i.e., CPAP or pressure support of 5 cm H_2O or less.
4. Decreased work of breathing; respiratory rate of less than 40/min
5. Ability to maintain respiratory function (respiratory rate, tidal volume, rapid shallow breathing index of less than eighty off mechanical support)
6. Adequate oxygenation at an F_{IO_2} of 0.5
7. Minute ventilation of less than 10 L/min off ventilator

After Intubation

Sedation after intubation should be used to assist in mechanical ventilation. Propofol, benzodiazepines, or narcotics may be used. Lidocaine, 0.5 to 1.0 mg/kg may be used to block the stimulation of the oral pharynx during extubation.

SUMMARY

Sedation and pain control play a very important role in the management of patients in the ICU. These drugs account for a large portion of the ICU pharmacy budget and greatly impact on the length of stay of patients in the ICU. Our ability to reach proper levels of sedation and pain control with sedation and pain control scales not only impacts on patient comfort but also on staffing and patient care maps and guidelines. Neuromuscular blockers still play an important role in the management of complex cases. They however are given with greater care than in the past for much shorter periods. The health care professionals managing patients who need sedation, pain control, and paralysis should be expert in airway management skills both for patient care and for hospital privileging guidelines.

SUGGESTED READINGS

Shapiro BA, Warren J, Egol AB, et al. Practice parameters for intravenous analgesia and sedation for adult patients in the intensive care unit. An executive summary. *Crit Care Med* 1995; 9:1596–1600.

Avramov MN, White PF. Methods for monitoring the levels of sedation. *Crit Care Med* 1995; 11:803–826.

Swart EL, Van Schijndel RJ, Van Loenen AC, et al. Continuous infusion of lorazepam vs. midazolam in patients in the intensive care unit. *Crit Care Med* 1999; 27(8):1461–1465.

Kress JP, O'Connor MF, Pohlman AS, et al. Sedation of critically ill patients during mechanical ventilation. *Am J Respir Crit Care Med* 1996; 153:1012–1018.

Shuster DR. A physiological approach to initiating, maintaining, and withdrawing mechanical ventilatory support during acute respiratory failure. *Am J Med* 1990; 88:268–278.

Gora-Harper ML. *The injectable drug reference.* Society of Critical Care Medicine, Bio-Scientific Resources, Princeton, NJ, 1998.

Papadakos PJ, Early M. Physician and nurse considerations of receiving a "fast track" patient in the ICU. *J of Cardiothor Anesth* 1995; 9(suppl):21–23.

Index

Page numbers followed by an "f" indicate figures; numbers followed by a "t" indicate tables.

A

A-a oxygen gradient. *See* Alveolar-arterial oxygen gradient
ABCD. *See* Amphotericin B cholesteryl sulfate complex
Abciximab, for acute myocardial infarction, 219
Abdominal examination:
in coma, 330
ultrasonography in renal failure, 108
Abdominal pressure, increased, 276
ABG analysis. *See* Arterial blood gas analysis
ABLC. *See* Amphotericin B lipid complex
Abulia, 325
ACE inhibitors. *See* Angiotensin-converting enzyme inhibitors
Acetaminophen:
hepatotoxicity of, 268, 270–271
premedication for transfusion, 316
Acetazolamide, for metabolic alkalosis, 114
N-Acetylcysteine, for acetaminophen intoxication, 270
Acid-base abnormalities, 112–115, 112t
Acid-peptic disease, 247–248, 250

Acidosis, 10. *See also* Metabolic acidosis; Respiratory acidosis
local, 52
Acinetobacter baumanii, 156
Acquired thrombocytopenia, 302, 303t
ACTH. *See* Corticotropin hormone
Activated partial thromboplastin time, 300
Acute respiratory distress syndrome, 2t, 9, 62, 107, 122t, 130t
in acute liver failure, 271
mechanical ventilation in, 81, 86–87
pulmonary capillary wedge pressure and, 41–42
Acute tubular necrosis, 106–108, 272, 339
ACV. *See* Assist-control ventilation
Addison's disease, 328, 329t
Adenosine:
for arrhythmias, 210t
arrhythmias and, 205t
for diagnosis of arrhythmias, 204
for reentrant supraventricular tachycardia, 198–199
ADH. *See* Antidiuretic hormone
Adrenal failure:
primary, 234, 237
secondary, 234, 237–238

Captopril, for acute myocardial
infarction, 221
Carbipenem, prescribing in renal
failure, 111
Carbohydrates:
composition of parenteral and
enteral formulations, 173t
daily requirement for, 174t, 175
dietary, 178
Carbon dioxide:
in exhaled air, 52–53
increased production of, 2t
production of, 9, 171–172
retention of, 7
Carbon monoxide poisoning, 329t
Carboxyhemoglobinemia, 28
Cardiac arrest, 268, 343, 344f
Cardiac arrhythmias. *See*
Arrhythmias
Cardiac catheterization, 64
Cardiac glycosides, for shock, 68
Cardiac indexes, 38, 46t
derived, 43–45
Cardiac markers, 64, 215
Cardiac output, 10–11, 26, 49, 51
in anemia, 312
continuous, 48
effect of positive pressure
ventilation, 88–89f
oxygen delivery and, 11–12
thermodilution, 42–43, 43f
Cardiac pharmacologic intervention,
assessment of, 45–47
Cardiac rehabilitation program, 224
Cardiac tamponade, 41, 51, 60, 63
Cardiogenic pulmonary edema, 82,
87–88, 88f
Cardiogenic shock, 222–224
differential diagnosis of, 63–64
hemodynamic profile in, 57, 57t
management of, 223
patient history in, 58
treatment of, 68
Cardiomyopathy, 63, 202, 268

Cardiopulmonary interaction, assessment of, 47–48
Cardiothoracic surgery, nutritional
support for, 175t
Cardiovascular system:
infection of, 120t
in shock, 58–59t
Cardioversion, 196, 203, 208–209,
209t
for atrial fibrillation, 209t
for atrial flutter, 209t
for reentrant supraventricular
tachycardia, 209t
for torsades de pointes, 204
for ventricular fibrillation,
208–209, 209t
for ventricular tachycardia, 209t
Carotid sinus massage, 198–199
Catheter. *See also specific types of
catheters*
gauge of, 20
insertion site, 137
patency of, 20
Catheter colonization, 138–139,
138t
Catheter infection, 18–19
without bacteremia, 19
bloodstream, 19, 124, 135–140
antibiotic therapy for, 127t,
139
catheter type and, 136–137
causative microorganisms, 139,
139t
definition of, 138t
diagnosis of, 137–139, 138t
insertion and maintenance of
catheter, 137
prevention of, 136–137
risk factors for, 135–136
therapy for, 139–140
local, 138t
microbiologic methods for evaluation of, 138t
pulmonary infiltrate in, 130t

ISBN 0-07-006696-5

90000

9 780070 066960

APOSTOLAKOS/INT
CARE MANUAL